Social Cognition: Impact on Social Psychology

Edited by

Patricia G. Devine
Department of Psychology
University of Wisconsin
Madison, Wisconsin

David L. Hamilton
Department of Psychology
University of California
Santa Barbara, California

Thomas M. Ostrom
Department of Psychology
Ohio State University
Columbus, Ohio

ACADEMIC PRESS
San Diego New York Boston London Sydney Tokyo Toronto

This book is printed on acid-free paper. ♾

Academic Press, Inc.
A Division of Harcourt Brace & Company
525 B Street, Suite 1900, San Diego, California 92101-4495

United Kingdom Edition published by
Academic Press Limited
24–28 Oval Road, London NW1 7DX

Library of Congress Cataloging-in-Publication Data

Social cognition : impact on social psychology / edited by
Patricia G. Devine, David L. Hamilton, Thomas M. Ostrom.
p. cm.
Includes index.
ISBN 0-12-213630-6
1. Social psychology. 2. Cognition--Social aspects. 3. Social perception. I. Devine, Patricia G. II. Hamilton, David L. (David Lewis), DATE. III. Ostrom, Thomas M., DATE.
HM251.S671149 1994
302--dc20 93-47061
CIP

PRINTED IN THE UNITED STATES OF AMERICA
94 95 96 97 98 99 QW 9 8 7 6 5 4 3 2 1

Social Cognition: Impact on Social Psychology

Contents

Contributors ix
Preface xi

1

Social Cognition and Classic Issues in Social Psychology

David L. Hamilton, Patricia G. Devine, and Thomas M. Ostrom

What Is Social Cognition? 2
Goals of the Volume and Chapter Previews 6
References 12

2

A Personal Perspective on Social Cognition

Robert P. Abelson

How Early Social Psychology Kept Its Mind 15
Behaviorism Nevertheless Had an Indirect Influence 18
Where Had All the Phenomenology Gone? A Personal Detour 19
A New Focus in Social Cognition: Coacting Subsystems 24
Inconsistency between Subsystems 27
How Many Subsystems? 28
Subsystems Based on Differences in Levels of Abstraction 29
Poor Subsystem Communication and the Analysis of Prejudice 29
Recapitulation 32
References 32

3

Impression Formation: From Recitals to Symphonie Fantastique

Jacques-Philippe Leyens and Susan T. Fiske

Asch's Theme 40
Implicit Personality Theory: A Major Variation on Asch's Theme 41
Anderson's Opposing Theme 43
Social Cognition and Process: Fantasia 43
Synthesis of the Opening Themes 55
Finis 65
References 66

4

Social Cognition Contributions to Attribution Theory and Research

Eliot R. Smith

Trends in Attribution Research 78
Three Threads of Attribution Research Today 85
Summary: What Has Social Cognition Done for Attribution? 100
References 102

5

The Role of Trait Constructs in Person Perception: A Historical Perspective

Robert S. Wyer Jr. and Alan J. Lambert

Inferences of Other's Traits from Their Behavior 113
Effects of Trait Descriptions on Evaluations of Others 119
Inferences of Traits from Evaluative Concepts 125
The Prediction of Behaviors from Trait Information 129
The Role of Traits in Perceptions and Judgments of Oneself 131
Concluding Remarks 135
References 136

6

Social Cognition of the Self

Patricia W. Linville and Donal E. Carlston

Historical View of the Self 144

Impact of Social Cognition on Enduring Issues of Self 147
Impact of Social Cognition on Emerging Issues of Self 172
Contributions of Social Cognition to the Study of Self 180
References 184

7

The Cognitive Foundations of Attitudes: It's a Wonderful Construct

Thomas M. Ostrom, John J. Skowronski, and Andrzej Nowak

Objectives of the Chapter 196
Attitude as a Traditional Latent Variable 197
Recent Advances in the Cognitive Analysis of Attitudes 199
Cognitive Codes, Structures, and Processes: A New Look at Attitudes 203
Emerging Conceptions of Cognition 239
Final Thoughts 248
References 249

8

The Social Cognition Analysis of Social Influence: Contributions to the Understanding of Persuasion and Conformity

Diane M. Mackie and John J. Skelly

Introduction 259
Persuasion 261
Conformity 272
Concluding Remarks 279
References 281

9

Social Cognition and the Study of Stereotyping

David L. Hamilton, Steven J. Stroessner, and Denise M. Driscoll

Stereotype Theory and Research: Historical Context 292
The Social Cognition Analysis: New Directions 298
Extending the Social Cognition Analysis 308
A Concluding Perspective 315
References 316

10

Prejudice and Prejudice Reduction: Classic Challenges, Contemporary Approaches

Margo J. Monteith, Julia R. Zuwerink, and Patricia G. Devine

Classic Theories and Change Strategies: An Overview 324
Contemporary Analyses of Prejudice 328
Reducing Contemporary Forms of Prejudice 336
References 342

11

Cognitive Processes and Intergroup Relations: A Historical Perspective

Myron Rothbart and Scott Lewis

Introduction 347
The Cognitive Revolution and Social Psychology 347
Zawadski's Critique 348
Lippmann's *Public Opinion* 351
Allport's *The Nature of Prejudice* 353
Sherif's Robbers' Cave Experiments 354
Levine and Campbell's *Ethnocentrism* 357
Tajfel's Cognitive Aspects of Prejudice 363
Social Categorization and the Minimal Group Paradigm 364
Perception of Intragroup Variability 368
The Contact Hypothesis and Category-Exemplar Dynamics 371
Problems and Prospects for the Cognitive Approach to Intergroup Relations 376
References 378

Author Index 383
Subject Index 399

Contributors

Numbers in parentheses indicate the chapter numbers of the authors' contributions.

Robert P. Abelson (2), Department of Psychology, Yale University, New Haven, Connecticut 06520

Donal E. Carlston (6), Department of Psychological Sciences, Purdue University, West Lafayette, Indiana 47907

Patricia G. Devine (1, 10), Department of Psychological Sciences, Purdue University, West Lafayette, Indiana 47907

Denise M. Driscoll (9), Department of Psychological Sciences, Purdue University, Lafayette, Indiana 47907

Susan T. Fiske (3), Department of Psychology, University of Massachusetts at Amherst, Amherst, Massachusetts 01003

David L. Hamilton (1, 9), Department of Psychology, University of California, Santa Barbara, Santa Barbara, California 93106

Alan J. Lambert (5), Department of Psychology, University of Illinois, Champaign, Champaign-Urbana, Illinois 61820

Scott H. Lewis (11), AT&T, Dallas, Texas 75240

Jacques-Philippe Leyens (3), Universitat Catholique de Louvain, Faculte de Psychologie, Belgium

Patricia W. Linville (6), Duke University, Center for Decision Studies, Fuqua School of Business, Durham, North Carolina 27706

Diane M. Mackie (8), Department of Psychology, University of California, Santa Barbara, Santa Barbara, California 93106

Margo J. Monteith (10), Department of Psychology, Texas Tech University, Lubbock, Texas 79409

Andrzej Nowak (7), Department of Psychology, University of Warsaw, Warsaw, Poland

Thomas M. Ostrom (1, 7), Department of Psychology, Ohio State University, Columbus, Ohio 43210

Myron Rothbart (11), Department of Psychology, University of Oregon, Eugene, Oregon 97403

John J. Skelly (8), Department of Psychology, Ohio State University, Columbus, Ohio 43210
John J. Skowronski (7), Department of Psychology, Ohio State University, Newark, Ohio 43055
Eliot R. Smith (4), Department of Psychological Sciences, Purdue University, West Lafayette, Indiana 47907
Steven J. Stroessner (9), Department of Psychology, Banard College, Columbia University, New York, New York 10027
Robert S. Wyer Jr. (5), Department of Psychology, University of Illinois, Champaign, Champaign-Urbana, Illinois 61820
Julia R. Zuwerink (10), Department of Psychology, University of Wisconsin, Madison, Wisconsin 53706

Preface

This book is about the contributions of social cognition analyses to the understanding of issues of classic and contemporary interest to social psychologists. Many of the issues of enduring concern to social psychology have benifited from the creative and productive efforts of many of our colleagues who took on the challenge of exploring the cognitive underpinnings of core social psychological phenomena. Over the years, we have been excited and impressed by the power of social cognitive analyses to reveal insights concerning social psychological phenomena and we have been inspired by the creativity and imagination of those who have investigated and continue to investigate the cognitive processes underlying social thought and behavior.

The idea for this volume evolved from a symposium at the 1987 meeting of the American Psychological Association, the theme of which was the contributions of social cognition to our understanding of classic issues in social psychology. Each of us participated in the symposium. Based on the clarity of the presentations and the positive reception from the audience members (many of whom were skeptics), we decided to organize this volume as a way to share these contributions with the field more broadly. The talks at the symposium represented broad overviews of development in specific areas and, although each speaker had contributed to these developments, none of the speakers limited their talks to their own research programs. In developing the concept for this volume, our goal was to have chapters that would accomplish what the symposium speakers had done so effectively. We were impressed with the enthusiasm with which our authors took on this challenge. Ultimately, we were able to bring together an outstanding group of authors whose chapters are outstanding examples of clear thinking and scholarship. Each chapter places the contributions of social cognition to specific research areas in historical context and, as such, brings the field up to date. In addition, the chapter authors have outlined new challenges and directions for future research.

This book is intended for a wide audience. We hope that our colleagues will find the reviews of specific contributions of social cognition useful and that they will serve to raise new research questions and directions. The book will also be useful in graduate seminars and advanced undergraduate courses for a comprehensive review of the contributions of social cognitive analyses to a wide range of social psychological phenomena. We hope that the book will be useful not only to sympathizers of the social cognition approach, but also to the skeptics who have been reluctant to embrace social cognitive analyses of social psychological phenomena. We believe that skeptics will be impressed with the balance with which our authors review the strengths and shortcomings of social cognitive analyses of social thought and behavior.

We would like to thank the staff at Academic Press, in particular Nikki Fine and Mike Rutherford, for their efforts in making this volume a success. Their attention to detail and their efficiency are greatly appreciated.

1

Social Cognition and Classic Issues in Social Psychology

David L. Hamilton
Patricia G. Devine
Thomas M. Ostrom

At some point in the mid-1970s something new began to evolve in social psychology; there emerged a way of thinking, theorizing, and experimenting that came to be known as social cognition. This new approach to studying social psychological phenomena quickly captured the attention and the interest of researchers across the spectrum of social psychology, and social cognition became a central, if not dominant, thrust in the discipline. In many respects it has defined and shaped the nature of social psychological inquiry during the last fifteen years. Just as the 1960s can be thought of as the era of consistency theories, and the 1970s as the decade of attribution, the 1980s became a period in which social cognition, having taken root during the late 1970s, now grew and flourished, extending its branches in numerous directions, bearing fruit that planted new seeds throughout the fertile grounds of social psychology.

Social cognition's products are now seen everywhere. Our journals are filled with research reflecting this approach; the *Journal of Personality and Social Psychology,* when it divided into three parts, adopted "social cognition" in the title of one of its sections; the term also became the title of a new journal, *Social Cognition,* and the title of an important textbook (Fiske & Taylor, 1984); by the mid-1980s many introductory social psychology texts included a chapter on social cognition; 1984 saw the publication of a three-volume *Handbook of Social Cognition* (Wyer & Srull, 1984), a second edition of which has recently been published (Wyer & Srull, 1994). The rapid development and spread of this new approach was unmistakable.

This enthusiasm was not shared by all, however. There were some who viewed these developments with alarm, while others viewed them with bemusement. Among the former, the concern was that social psychology was no longer "social" but instead had become overly mentalistic, indistinguishable from the newly emerged field of cognitive psychology. In contrast, and somewhat ironically, the predominant view among the latter was that this "new" development wasn't really all that new, that social psychology had always had an emphasis on the cognitive underpinnings of social behavior.

Social cognition, then, generated both broad enthusiasm and serious reservations within the social psychological community. What, then, is this "thing" that fostered such diverse reactions?

WHAT IS SOCIAL COGNITION?

In general terms, social cognition is a conceptual and empirical approach to understanding social psychological phenomena by investigating the cognitive structures and processes by which they operate (Sherman, Judd, & Park, 1989). As will become evident in the chapters comprising this volume, there are many ways of defining and describing social cognition and what it entails. At this point we can elaborate on this definition by developing several distinct, but related, points.

1. *The social cognition approach focuses on the direct investigation of the cognitive underpinnings of whatever social phenomenon is being studied.* It is certainly true, as emphasized by the second group of skeptics noted earlier, that "social psychology has always been cognitive," and in Chapter 2 of this volume Robert Abelson summarizes well the unique and important role social psychology played in perpetuating the importance of mentalistic concepts in an American psychology that was otherwise hostile to such thinking. The language of social psychology has always focused on concepts referring to cognitive structures (e.g., attitudes, beliefs, stereotypes, implicit personality theories) and cognitive processes (e.g., attitude change, impression formation, social comparison, attribution, decision making). To a considerable extent, however, these terms have had the status of mediating variables that help us explain the judgments, feelings, or behaviors of our subjects. What is new in social cognition is the extent to which these structures and processes become the focus of investigation. So, for example, the study of impression formation is not limited to assessing how much subjects like a target person, but instead investigates how that impression is mentally represented and what aspects of it are used in making the evaluative judgment. The study of attributions is not concerned solely with how the perceiver deviates from the prescriptions of a normative model, but instead inquires how causal knowledge is acquired, stored, and used in the attribution process. Similar distinctions can be made for other content areas.

It is important to acknowledge that this difference in the focus of inquiry is largely quantitative, not qualitative. For example, there is a long history of research investigating the structure of attitudes (McGuire, 1985); consistency theories were concerned with the relations among cognitive elements (Festinger, 1957; Heider, 1958); and the implicit personality theory literature of the 1960s was almost totally focused on determining the structure of perceivers' beliefs about personality (Schneider, 1973). Similarly, it would be unfair (as well as inaccurate) to imply that social psychological research was not interested in issues of process; in some sense, it always has been. Again, several examples of this type of analysis can be cited. There was, for example, Cartwright's (1941) research measuring decision times as a means of evaluating conflict between alternatives; Zajonc's (1960) research on cognitive tuning, which investigated the effect of processing goals on the structural relations among the elements of a mental representation; and the Yale attitude change program (Hovland, Janis, & Kelley, 1953), which was organized around an information processing analysis of several mediating stages in the persuasion process (attention, comprehension, acceptance). The reader undoubtedly can supply other examples. Finally, it is noteworthy that one of the important early textbooks of social psychology (Krech & Crutchfield, 1948) had a distinctly cognitive flavor. It set forth a number of "propositions" about fundamental processes, and then used those principles both in the analysis of basic social psychological issues and in applications to social problems.

With the advent of social cognition, however, this approach became a more systematic way of thinking about conceptual issues and research topics. In particular, two features differentiate social cognition research from previous approaches in this regard. First, in a social cognition approach structure and process are inherently intertwined, so that efforts to understand one require some attention to the other as well. Second, the emergence of social cognition research did not just "happen," but rather evolved as a consequence of the "cognitive revolution," a few years earlier, in experimental psychology. Because of the rapidly developing advances associated with that change, social cognition researchers were able to take advantage of new theoretical models and methodological tools developed in cognitive psychology and use them to address long-standing problems and issues in social psychology from a new perspective and with new experimental strategies. This link also leads us to a second feature of social cognition.

2. *The social cognition approach adopts an information-processing model as a means of understanding social phenomena.* The individual in the social context—the focus of social psychology—is viewed as one who is virtually always engaged in some form of information processing, however rudimentary. This statement applies whether the person is forming an impression of a stranger, chairing an important committee meeting, thinking back to one's high school prom, reacting to an interracial threat, flirting with the opposite sex, coping with a parent's life-threatening illness, or deciding which brand of deodorant to buy. In any circumstance, the person attends to

and encodes information from the (real or imagined) social context, interprets and elaborates on that information through evaluative, inferential, and attributional processes, and represents that elaborated "knowledge" in memory, from which it later can be retrieved for use in subsequent thought and judgment processes and for guiding behavior. This statement is not meant to imply that people routinely engage in a thorough, systematic analysis of the relevant information and its ramifications. On the contrary, in many cases people's "analyses" will be quite shallow, their processing will be quite superficial, and their responses will be based on arbitrary features of that information. The goal of the social cognition approach is to understand how these information processing mechanisms mediate the social perceptions and behaviors that have always been the grist of social psychology's mill.

3. *The social cognition approach assumes a communality across different content domains in psychology.* This communality is most evident in the close alignment of social cognition with cognitive psychology, reflecting the assumption that the same information processing principles apply in both the social and nonsocial domains. But social cognition is not simply an application of cognitive psychology to social psychological topics. On the contrary, this assumption of communality has a couple of important consequences. First, it allows the same set of constructs or principles to be used for the analysis of diverse phenomena. Second, and following from the first, it generates a basis for meaningful communications with researchers in related fields (e.g., personality, developmental psychology, communication). Thus, although some critics have accused social cognition of being narrow, it is anything but parochial in its underlying assumptions.

This shared focus on basic cognitive processes does not, however, imply a singular definition of the subject matter of psychology. As with any single approach or orientation, social cognition offers a particular perspective for analyzing substantive issues. It is not presented as a complete redefinition of what social psychology is or should be (as some critics have presumed). The phenomena to be understood are the heart of social psychology. Social cognition's role is to offer new explanatory constructs to explain these phenomena. It is clear that social cognition has already had a profound impact on the manner in which many social psychologists think about issues and do their research.

4. *Social cognition is an approach, not a content area.* Some of the roots of the "movement" now known as social cognition are found in research conducted in the mid-1970s on topics that traditionally were considered "social perception" (impression formation, stereotyping). Because of those origins, some misconceptions developed that social cognition was a new name for the traditional content area of person perception. This view was not only expressed by some of the critics of this new approach, but also was

reflected in some textbooks' treatment of social cognition. If this were true, then social cognition would be fairly limited in its range of applicability.

The erroneous nature of this view soon should have been apparent, as increasingly diverse social psychologists pursued their research topics within an information processing framework. By the early 1980s books had appeared applying this approach not only to impression formation (Hastie et al., 1980) and stereotyping (Hamilton, 1981) but also to personality issues (Cantor & Kihlstrom, 1981) and a broad range of topics in social psychology, including attribution, social communication, affect, judgment processes, and the self (Higgins, Herman, & Zanna, 1981; Wyer & Srull, 1984).

Social cognition is not defined by any particular content or substantive issue, but rather by an *approach to* one's content or issues. As already discussed, that approach rests on an information processing analysis that guides one's conceptual and empirical investigation of the cognitive processes underlying one's topic. As such, its application is not constrained by content; it can be adopted in the study of any topic in social psychology. In fact, one of the central goals of this volume is to document the range of classic topics in social psychology that have benefitted from the application of this approach.

These features summarize the primary elements of a social cognition approach to social psychology. Its development and application during the last fifteen years has changed the way social psychologists think theoretically about their favorite topics and the way they conduct their research. But how has it changed social psychology? And has it all been beneficial? What has it contributed to our understanding of some of the classic topic areas in the field? Assuming it has benefitted our discipline, what has been neglected as this approach has risen to its preeminent place during this period? And what is its potential role in the future of social psychology?

A few years ago, at the annual American Psychological Association Convention, there was a symposium (organized by Patricia Devine) in which the four participants were asked to address these questions for their respective areas of research. Subsequently, the three of us decided that a broader, more thorough treatment of this topic was appropriate. Social cognition has become a household term in psychology and has had some influence for over fifteen years. It has been the catalyst for fresh theoretical perspectives and new empirical work that have significantly expanded our knowledge of traditional topics in social psychology, and it has spawned new directions of inquiry. Moreover, several years' worth of students have been passing through our graduate programs with little opportunity to appreciate the extent of change generated by this approach during this period. It seemed timely to take stock and to evaluate the impact of this intellectual adventure. Therefore, we launched this volume, and we did so with specific goals in mind.

GOALS OF THE VOLUME AND CHAPTER PREVIEWS

The primary purpose of this volume is to document the contribution of social cognition to the study of classic issues in social psychology. It is important to recognize that our reference to "contribution" does not mean to imply that all of the ideas presented are "new." Nor does it mean that the "old" social psychological theories are wrong or even forgotten. Indeed, we believe that the strength of the social cognitive approach to studying social psychological issues is most clearly illuminated when it builds on and is integrated with classic work in social psychology. In fact, this was the spirit in which the present volume was conceived.

To achieve this goal, we decided to develop a volume in which each chapter would be concerned with a different historically important content area in social psychology. The authors of these chapters, experts in their respective topic domains, were asked to evaluate the impact of social cognition in their area. Specifically, we presented authors with three broad goals to keep in mind in preparing their chapters. First, they were to summarize "the way things were" in their area before social cognition, as a systematic approach, developed. This summary might articulate the classic issues, the theoretical approaches, and the empirical controversies that predominated prior to the mid-1970s. Second, we asked them to document the impact that social cognition has had in their areas during the last two decades. This assessment might include discussion of the theoretical models, methodological changes, and major empirical advances that have occurred during this period, due (at least in part) to social cognition's influence. Third, we asked the authors to consider the implications of this work for the future. This aspect might include discussion of the potential of social cognition to propel theorizing and research in new directions; it might include consideration of the limitations of this approach, the "blind spots" that derive from wearing the social cognition lenses; and it might include consideration of how this approach could profitably interface with other approaches to these classic topic areas in social psychology, thereby providing a broader, more comprehensive understanding of these issues.

Our authors tackled these objectives in different ways, some focusing on one of these goals, others emphasizing another, still others explicitly addressing all of them in balanced fashion. Regardless of these differences, all of the authors took seriously the charge to adopt a broad perspective and to reflect on how social cognition has influenced research and theorizing in their respective areas. The result is a volume that effectively documents social cognition's impact and illustrates how the social cognition approach can provide theoretical leverage for illuminating a variety of classic topics in social psychology. Together they reveal that social cognition has had a broader, more pervasive effect on social psychology than many have recognized. In sum, the chapters provide a coherent statement of what social cognition is today, both theoretically and empirically, and an evaluation of its role in social psychology.

Although most of our authors were given the general guidelines we outlined earlier, there was one exception to this general rule. We felt that the career-long contributions of Robert P. Abelson had, in many important ways, both anticipated and laid the foundation for many of the developments that ultimately came to be described as "social cognition." Therefore we invited Abelson to write a different kind of chapter, one in which he commented, from his own personal experiences, on the developments that have transpired in social psychology during the forty-year period spanned by his career. We asked him to discuss the historical background from which contemporary social cognition emerged, to share how his own thinking developed during these years, and to comment on both the contributions and limitations of present-day social cognition theory and research. Fortunately, Abelson agreed to our invitation, and the result is a unique and engaging chapter, dotted with personal anecdotes, providing not only a historical account but also an intriguing window into the thinking of one of social psychology's creative geniuses. Our book opens with this chapter (Chapter 2) in recognition of the contribution that Abelson's thinking has made to developments in virtually all of the content areas covered in subsequent chapters.

Abelson's personal retrospective provides readers with a fascinating glimpse of the challenges faced by those who believed that mentalistic analyses would contribute to our understanding of social psychological phenomena. Although modern social psychology has clearly had a strong cognitive tradition, early efforts to explore mentalistic concepts went against the dominant behavioristic grain of the times. Placed in this context, Abelson's review of important developments is informative for those who have "grown up" intellectually in the more recent cognitive tradition. Seeing these developments through Abelson's eyes is both delightful and enlightening. For example, Abelson acknowledges the often elegant research designs and precise methods that characterize social cognition research. However, he also challenges social cognition researchers to move beyond "Neat research," which emphasizes simplicity and orderliness, to take on the challenges of "Scruffy approaches," which confront the disorder of complex phenomena rather than suppressing it. Complex social phenomena, such as prejudice, will not likely give way to "Neat" analyses alone. Abelson characterizes one of the recent, influential developments in social psychology as the proliferation of "coacting central subsystems." Abelson contrasts such two-system models with classic single-system consistency theories, identifies some of the potential limitations of the current models, and outlines new directions for theoretical elaboration of such models. As such, Abelson continues to set theoretical and empirical agendas for the field. And we are the better off for it.

Several of the chapters provide analyses of the contribution of social cognition to various intrapersonal phenomena. For example, Jacques-Philippe Leyens and Susan Fiske (Chapter 3) discuss the contribution of social cognition to the study of person impressions. As they note, "the study of impression formation should be an area of research par excellence in which to evaluate the progress of social cognition research" (p. 2); as their review indicates, it clearly is. Leyens and Fiske nicely illustrate how both traditionalists (seeking connection with the classic research) and innovators (seeking novelty) can find comfort with the work on person perception and impression formation. In their efforts to illustrate both continuity and change in the theoretical and empirical work in this domain, they use the metaphor of a classical sonata form of a symphony's first movement. Music aficionados will see that the metaphor works well. For nonaficionados, Leyens and Fiske do a nice job of setting the stage for their metaphor, and of placing the contributions of social cognition in historical context as well as identifying fruitful research directions.

Identifying the causes of behaviors by making attributional judgments has been one of the most extensively researched topics in social psychology. Eliot Smith (Chapter 4) analyzes the classic work on attribution and the challenges it created for researchers approaching the study of attribution from a social cognition analysis. Smith reviews some of the major trends in attribution research and illustrates how these changes parallel developments in cognitive psychology. In addition, Smith shows that current attribution theorists have attempted to place attribution in the context of broader theoretical models that attempt to integrate a range of research paradigms and dependent variables and to link work across a variety of domains (e.g., social, cognitive, developmental, clinical, and personality psychology). Smith then outlines three streams of attribution research today, including new perspectives on Kelley's (1967) ANOVA model, linguistic influences on attribution, and cognitive processes and memory structures involved in attribution. In each case, Smith illustrates how social cognition has influenced the direction of theoretical and empirical developments. Smith concludes his chapter by outlining what he sees as the specific contributions of social cognition to the area of attribution and offers some tentative prognostications for future attribution work.

Social psychologists have long been concerned with the issue of how social perceivers make trait inferences. Robert Wyer and Alan Lambert (Chapter 5) observe that perceivers have a proclivity to use trait adjectives in describing their impressions of others. They further observe that personality traits have been central in the language of personality and social psychologists, both historically and contemporaneously. The goal of Wyer and Lambert's chapter is to review social cognition's influence on the way that personality and social psychologists think about trait constructs. In doing so, they delineate the cognitive processes involved in making trait inferences (e.g., how trait inferences are made from behavior, the role of trait concepts in organizing social information, the structure and use of person representations). Wyer and Lambert effectively use an interplay between the "then" and the "now" for a variety of issues in the trait inference literature, an analysis that sensitizes the reader to social cognition's contributions to this research domain.

Patricia Linville and Donal Carlston's Chapter 6 concerns the concept of self, which has long had a central role in social psychology. These authors provide a comprehensive analysis of issues that challenged William James and his contemporaries and discuss how social cognition has advanced our understanding of the role of the self in social psychology. Their review centers on the progress made with regard to three enduring issues: (1) whether the self is best construed as a single structure or as consisting of multiple components; (2) the distinction between declarative-based (factual) knowledge and procedural-based (rule) self-knowledge; and (3) the stability versus malleability of the self. Linville and Carlston illustrate how social cognition both provides a new perspective for thinking about these classic issues and raises questions that are made tractable because of the theoretical and methodological advances associated with this approach.

In a now-classic statement, Gordon Allport (1935) once argued that the central theoretical construct of social psychology is the attitude. Thomas Ostrom, John Skowronski, and Andrzej Nowak (Chapter 7) ask us to consider the world of social psychology without the attitude construct and, having done so, they conclude that it continues to be "a wonderful construct." They illustrate how social cognition has enriched classic information processing approaches to the study of attitudes and persuasion. The cognitive perspective allows us to analyze past conceptual work on attitudes into issues regarding cognitive code, structure, and process. In their analysis, however, attitude theory and research is also a field ripe for future advances from a social cognitive perspective. Ostrom, Skowronski, and Nowak delineate the ways in which existing cognitive theorizing can be fruitfully mined in efforts to develop a more complete understanding of the way in which attitudes are represented and the processes by which they exert their influence on thought and behavior.

Diane Mackie and John Skelly (Chapter 8) examine the impact of social cognition on the study of social influence, specifically in the areas of persuasion and conformity. In doing so, Mackie and Skelly also reveal social cognition's potential for contributing to analyses of important interpersonal phenomena. Although persuasion and conformity historically have been separate areas of research, each with its own theories and methods, Mackie and Skelly effectively argue that the separation is more apparent than real. The goal of their chapter is to review how social cognition has affected each area separately and then to illustrate how the two areas can be conceptually integrated through a social cognition analysis. Their central point is that, to understand any form of social influence, it is important to develop an analysis of the proximal intrapersonal processes involved in responding to distal influence factors (e.g., persuasive argument, pressure from other people). It is with regard to this issue that social cognition analyses have made direct and explicit contributions. This chapter identifies important new directions for research (e.g., determining how validity is conferred on persuasive arguments or social indicators; exploring the integration of motivation and goals with cognitive factors in social influence) and suggests that progress on these fronts can build on the foundation developed through the application of social cognition principles to social influence.

The final section of the volume concerns contributions of social cognition in the interrelated areas stereotypes, prejudice, and intergroup relations. These chapters substantiate Gordon Allport's (1954) early suggestion that cognitive processes are important in intergroup phenomena. For a long time Allport's analyses remained at the level of speculation. However, the theoretical insights and tools provided by advances in cognitive psychology have enabled the systematic testing of some of his hypotheses and have paved the way for advances not anticipated by Allport. Each of these chapters effectively integrates historical challenges with contemporary work. The chapters illustrate continuity of current developments with past research, as well as highlight the progress and new directions spawned by the application of social cognition to these areas.

David Hamilton, Steven Stroessner, and Denise Driscoll (Chapter 9) discuss how social cognition has affected the way social psychologists think about and do research on stereotypes. They emphasize that a social cognition analysis attempts to understand how stereotypes, as cognitive structures, are represented in perceivers' minds and how they guide information processing to affect perceivers' perceptions of groups and group members. One important benefit of this approach is that it has brought the study of stereotypes into mainstream social psychology. Hamilton, Stroessner, and Driscoll outline an agenda for future research exploring the role of cognitive processes in some long-standing yet unresolved issues in the stereotype literature (e.g., stereotype assessment, stereotype change). They also argue that social cognition's emphasis on information processing provides a useful foundation for extending analyses to include motivational and affective factors.

Margo Monteith, Julia Zuwerink, and Patricia Devine's Chapter 10 focuses on the challenges associated with trying to reduce prejudice. The classic work on this topic indicates that developing effective techniques for prejudice reduction has produced only mixed success. According to Monteith, Zuwerink, and Devine, one of the key difficulties with past research was its largely atheoretical nature and its failure to adequately delineate the theoretical processes involved in prejudice reduction. It is here that the authors see the clearest contributions of social cognition. Their chapter considers the various social cognitive analyses for the so-called modern forms of prejudice, in which many people experience individual-level conflict or ambivalence (i.e., inconsistency between egalitarian attitudes and prejudiced responses). Based on this analysis, the authors outline the potential of a social cognition approach to promoting change.

Myron Rothbart and Scott Lewis (Chapter 11) review the contributions of social cognition to the study of intergroup relations and the prospects for ameliorating intergroup tensions. They argue that the conceptualization of the limited-capacity processor who needs to simplify the complex stimulus world is central to an understanding of intergroup perception and intergroup conflict. Rothbart and Lewis argue that research into the nature and function of categorization processes has been a major contribution of the cognitive approach to intergroup relations. They also consider the implications of social cognitive analyses for work on the minimal-group situation, social identity theory, differential perception of ingroup and outgroup characteristics, and the contact hypothesis. Although Rothbart and Lewis view the contributions of social cognition as liberating conceptual analyses in this area (e.g., away from the psychodynamic perspective), they caution students of intergroup relations against being limited by a purely cognitive analysis, for phenomena as complicated as intergroup violence are unlikely to be solely cognitive in nature.

The chapters in this volume cover a broad range of topics, spanning the intrapersonal, interpersonal, and intergroup levels of analysis. Even this coverage, however, provides an incomplete sampling of the topics that have usefully been addressed by those adopting a social cognition perspective. Recent research on aggression (Berkowitz, 1990; Dodge, Pettit, McClaskey, & Brown, 1986), affect (Forgas, 1990; Mackie & Hamilton, 1993; Ortony, Clore, & Collins, 1988; Srull, 1983), group decision making (Pennington & Hastie, 1992), and survey methodology (Hippler, Schwarz & Sudman, 1987; Schwarz & Strack, 1991; Tourangeau & Raskinski, 1988) provides other examples of the impact of social cognition on topics and issues of central importance in social psychology. All of this work illustrates a point we stressed earlier in this chapter, that social cognition is not a content area but rather an approach to the conceptual and empirical analysis of any content area in our discipline.

Although social cognition has often been described, with some validity, as a "new" approach to social psychology, we believe that this feature has been overemphasized. An important theme that we hope the reader will discern in this volume is that social cognition has more continuity with the past than sometimes is apparent in the literature. It is certainly true that we are impressed by the progress that has been made by applying this approach to social psychological phenomena during the last fifteen years. At the same time, however, it is important to recognize that this progress builds on foundations that were established in previous decades. In addition, we are optimistic about this approach's potential for future developments, as anticipated in virtually every chapter of this volume. We invite our readers to take on the challenges outlined in these chapters as social cognition evolves in new directions, extending our theorizing and our research beyond the achievements documented here.

ACKNOWLEDGMENTS

Preparation of this chapter was supported in part by NIMH Grant MH 40058 to the first author. The authors are grateful to Diane M. Mackie for her comments on a preliminary version of this chapter.

REFERENCES

Allport, G. W. (1935). Attitudes. In C. Murchison (Ed.), *Handbook of social psychology* (pp. 798–844). Worcester, MA: Clark University Press.
Allport, G. W. (1954). *The nature of prejudice.* Reading, MA: Addison-Wesley.
Berkowitz, L. (1990). On the formation and regulation of anger and aggression: A cognitive-neoassociationistic analysis. *American Psychologist, 45,* 494–503.
Cantor, N., & Kihlstrom, J. F. (Eds.). (1981). *Personality, cognition, and social interaction.* Hillsdale, NJ: Erlbaum.
Cartwright, D. (1941). Relation of decision time to the categories of response. *American Journal of Psychology, 54,* 174–196.
Dodge, K. A., Pettit, G. S., McClaskey, C. L., & Brown, M. M. (1986). Social competence in children. *Monographs of the Society for Research in Child Development,* Serial No. 213.
Festinger, L. (1957). *A theory of cognitive dissonance.* Palo Alto, CA: Stanford University Press.
Fiske, S. T., & Taylor, S. E. (1984). *Social cognition.* Reading, MA: Addison-Wesley.
Forgas, J. P. (Ed.). (1990). *Emotion and social judgments.* Oxford: Pergamon Press.
Hamilton, D. L. (Ed.). (1981). *Cognitive processes in stereotyping and intergroup behavior.* Hillsdale, NJ: Erlbaum.
Hastie, R., Ostrom, T. M., Ebbesen, E. B., Wyer, R. S., Jr., Hamilton, D. L., & Carlston, D. E. (Eds.). (1980). *Person memory: The cognitive basis of social perception.* Hillsdale, NJ: Erlbaum.
Heider, F. (1958). *The psychology of interpersonal relations.* New York: Wiley.
Higgins, E. T., Herman, P. C., & Zanna, M. P. (Eds.). (1981). *Social cognition: The Ontario symposium.* Hillsdale, NJ: Erlbaum.
Hippler, H. J., Schwarz, N., & Sudman, S. (Eds.). (1987). *Social information processing and survey methodology.* New York: Springer-Verlag.
Hovland, C. I., Janis, I. L., & Kelley, H. H. (1953). *Communication and persuasion.* New Haven, CT: Yale University Press.
Kelley, H. H. (1967). Attribution theory in social psychology. In D. Levine (Ed.), *Nebraska symposium on motivation* (Vol. 15, pp. 192–240). Lincoln: University of Nebraska Press.
Krech, D., & Crutchfield, R. S. (1948). *Theory and problems of social psychology.* New York: McGraw-Hill.
McGuire, W. J. (1985). Attitudes and attitude change. In G. Lindzey & E. Aronson (Eds.), *The handbook of social psychology* (3rd ed.), (Vol. 2, pp. 233–46). New York: Random House.
Mackie, D. M., & Hamilton, D. L. (Eds.). (1993). *Affect, cognition, and stereotyping: Interactive processes in group perception.* San Diego, CA: Academic Press.

Ortony, A., Clore, G. L., & Collins, A. (1988). *The cognitive structure of emotions*. New York, NY: Cambridge University Press.

Pennington, N., & Hastie, R. (1992). Explaining the evidence: Tests of the story model for juror decision making. *Journal of Personality and Social Psychology, 62,* 189–206.

Schneider, D. J. (1973). Implicit personality theory: A review. *Psychological Bulletin, 79,* 294–309.

Schwarz, N., & Strack, F. (1991). Context effects in attitude surveys: Applying cognitive theory to social research. In W. Stroebe & M. Hewstone (Eds.), *European review of social psychology* (Vol. 2, pp. 31–50). Chichester, England: Wiley.

Sherman, S. J., Judd, C. M., & Park, B. (1989). Social cognition. In M. R. Rosenzweig & L. W. Porter (Eds.), *Annual review of psychology* (Vol. 40, pp. 281–286). Palo Alto, CA: Annual Reviews.

Srull, T. K. (1983). Affect and memory: The impact of affective reactions in advertising on the representation of product information in memory. In R. Bagozzi & A. Tybout (Eds.), *Advances in consumer research* (Vol. 10, pp. 520–525). Ann Arbor, MI: Association for Consumer Research.

Tourangeau, R., & Raskinski, K. A. (1988). Cognitive processes underlying context effects in attitude measurement. *Psychological Bulletin, 103,* 299–314.

Wyer, R. S., Jr., & Srull, T. K. (Eds.). (1984). *Handbook of social cognition*. Hillsdale, NJ: Erlbaum.

Wyer, R. S., Jr., & Srull, T. K. (Eds.). (1994). *Handbook of social cognition*(2nd ed.). Hillsdale, NJ: Erlbaum.

Zajonc, R. B. (1960). The process of cognitive tuning in communication. *Journal of Abnormal and Social Psychology, 51,* 159–167.

2

A Personal Perspective on Social Cognition

Robert P. Abelson

The editors of this volume asked me to write a personal perspective on developments in social cognition over the past forty years. My perspective is idiosyncratic. The information explosion has blown me away; so, like the prototypical limited information processor, I selectively highlight bits and pieces of the vast scene. Specifically, I comment on some slices of social psychology's history in which there was a struggle to develop mentalistic concepts in an unsympathetic behaviorist environment. I note a few behavioristic presuppositions that social psychology—and later, social cognition—inherited from this struggle. I then relate how I tried to depart from this legacy in the development of some of my own views. Last, I discuss a recent trend in social cognition that is extremely rich in its potential to do justice to the complexities of mental life and of intergroup relations.

HOW EARLY SOCIAL PSYCHOLOGY KEPT ITS MIND

Modern social psychology has always had a strongly cognitive orientation. As Ross and Nisbett (1991) put it, "[An] . . . enduring contribution of social psychology is . . . [that] the impact of any 'objective' stimulus situation depends upon the personal and subjective meaning that the actor attaches to that situation" (p. 11). This seems quite noncontroversial to social psychologists, and it is hard to appreciate the historical fact that as recently as thirty-five years ago it was virtually taboo in mainstream American psychology to indulge in such subjectivism. From the mid-1920s through the mid-1950s, behaviorism, with its ideological resistance to any and all mentalistic theorizing, was almost totally dominant. During this period, cognitive psychology as we now know it had not yet gotten off the ground, and it fell to social psychology to provide an epistemological safety valve against behaviorism.

Accounts of the history of social psychology (Jones, 1985; McGuire, 1985; Patnoe, 1988) agree that the person most influential in launching modern social psychology in the 1940s was Kurt Lewin. A lesser, but nonetheless important, role was played by Solomon Asch. Both men came out of a European tradition antithetical to behaviorism; both studied group behavior, yet focused on the mind of the individual—Asch (1940, 1946) in terms of how others were perceived and why their behavior was influential, and Lewin (1938) in his "life spaces" containing regions and barriers near desired goal states.[1]

Lewin's major influence was through his extraordinary group of students, and his exemplary demonstrations of the possibility of controlled experimentation on important group phenomena. After Lewin died in 1947, his students (Festinger, Schachter, Kelley, Thibaut, and Deutsch, among others) carried on his tradition of interrelating small group behaviors with the mental lives of group members. This research tradition grew up independent of behaviorism, but could not indefinitely avoid contact with it.

What happened in the 1950s when the cognitivist suppositions of emerging social psychology encountered the rigid behaviorist constraints on permissible psychological discourse? As with other examples of interactions between a minority subculture and a dominant culture, there was more than one way for the embattled minority to cope. One possibility was surface conformity to the majority, while still keeping one's own counsel.

A critical example of such a strategy occurred at Yale in the early 1950s. (I began my career at Yale in 1952.) Carl Hovland had established his research group on persuasive communication in the very department where Clark Hull was preaching his hypothetico-deductive theories of learning. There was no doubt that Hull was a revered figure whose legacy was felt long after his death in 1951. In fact, learning theory was a required course for first-year graduate students for more than a decade thereafter, and the phrase "experimental psychology" was largely taken to refer to animal learning experiments. (When Tex Garner arrived in 1966 to lead a cognitive psychology group, he offered the advice, "You still need to scrape Clark Hull off the walls in here.")

How did Hovland's group deal with the competing traditions? A close reading of the classic volume *Communication and Persuasion* (Hovland, Janis, & Kelley, 1952) reveals the answer. Hovland et al. indeed spoke the language of behaviorism, but in fact used other theoretical traditions for

[1]Lewin's life spaces were formulated in a pseudo-mathematical style that had no pertinent body of mathematical theory to back it up, and thus proved infertile as anything but a metaphor. However, a Finnish psychologist named Kullervo Rainio, a writer of psychology textbooks popular in Finland, and a sometime member of the Finnish parliament, persevered in producing a treatise on Lewin's mathematics (Rainio, 1986) that he began nearly forty years ago.

their real reasoning. There were numerous references to the concepts of reinforcement, incentives, drive, and the like. The process of accepting the recommendations of a communicator was depicted as a kind of inner speech that could be strengthened by "rehearsal" until it was "learned." Yet, if you strip away the postured language in this book, you realize that the parts written by Irv Janis were anchored in psychodynamic thinking, those by Hal Kelley rooted in the Lewinian group tradition, and those by Carl Hovland colored by his interests in concept formation (Hovland, 1952).

Hovland and colleagues thus were closet cognitivists. The mentalist emphasis became overt when Hovland expanded the group. Brehm and Cohen (1962) championed dissonance theory, McGuire (1960) devised his model of syllogistic thinking, and Rosenberg and I theorized about belief structures (Abelson, 1959; Abelson & Rosenberg, 1958; Rosenberg & Abelson, 1960). Hovland's own cognitive proclivity was typified by his attendance at a month-long summer seminar on computer simulation of reasoning and problem solving run by Newell, Simon, and Shaw 1958. The overall style of the expanded group was a cacophonous expression of cognitivism. I think that Carl Hovland managed to get away with this because of his stature, and because the group did not launch a general campaign *opposed* to behaviorism. We simply went our own merry ways.

In the end, the best strategy for resisting behaviorist influence was complete obliviousness. A master of this art was Fritz Heider, who came to the United States in 1930 with a European philosophical background.[2] His book, *The Psychology of Interpersonal Relations* (Heider, 1958), was a smash hit in social psychology, though it did not say a thing about actual interpersonal relations, only people's conceptions of generic social events. Even such a tough critic as Leon Festinger liked it, because it was so closely and elegantly reasoned. Heider's "balance theory" saw a number of applications, and his early papers on social attribution were the foundation for all the attribution work that came after. Heider's 1958 book can be seen as a precursor of the modern fascination with the concept of schemas.

I had the privilege of meeting Heider on several occasions. In 1977, I was driving him and his wife, Grace, from New Hampshire to New Haven, and the radiator was boiling over every ten minutes, requiring a refill from one of the many gallon jugs of water I had stashed in the trunk. Fortunately, Fritz was full of stories, including a surprising tale of interaction between Clark Hull and the Heiders in the 1940s. It seems that Hull had invited them to join his faculty/student seminar, and every week for a whole semester the Heiders drove from Amherst to New Haven to attend. I was fascinated to hear this, and I said, "But how did you react to their point of view, which

[2]Heider's (1927) dissertation at Graz was concerned with the then burning issue: How come when we have our glasses on and look out the window at, say, a tree, we perceive the tree but (typically) not our glasses or the window frame?

seems so different from yours?" In his lyrical Austrian accent he quietly replied, "Oh, I just listened. I knew it was all nonsense, but they were so enthusiastic."

BEHAVIORISM NEVERTHELESS HAD AN INDIRECT INFLUENCE

Social psychology never succumbed to behaviorism, but it was influenced in content and in method by some of behaviorism's suppositions. Even though the famous Festinger and Carlsmith (1959) experiment obtained results inimical to reinforcement theory, Festinger (1957) had made his account of dissonance reduction sound like drive reduction. This was an appeal to the staple motivating circumstance in learning theory (albeit Festinger never concerned himself with the learning of dissonance reduction strategies).[3]

Another, more general, continuity between behaviorism and cognitive social psychology is the faith in reductionism in formulating an experimental agenda. Since the beginnings of experimental social psychology, researchers have tried to represent social stimuli with single words or lists of words, rather than with sentences, propositions, or higher level constructs. The notion was that if one understood the psychological processes involved in the simplest tasks with the simplest stimuli, then and only then could one synthesize an understanding of more complex situations.[4] To many psychologists, even nonbehaviorists, this strategy seemed (and still seems) sufficiently self-evident as not to require justification.

I will use the term *logotropism* to denote the attachment of psychologists to the use of isolated words or phrases as stimulus materials. Social psychologists were logotropes during the historical period when they otherwise escaped the influence of behaviorism. An obvious example is Solomon Asch's famous demonstration of the effect of "central" traits on impression formation, by noting the large difference made by substituting *cold* for *warm* in a list of intellectual trait words (Asch, 1946). Critics of Asch's centrality concept stayed on the word level, too. Rosenberg, Nelson, and Vivekananthan (1968) did a multidimensional scaling of trait words, and argued that "warm" and "cold" were so distant from each other on the social dimension of the two-dimensional trait space that when respectively aver-

[3]Festinger later regretted that he had endowed dissonance with the aversive properties of a drive state. He said privately that he should have simply postulated a *formal* link between dissonance and the use of dissonance reduction strategies. As it has turned out, he was right the first time. Aversive arousal, according to Cooper and Fazio (1984), proves crucial in distinguishing dissonance theory from its rival, self-perception theory.

[4]The most radical version of this notion is that elemental analysis is *sufficient* to explain all seemingly higher level phenomena. Endel Tulving once remarked to me, "There is nothing you can learn about the psychology of language that you can't find out by studying words."

aged in with a redundant cluster of intellectual trait words, they would obviously pull the impressions far apart. Norman Anderson (1966) pitched into the battle with his "information integration" models, for which his famous list of the favorability ratings of 555 trait words (Anderson, 1968) was a convenient research weapon.

Logotropism was further enhanced by the popularity of the book *The Measurement of Meaning* (Osgood, Suci, & Tannenbaum, 1957) and its accompanying research tool, the Semantic Differential. The meaning of the stimulus word (e.g., mother, statue, policeman) was specified by reference to bipolar scales with a word on each end: good/bad, strong/weak, active/passive, and their variants. This system had great appeal; it was simple and commonsensical, and it kept popping up in different contexts. Its benefits are clear, but its downside—and to some extent the downside of logotropic methods in general—is a bit less obvious.

WHERE HAD ALL THE PHENOMENOLOGY GONE? A PERSONAL DETOUR

Even though I and many others made use of Osgood's semantic dimensions (e.g., in Abelson & Sermat, 1962), I was never very happy with its limited conception of meaning. One problem was that Osgood's system dealt only with connotative meaning, and I wanted some way to deal with *denotative* meaning. One can locate STATUE on his three dimensions, for example, as somewhat good, rather strong, and totally inactive, without capturing at all that statues are usually downtown on stone pedestals, that they honor war heroes, that they are created by sculptors, and so on. A second problem was that the semantic differential was forever being used to scale *nouns,*[5] and nobody seemed to care about *verbs,* not to mention propositions combining nouns *and* verbs. The result was a static picture of mental life. It was not easy to scale verbs, I knew (a multidimensional scaling solution for verb similarity judgments yields a mess, as David Kanouse and I once discovered), but nobody was even trying.

In my view, the key ingredients in representations of social reality are collocations of propositions about social actions: for example, persons of type X are prone to take actions A,B,C in situations of type Q; if group G takes political action P, then we should reply with response R; the appropriate sequence of actions in environment E comprises U,V,W . . . , and so on.

Furthermore, it is important for these propositions to have rather con-

[5]Experimental cognitive psychologists were noun oriented, as well. James Deese (1962), for example, published a theoretical account of the semantic similarities of concepts in which the concepts were all nouns. It was easy to slip into a verbless depiction because of the emphasis in cognitive psychology on the nounish notion of stimulus *categories*.

crete referents, an insight that gradually dawned on me from my experience in trying to design a computer simulation of the operation of an ideological belief system. The utterances of ideologues are highly predictable (one might even say "scripted"), and this led me some years ago (Abelson & Carroll, 1965) to attempt to simulate the foreign policy views of Senator Barry Goldwater, the most single-minded hawk of the early 1960s. At the time, I was guided by a version of Heider's (1958) balance theory (Abelson & Rosenberg, 1958; Rosenberg & Abelson, 1960), which rested on the subjective propositions that good guys do good things and bad guys do bad things. In the true believer's mental world, any assertions to the contrary should be transformed to fit these comfortable propositions.

Senator Goldwater's public statements formed a tight, balanced system: Communists were responsible for all evil around the globe, while America and the Free World had the values and the capability to defeat evil and promote good. Our computer model was intended to imitate what Goldwater might say if confronted with potential news developments. Thus, if a Communist nation or group threatened or damaged a Free World nation, the model would output a statement of outrage and condemnation; any military action that America might take to prevent or block such a development was warmly endorsed. By categorizing actors as them or us, and actions as helpful or harmful to them or us, the model was prepared to emit one or another stock cliché from its one-dimensional storehouse of declamations.

If an imbalanced "news item" such as "American troops kill innocent Vietnamese civilians" were presented to the model, it would struggle to reinterpret the item within its world view (e.g., by asserting that the Vietnamese were not in fact innocent civilians). (In a pair of prior articles [Abelson, 1959, 1963], I had outlined a set of mechanisms for restoring balance to imbalanced propositions.)

The computer simulation of Goldwater's style and content worked tolerably well except for one glaring defect. The model would accept nonsensical input, as long as it was cognitively balanced. Thus to the news item, "Fidel Castro throws eggs at Taiwan," the model would cheerfully react with one of its stock phrases for Communist evildoing, such as "Yes, that's the kind of provocation against a Free World nation you would expect from a Communist government." There was no representation in the model for mundane realities such as the logistical impossibility of throwing eggs halfway around the world, much less the semantic incongruity of throwing eggs at a country. The lesson here is that the belief systems of sane ideologues cannot be entirely governed by a cognitive balance principle; real-world knowledge always constrains the set of assertions believed true by the system. Again, we have the theme that connotative meaning is insufficient—denotative meaning is important, too.

My concern with this defect in the Goldwater model, along with my hankering for verb representations and attention to event sequences, led me to develop the script concept (Abelson, 1973, 1976, 1981a; Schank & Abelson, 1977). In a revised model of Goldwater's world view (Abelson, 1973), Communist schemes were concretized into a number of subtypes: military takeover, internal subversion, and tricking us into disarmament, for example. All of these were more or less routinized sequences of events, often with sequences of microevents embedded within them. Internal subversion of a country comprised radical student agitation, infiltration of labor unions, placement of "fellow travelers" in key government posts, the smuggled entry of arms from neighboring Communist countries, and finally a coup taking over the government. The throwing of eggs was understood within a script concerning radical student agitation against Free World visitors to neutral countries, but occurred nowhere else in the system. Thus the system could recognize egg throwing as a hostile Communist action, and at the same time be capable of rejecting the premise that Castro throws eggs at Taiwan. Castro, after all, is not a student, nor is Taiwan a Free World figure visiting Havana.[6]

At the time I first grappled with this representation of a large albeit relatively simple belief system, my approach was probably seen as eccentric. I was trying to fill a big system with little pieces, whereas everyone else was trying to understand the workings of pieces in isolation. In the 1960s, the "cognitive consistency" theories—dissonance, balance, and incongruity—preoccupied social psychologists (Abelson et al., 1968). (I shall have more to say about cognitive consistency later.) In the 1970s, the dominant topic was attribution theory. True to the habit in social psychology, the popular topics of both decades focused on cognition. They were less logotropic than the topics of the 1950s, but rather modest in the complexity of belief structures they were willing to deal with. Instead of word lists, we had small clusters of events or propositions demanding resolution or inference by the individual (*Imbalance:* I like O; O did X; I dislike X. *Dissonance:* I believe X; I am saying not X; no reward or threat is present. *Attribution:* P does X in response to S; P does not do X in response to other S's; other P's also do X in response to S.)

Other eccentrics came out in the 1970s with even more general models of knowledge representation and manipulation: Anderson's (1976) ACT model; Newell and Simon's (1972) comprehensive and influential view of human information processing; Minsky's (1975) concept of "frames"; Norman and Rumelhart's (1975) propositional network models; and Schank's (1972) "conceptual dependency" system. These people are remote from social psychology (comprising a mix of cognitive psychologists and computer scientists interested in artificial intelligence), but their influence hopped across

[6]Even with the clarification provided by scripts, my Goldwater Machine still had some bugs. Years later, Yale Computer Science student Jaime Carbonell (1978) used better programming techniques to formulate general simulations of foreign policy ideologies.

disciplinary boundaries. Perhaps my book with Roger Schank (Schank & Abelson, 1977) helped provide a bridge across these boundaries.

At any rate, in the 1980s there emerged as "social cognition" the loose union of a broad system conception with a focused miniprocess approach in social psychology. It was characterized by two somewhat contradictory impulses. On one hand, it tried to capture some of the complexities of real belief and knowledge structures; on the other, it still embraced the logotropic methods of laboratory cognitive psychology.

In the early 1980s, the concept of a cognitive schema was adopted as a kind of mascot in social cognition. Roughly speaking, a schema is a manageable package of knowledge or beliefs that serves to organize perception and cognition when activated. This concept was used so much as to create lengthy discussion about the conditions for its appropriate employment (Fiske & Linville, 1980), and debate has continued into the 1990s (Kuklinski, Luskin, & Bolland, 1991).

I myself was concerned from way back that schemas were being invoked too narrowly. In social cognition work, schemas were often exemplified by prototypes and stereotypes, operationalized as *lists* of characteristic attributes (e.g., Cantor & Mischel, 1979; Weber & Crocker, 1983). This is no condemnation of the interesting research on prototypes and stereotypes. Rather, I am doubting the theoretical usefulness of any kind of "schematic" structures in cases when semantic clusters—word lists, in essence—will do. (Note the continued survival of logotropism.) Schemas are only interesting when they consist of *interrelated propositions that permit nontrivial inferences* about a given situation.

Some of the simplest representations that are usefully construed as schemas are: for events, *scripts* of typical event sequences (Schank & Abelson, 1977), *plot units* (Lehnert, 1981) such as "broken promise," *thematic affect units* (Dyer, 1983) like "Don't count your chickens before they are hatched"; for objects, *frames* (Minsky, 1975) such as "a room," and systems of object attributes and relations (Gentner, 1983) such as "the solar system." Schemas of these sorts all have the property that assertions about any of their parts have implications for particular other parts: if, in the restaurant script, the waiter brings something other than what the customer ordered, subsequent events follow an alternative to the usual path; if, in a room, a wall is six feet high at one end and eight feet high at the other, this has consequences for how the other walls might be configured.

True, prototypes and stereotypes might be said to permit inferences, too, but these inferences are usually of the form "more of the same." If we are told that Alice engaged in dependent behavior A and dependent behavior B, we may conclude that Alice is dependent, and predict she will perform dependent behavior C. These inferences are dull—except when they are wrong. Trait-based representations, as presently conceptualized by social psychologists, tend to be all or none; for example, the stereotypic librarian is female, introverted, bookish, and neat. When subjects are presented with nonbookish librarians, we know that this ought to shake them up a bit, but we do not know quite how to model the resulting cognitive processes. The stereotype has no moving parts. Cases inconsistent with the stereotype may weaken it, but there is (as yet) no coherent account of the details of the process by which this happens. (*Subtyping* [Weber & Crocker, 1983; Brewer, 1988] is a potentially interesting process for handling exceptions to stereotypes, but the details of such a process also remain unclear.) Prototypes and stereotypes might be interesting as schematic structures, but only if the interconnections of their component parts could be articulated.

To make my own point of view distinctive, I have downplayed the contribution of elegant experimental methods to social cognition, but not from want of respect for them. Such methods have been essential to the research explosion catalyzed by widely cited paradigmatic studies: the use of recall measures by Hastie and Kumar (1979), Bargh and Thein (1985), and many others to study the organization of person percepts, and by Hamilton and Gifford (1976) to support a cognitive interpretation of stereotyping; the employment of priming paradigms by Higgins, Rholes, and Jones (1977) and Banaji et al. (1993), and reaction time measures by Fazio (1990) and Dovidio and Gaertner (1990) in the indirect assessment of attitudes; and a host of others reviewed in Fiske and Taylor (1991), Wyer and Srull (1985), and the present volume.

Nevertheless, I hope that the field of social cognition will not rely entirely on stock paradigms with very simple stimuli. Intellectual inquiry, like all fields of human endeavor, admits of alternative styles of approach. One of my early mentors, Silvan Tomkins, nicely laid out the contrast between what he called normative and humanistic approaches (Tomkins, 1992). Following a terminological suggestion by Roger Schank, I prefer allusion to the "neat" versus the "scruffy" styles of inquiry. Neat research and scholarship emphasize simplicity and orderliness. It presupposes an underlying logical structure in the phenomenon under study, and takes its task to be the discovery of nature's principles. Scruffy approaches, by contrast, are more oriented toward modeling interesting complexities, taking the task to be the confrontation with disorder instead of the suppression of it.

In these terms, the strands of history I have reviewed might be caricatured as a battle between Neats and Scruffies (Abelson, 1981b). The behaviorists, of course, take the role of Neats, and the cognitivists such as myself, interested in knowledge and belief structures, play the part of the Scruffies.

The field of social cognition is positioned somewhere in between, though it is disposed like all scientific disciplines to be more comfortable when research is designed and comes out as the Neats would have it. There tends to be substantial difficulty translating the ideas of Scruffies[7] into tight re-

[7]Readers curious about further ideas in the Schank and Abelson mold will find books by

search paradigms, although there have been elegant experimental studies of script activation and deactivation (Sharkey, 1985), and of the propensity for social episodes to remind individuals of thematically similar episodes (Seifert et al., 1986), among others. Meanwhile, there has been a renewed interest in computer simulation as an alternative or supplemental approach to laboratory research (Ostrom, 1988; Greenwald & Banaji, 1989; Nowak, Szamrej, & Latane, 1990; Smith, 1991).

A NEW FOCUS IN SOCIAL COGNITION: COACTING SUBSYSTEMS

In a recent set of developments in social cognition (and related fields), a higher level of realistic complexity has been acknowledged than has heretofore been the case. If the complexities can be handled, the modeling of mind will be significantly enhanced. I refer to the hypothesized existence of *coacting central subsystems*—that is, qualitatively distinct cognitive (or motivational) activities that are carried out in parallel. It is remarkable how many theories have appeared recently with the claim that there are two subsystems—especially since the respective claimants invoke different twosomes, and often do not refer to one another's dichotomies. I will trot breathlessly through a number of these, lining them up in Table 1 in two parallel columns, and then discuss some general threads running through them. (I have not attempted to include every important dichotomy; for example, Petty and Cacioppo's [1986] central vs. peripheral process distinction is omitted because it is qualitatively different from the others listed.) The upper half of the table concerns dichotomies based on process distinctions, and the lower half, on content distinctions.

The most influential example of a two-process theory in social psychology has been Zajonc's (1980) formulation that the affective response to a stimulus is activated independently of, and prior to, the cognitive response. Liking or disliking can thus occur before a stimulus is consciously recognized (if, indeed, it is recognized at all). Broadly speaking, the distinction here is between *judgmental* and *affective* processing. With a rather different emphasis, Langer (1989) uses her distinction between *mindful* and *mindless* stimulus processing to organize a body of research on the decision consequences of inducing subjects to think carefully about what they observe.

Other versions of two-tiered response systems have been applied to the analysis of racial prejudice. Devine (1989) writes of the struggle between the

---

Schank (1982, 1986, 1990) of interest. These explore memory organization, learning from experience, the psychological functions of storytelling, and common sense explanation. Other projects of special note are Seifert's (1987) model of an "advice to the lovelorn" columnist, and incisive work in artificial intelligence on a central social cognition topic—the explanation of social events (Kass, 1990).

TABLE 1
Some Dichotomies in Social Cognition

Source	System A	System B
Process Dichotomies		
Zajonc (1980)	Judgmental	Affective
Langer (1989)	Mindful	Mindless
Devine (1989)	Self-conscious	Habitual
Dovidio & Fazio (1992)	Deliberate	Spontaneous
Schneider & Shiffrin (1977)	Controlled	Automatic
Uleman & Bargh (1989)	Intended	Unintended
Banaji & Greenwald (1993)	Explicit	Implicit
Thaler (1980)	Planned	Impulsive
Kinder & Sears (1985)	Self-interested	Symbolic
Katz (1960); Herek (1987)	Instrumental	Expressive
Bruner (1986)	Logical	Narrative
Nemeroff & Rozin (1990)	Rational	Metaphorical
Content Dichotomies		
Fiske & Neuberg (1990)	Category based	Piecemeal
Brewer (1988)	Category based	Person based
Jones & McGillis (1976)	Category based	Target based
Crosby (1982); Chira (1991)	General	Particular
Sears (1983)	Categorical	Personal
Sears & Lau (1983)	Political	Personal

self-conscious activation of egalitarian values and the *habitual* rush of negative feelings intruding into racial judgments and behavior. Dovidio and Fazio (1992) make a related distinction between *deliberate* and *spontaneous* responses to racial stimuli, and Fazio (1990) uses this response distinction to apply generally to all attitude objects. The granddaddy of these two-process models of cognition is Schneider and Shiffrin's (1977) analysis of *controlled* versus *automatic* processes, though these terms have gone somewhat out of fashion. Uleman and Bargh (1989) opt instead for the dichotomy between *intended* and *unintended* cognition, and Banaji and Greenwald (1993) for *explicit* versus *implicit* cognitive processes.

A cognate distinction has been made by political scientists and economists (Elster, 1979; Schelling, 1984) who have postulated "multiple selves" to deal with situations in which self-control is endangered through indulgence in temptation. Elster's famous example is of Ulysses, who ordered his crew to lash him to the mast so that when the ship approached the Sirens, he could not succumb to their call. In such cases, the *planning* self must cleverly anticipate the impulsive behavior of the *doing* self (Thaler, 1980; Shefrin & Thaler, 1993) in order to maintain the long-term interests of the individual. As a less exotic example, the planner may pay a fee to join a financially useless Christmas Club merely to guarantee protection of the planner from the spendthrift doer by obligatory deposits into a closed savings account.

Another type of dichotomy arises from the distinction between *self-interest* politics and *symbolic* politics (Kinder & Sears, 1985), that is, whether people support candidates or causes because there is something in it for them (monetary or material gain) or whether support arises from a symbolic attachment—a gut feeling. An even broader differentiation is captured by the contrast between the *instrumental* function of attitudes and the *expressive* function (Katz, 1960; Herek, 1987; Abelson & Prentice, 1989; Shavitt, 1989).

Still other theorists have proposed two-category modes of cognitive operation somewhat parallel to the instrumental/expressive distinction. Bruner (1986) contrasts the *logical* and the *narrative* modes. Nemeroff and Rozin (1990), in an analysis of people's models of social contagion, contrast *rational* models based on the spread of germs with *metaphorical* models, in which some symbolic essence is transferred from one person to another, via articles of clothing or by touching. Thus many people would be thrilled to wear Elvis Presley's boots, and would feel creepy wearing Hitler's. More pointedly, the fear of contact with AIDS victims seems often due to the fear of "catching" homosexuality, as it were, more than the fear of contracting the virus.

Meanwhile, there has arisen another cluster of dichotomies, based on distinctions between levels of generality of stimulus objects. Fiske and Neuberg (1990) have modeled attitude structures in which evaluations of person *categories* may differ from attitudes toward specific *members*. Brewer (1988) makes a similar distinction (along with a fourfold set of process types that I have not attempted to squeeze into Table 1). Jones and McGillis (1976) have analyzed the different consequences of *category-based* versus *target-based* expectancies. Crosby (1982) has noted the apparent paradox that women perceive *general* gender discrimination in the world of work, but tend to deny any trace of bias in their own *particular* job situations. In a comparable paradox, members of the general public give the United States school system an average grade of C, but grades of A or B to their local schools (Chira, 1991). These phenomena seem closely related to Sears's (1983) "person positivity" effect, in which respondents are wont to criticize politicians (or professors, etc.) in *categorical* fashion, but to view almost all particular politicians (professors, etc.) in favorable *personal* terms.[8] These disparities may make sense if one realizes that for most people, the workaday world of personal reality does not often connect directly with the world of political issues. These worlds "do not share the same vicissitudes,"[9] as it were. Thus,

[8]It is not true, by the way, that *negative* abstract categories are always pitted against positive exemplars. Surveys of public opinion find that many individuals who support the abstract ideal of free speech also reject such freedom for members of disliked groups (Nunn, Crockett, & Williams, 1978).

[9]I heard this charming Gestaltist phrase used by Nehemiah Jordan, a defender of Heider's balance principle, to discount refutations based on absurd examples such as "I like chicken," "Chickens like chicken feed," therefore, "I like chicken feed."

thinking about *political* matters can proceed independently of thinking about *personal* matters, and it takes special circumstances for one of these frames of reference to be brought to bear on events in the other (Sears & Lau, 1983).

INCONSISTENCY BETWEEN SUBSYSTEMS

Let us eyeball Table 1. In the *process* distinctions, self-conscious cognitive processes are contrasted with impulsive, affective processes. Of course, it is not a new idea that separate mental actors, as it were, might operate in ignorance of each other, or even in mutually subversive ways. Freud's (1901/1960) construction of psychodynamic process postulates a battle between the Id and the Superego, with poor Ego caught in the middle. Hilgard (1977), writing of the deceptions that hypnotized subjects can be induced to play on themselves, refers to "divided consciousness."

It is intriguing that the rash of coactive process ideas in social cognition has reached peak attention at the same time that "parallel distributed process" models (Rumelhart et al., 1986) are in ascendancy in cognitive science and neuroscience. At a minimum, such models invoke layered networks of real or hypothetical neural elements that have the capability of learning to select appropriate response categories to apply to heterogeneous stimulus inputs, that is, to perceive. Most of the work to date has been on what one might call *cooperative* parallel processing; that is, the various parts of the network together on a common task. There is no reason, however, why one cannot imagine *antagonistic* parallel processing, wherein subnetworks compete with each other for temporary or semipermanent control of the organism's perceptions and other responses. Over a decade ago, Greenwald (1982) argued eloquently for a "disunified" conception of personality, but his argument seems not to have had much impact. Meanwhile, artificial intelligence guru Marvin Minsky in his book *The Society of Mind* (1985) has argued that the mind (and brain) houses a rather boisterous crowd of actors furiously working obliquely or at cross-purposes, sending information, requests, and commands to one another, with emergent consequences that are sometimes rather unpredictable. There is real doubt as to "who's in charge here."

The understanding of independent, often antagonistic mental subsystems is, I believe, of great potential importance for social psychology, especially when viewed against the past emphasis on single-system consistency theories (Abelson et al., 1968). In the old-fashioned view, cognitive inconsistency was held to be an unstable, unpleasant state motivating the individual to restore cognitive balance, or reduce cognitive dissonance, by altering conscious belief(s). All of the cognitive elements in the inconsistency reduction process were assumed to be simultaneously present, and the resolution selected according to the relative changeability of the elements.

But this is rather too Neat. What if the elements belong to different subsystems that do not communicate well with one another? Then it seems quite possible for chronic inconsistencies to survive, or even become exaggerated through selective exercise of one subsystem over the other. Indeed, Timothy Wilson has convincingly shown that giving reasons for our feelings can readily disrupt attitude–behavior consistency (Wilson et al., 1989). This phenomenon seems to be caused by the lack of the ability to articulate our feelings. We cannot really say why we feel the way we do, and when asked, we give stock justifications that carry us even further from our true inner states.

When mental subsystems work at cross-purposes, social cognitionists often seem to root for one of the subsystems to win out over the other. One of the subsystems is seen as the appropriate process, and the other as an interference, a nuisance to be overcome. The Wilson reason-giving phenomenon aside, it is usually the deliberate, self-conscious, or rational process—the one in the System A column of Table 1—that is the good guy, while the mindless, habitual, or symbolic process is the bad guy. This may be partly due to the fairly slow arrival of affect onto the agenda of social psychologists, partly because of a bias toward rational instrumentalism in Western thought, and partly because in the major topic pitting reason against impulse—racial prejudice—is an area in which the self-conscious, rational self is a socially desirable egalitarian, fighting against the habitual negative feelings of a prejudiced inner self. This is quite explicit in Devine's (1989) analysis. For Sears, Huddy, and Schaffer (1986), negative racial feelings are seen as the result of early emotional conditioning to symbols associated with race, a process unrelated to the rational, instrumental concerns of the individual.

HOW MANY SUBSYSTEMS?

Inconsistency between subsystems may be quite resistant to resolution. The very existence of separate subsystems would suggest that they perform nonredundant functions for the individual. The organism, like the slick politician, may be well served by adopting contradictory positions in different circumstances, possibly without even realizing it.

To get a handle on the possibilities here, the different dichotomies have to be cleaned up (a good task for Neats). The dichotomies are not going to turn out to be the same. Typically in psychology, seemingly one-dimensional constructs become two- to four-dimensional on closer scrutiny. To see finer distinctions between the two columns in the upper half of Table 1, one can try to imagine cross-tabulations of pairs of dichotomies. For example, consider the 2 × 2 table crossing self-interested/symbolic with explicit/implicit. These two pairings (like other pairs of pairings in Table 1) may seem to line up with one another, so that explicit self-interest is contrasted with implicit symbolism. But is this fusion warranted?

Self-interested cognitions have to do with decision making for material gain, with finding and assigning cost to various means to an end. Since material gains are typically articulated consciously, self-interested mental activity is typically explicit. In fact, it is not altogether easy to imagine implicit self-interest. The absence of this cell in the 2 × 2 tempts one to presuppose that the opposite cell—explicit symbolic activity—is also empty. However, this is clearly not the case, as response to symbols (such as national flags) can be quite overt.

In general, the image of conscious reasoning pitted against unconscious feelings blends two distinguishable process factors. Feelings need not be unconscious, nor for that matter need reasoning be conscious (albeit reasoning about material gains is often taken to be so). Fourfold rather than twofold categorizations of subsystems may thus arise from various pairs of pairs.

SUBSYSTEMS BASED ON DIFFERENCES IN LEVELS OF ABSTRACTION

I have not yet commented on the dichotomies in the bottom half of Table 1. These distinctions are based on content rather than process; specifically, they depend on the level of abstraction of the stimuli being processed. All six dichotomies refer in one way or another to the contrast between the particular and the abstract, or, alternatively put, between things experienced and things mediated.

Again, there is the conceptual problem of analyzing the apparent overlap between pairs of distinctions, for example, whether category based versus piecemeal refers to the same differentiation as general versus particular. I will not dwell on this repeated 2 × 2 exercise, to say nothing of the attempt to line up these content distinctions with the process distinctions previously discussed. Rather, I want to call attention to the way a content dichotomy applies to the social cognition analysis of stereotyping.

POOR SUBSYSTEM COMMUNICATION AND THE ANALYSIS OF PREJUDICE

The distinctions in Table 1 based on levels of abstraction arose largely because of the empirical discovery of manifest inconsistencies of response: people dislike politicians in general, but like most particular politicians; working women see discriminatory treatment of women at large, but not (usually) in their own situations; and so on. Such inconsistencies have been greeted with some surprise by psychologists. It is intuitively compelling that reason and impulse can often conflict with each other, but it is not so clear that a generalization can readily be at odds with its exemplifications. The latter seems illogical,[10] without any obvious motivation.

This impression of illogic presupposes that the cognitive subsystems working on generalities and on particularities communicate well with each other, and therein lies our sense of surprise, since it turns out that such communication is apparently rather poor. We should not have been surprised, however. The subsystem distinction here is between reasoning by general principles and reasoning by example. The architecture of these two forms of reasoning can be very different, as can be appreciated from the artificial intelligence literature on expert systems. "Case-based" expert systems (Riesbeck & Schank, 1989), which approach problem situations by modifying the advice given for particular past situations, usually have different memory organizations and different processing styles from expert systems that apply logical rules.

We are likewise surprised when a person with bigoted attitudes toward group X claims to have good friends who are X's. We tend privately to regard this as hypocrisy, and, when wearing our social psychology hats, to invent special mechanisms such as subtyping (Weber & Crocker, 1983) to account for the inconsistency. However, there is quite a different way to look at this. We can recognize that attitudes and behaviors toward groups are naturally separate in an individual's repertoire from attitudes and behaviors toward individuals.[11] The bigot's representation of a scorned group is oriented toward what "they" do and cause—"they always sit together in the dining hall and make a lot of noise"; "they are taking over the neighborhood;" "they are getting special privileges from the government." The outgroup is represented cognitively not just as a category, but more importantly *as an actor* (nouns *and verbs!*). By contrast, the representation of individual X's with whom the bigot interacts directly is probably couched in terms of interper-

[10]Amos Tversky tells the true anecdote of the 4-year-old girl who was separated from her parents in a large public building. The parents asked an official in the lobby if he had seen a 4-year-old girl in the previous ten minutes. "No," he said. "No little girl at all?!" "Sorry, no." "Well," (getting excited) "she's wearing a red dress, and carrying yellow flowers." "Oh," came the reply, "why didn't you say so? Of course I've seen her!"

[11]A similar disparity may hold between negative attitudes toward the leaders of enemy countries (e.g., the Soviet Union, or Iraq) and positive attitudes toward "the people" of those countries, a phenomenon that Ralph White (1969) called the "blacktop illusion." I once asked Barry Goldwater (during a reception at Yale in 1962) whether European disarmament would help reduce Communist use of military threat as a political tactic. His reply (honest!) was, "Oh, they're not so threatening. I know a couple of East German fighter pilots, and they're nice guys." (My Goldwater simulation was totally unable to capture such personalizations!)

sonal relationships (perhaps heavily "scripted" [Abelson, 1981a], but interpersonal nonetheless).

The much analyzed LaPiere (1934) study is a case in point. After traveling extensively with a presentable young Chinese couple and being received without incident at all but one of 200 restaurants and motels, LaPiere's subsequent letters to these establishments asked the question, "Do you accept members of the Chinese race as guests?" That 90% of those who answered said "No" was his celebrated challenge to social scientists trying to predict behavior from attitude statements. A great many possible explanations of the disparity between the negative statements and the positive behaviors have been put forward (e.g., the Chinese couple were more polite and charming than stereotypical Chinese). To these I would simply add the observation that LaPiere's question was pluralized, and the respondents may have imagined—and dreaded—having a *group* of Chinese as guests.

The reader may wonder what other kinds of negative behaviors an individual can exercise toward groups. The group-oriented behaviors I have in mind can be largely characterized as *political* responses: organizing protests against the X's moving in; gossiping with neighbors about what can be done; protesting to authorities; colluding in discriminatory practices; voting against candidates who are X's; participating in demonstrations, boycotts, or bias crimes; and so on. Ordinarily, of course, individuals do not act alone against a target outgroup. They organize collectively, activating the collective "we" to respond to the collective "them." What I am proposing is that the distinction between the personal subsystem and the political subsystem be taken seriously, allowing the possibility that the two subsystems communicate poorly.

It is striking that social psychologists and social cognitionists have persistently defined prejudice as the application of a negative attitude toward a group to individual members of that group. What about the application of the negative attitude to behavior toward *the group itself?* The group-level connection between attitudes and behavior seems to me to be of greater relevance in understanding how to minimize intergroup antagonism than the present tortuous formula of correcting prejudice against group X by giving positive experiences with members of X and hoping this will generalize to the group. Positive experiences with individual group members may not readily lead to a more favorable view of the group (Rothbart & John, 1985; Wilder, 1986), but changing the perception of the outgroup's motives and activities as a group may be quite effective. Indeed, this very simple but powerful notion is implicit in the classical Sherif and Sherif (1953) Robbers' Cave study, but has gotten lost in social cognition's emphasis on presenting stimulus information about individuals to individuals. As always (Abelson, 1993), I am in the position of urging social cognition researchers to take the next step, to gradually improve our understanding of racial prejudice and other complex realities.

RECAPITULATION

I have traced parts of the history of social psychology and its offspring, social cognition, mainly those in which I was personally involved. My account was framed in terms of the predilection for tight experiments with simple stimuli, in competition with the desire to give a fairly rich account of the important social phenomena around us. That there are strong pressures in both directions I attributed partly to the historical struggle between behaviorism and phenomenology, but more generally to the never ending battle between Neats and Scruffies. My own approach comes down somewhat on the Scruffy side, but with an appreciation of the laboratory successes in social cognition.

My tendency has been to ask of bodies of theory and research what it is that they leave out, and in what direction further progress may lie. In this spirit, I have reviewed two batches of dichotomies that have variously appeared in the recent literature. One batch is addressed to the distinction(s) between processes of deliberate, explicit judgment and those of spontaneous feeling or implicit impulse. The second batch contrasts levels of abstraction of cognitive elements, pitting the particular against the abstract. As an example from the second batch, I briefly analyzed the distinction between negative orientations toward outgroup individuals, and toward the group itself. This distinction may have important implications for the study of racial prejudice, if we take seriously the prospect that the individual-oriented process and the group-oriented process may work at cross-purposes, communicating poorly with one another and producing inconsistencies.

Neatening up the two batches of dichotomies by pruning redundancies, and specifying the conditions for antagonism between processes present important agendas for social cognition.

REFERENCES

Abelson, R. P. (1959). Modes of resolution of belief dilemmas. *Journal of Conflict Resolution, 3*, 343–352.

Abelson, R. P. (1963). Computer simulation of 'hot' cognition. In S. S. Tomkins & S. Messick (Eds.), *Computer simulation of personality.* New York: Wiley.

Abelson, R. P. (1973). The structure of belief systems. In R. C. Schank and K. M. Colby (Eds.), *Computer models of thought language.* San Francisco: Freeman.

Abelson, R. P. (1976). Script processing in attitude formation and decision making. In J. S. Carroll & J. W. Payne (Eds.), *Cognition and social behavior.* Hillsdale, NJ: Erlbaum.

Abelson, R. P. (1981a). The psychological status of the script concept. *American Psychologist, 36*, 715–729.

Abelson, R. P. (1981b). Constraint, construal, and cognitive science. *Third Annual Conference of the Cognitive Science Society.* University of California at Berkeley.

Abelson, R. P. (1989). Beliefs as possessions: A functional perspective. In A. R. Pratkanis, S. J. Breckler, & A. G. Greenwald (Eds.), *Attitude structure and function* (pp. 361–381). Hillsdale, NJ: Erlbaum.

Abelson, R. P. (1994). Attitude extremity. In R. Petty and J. Krosnick (Eds.), *Attitude strength.* Hillsdale, NJ: Erlbaum.

Abelson, R. P., & Carroll, J. D. (1965). Computer simulation of individual belief systems. *American Behavioral Scientist, 8,* 24–30.

Abelson, R. P., & Prentice, D. A. (1988). Beliefs as possessions—A functional perspective. In A. R. Pratkanis, S. J. Breckler, & A. G. Greenwald (Eds.), *Attitude structure and function.* (pp. 361–382).Hillsdale NJ: Erlbaum.

Abelson, R. P., & Rosenberg, M. J. (1958). Symbolic psycho-logic: A model of attitudinal cognition. *Behavioral Science, 3,* 1–13.

Abelson, R. P., & Sermat, V. (1962). Multidimensional scaling of facial expressions. *Journal of Experimental Psychology, 63,* 546–554.

Abelson, R. P., Aronson, E., McGuire, W. J., Newcomb, T. N., Rosenberg, M. J., & Tannenbaum, P. H. (Eds.). (1968). *Theories of cognitive consistency: A sourcebook.* Chicago: Rand McNally.

Anderson, J. (1976). *Language, memory, and thought.* Hillsdale, NJ: Erlbaum.

Anderson, N. H. (1966). Component ratings in impression formation. *Psychonomic Science, 6,* 279–286.

Anderson, N. H. (1968). Likableness ratings of 555 personality-trait adjectives. *Journal of Personality and Social Psychology, 9,* 272–279.

Asch, S. E. (1940). Studies in the principles of judgments and attitudes: II. Determination of judgments by group and by ego standards. *Journal of Social Psychology, 12,* 433–465.

Asch, S. E. (1946). Forming impressions of personality. *Journal of Abnormal and Social Psychology, 41,* 258–290.

Banaji, M. R., & Greenwald, A. G. (1993). Implicit stereotyping and prejudice. In M. P. Zanna & J. M. Olson (Eds.), *The psychology of prejudice; The Ontario Symposium* (Vol. 7). Hillsdale, NJ: Erlbaum.

Banaji, M. R., Hardin, C., & Rothman, A. J. (1993). Implicit stereotyping in person judgment. *Journal of Personality and Social Psychology, 65,* 272–281.

Bargh, J. A., & Thein, R. D. (1985). Individual construct accessibility, person memory, and the recall-judgment link: The case of information overload. *American Psychologist, 49,* 1129–1146.

Brehm, J. W., & Cohen, A. R. (1962). *Explorations in cognitive dissonance.* New York: Wiley.

Brewer, M. B. (1988). A dual process model of impression formation. In T. K. Srull & R. S. Wyer, Jr. (Eds.), *Advances in social cognition* (Vol. 1, pp. 1–36). Hillsdale, NJ: Erlbaum.

Bruner, J. (1986). *Actual minds, possible worlds.* Cambridge, MA: Harvard University Press.

Cantor, N., & Mischel, W. (1979). Prototypes in person perception. In L. Berkowitz (Ed.), *Advances in experimental social psychology* (Vol. 12). New York: Academic Press.

Carbonell, J. (1978). POLITICS: Automated ideological reasoning. *Cognitive Science, 2,* 27–51.

Chira, S. (1991). How to translate the talk about school reform into action? *New York Times,* March 24, p. 4–1.

Cooper, J., & Fazio, R. H. (1984). A new look at dissonance theory. In L. Berkowitz (Ed.), *Advances in experimental social psychology* (Vol. 17, pp. 229–266). New York: Academic Press.

Crosby, F. (1982). *Relative deprivation and working women.* New York: Oxford University Press.

Deese, J. (1962). On the structure of associative meaning. *Psychological Review, 69,* 161–175.

Devine, P. G. (1989). Stereotypes and prejudice: Their automatic and controlled components. *Journal of Personality and Social Psychology, 56,* 5–18.

Dovidio, J., & Fazio, R. (1992). New technologies for the direct and indirect assessment of attitudes. In J. Tanur (Ed.), *Questions about survey questions.* New York: Russell Sage.

Dovidio, J. F., & Gaertner, S. L. (1990). Changes in the nature and expression of racial prejudice. In H. Knopke, J. Norrell, & R. Rogers (Eds.), *Opening doors: An appraisal of race relations in contemporary America.* Tuscaloosa, AL: University of Alabama Press.

Dyer, M. G. (1983). *In-depth understanding: A computer model of integrated processing for narrative comprehension.* Cambridge, MA: MIT Press.

Elster, J. (1979). *Ulysses and the Sirens.* Cambridge: Cambridge University Press.

Fazio, R. H. (1990). Multiple processes by which attitudes guide behavior: The MODE model as an integrative framework. In M. P. Zanna (Ed.), *Advances in experimental social psychology* (Vol. 23, pp. 75–110). New York: Academic Press.

Fazio, R. H., Sanbonmatsu, D. M., Powell, M. C., & Kardes, F. R. (1986). On the automatic activation of attitudes. *Journal of Personality and Social Psychology, 50,* 229–238.

Festinger, L. (1957). *A theory of cognitive dissonance.* Evanston, IL: Row, Peterson.

Festinger, L., & Carlsmith, J. M. (1959). Cognitive consequences of forced compliance. *Journal of Abnormal and Social Psychology, 58,* 203–211.

Fiske, S. T., & Linville, P. (1980). What does the schema concept buy us? *Personality and Social Psychology Bulletin, 6,* 543–557.

Fiske, S. T., & Neuberg, S. L. (1990). A continuum of impression formation, from category-based to individuating processes: Influences of information and motivation on attention and interpretation. In M. P. Zanna (Ed.), *Advances in experimental social psychology* (Vol. 23, pp. 1–74). San Diego, CA: Academic Press.

Fiske, S. T., & Taylor, S. E. (1991). *Social cognition* (2nd ed). New York: McGraw Hill.

Freud, S. (1901/1960). *The psychopathology of everyday life.* London: Hogarth.

Gentner, D. (1983). Structure-mapping: A theoretical framework for analogy. *Cognitive Science, 7,* 155–170.

Greenwald, A. G. (1982). Is anyone in charge? Personalysis versus the principle of personal unity. In J. Suls (Ed.), *Psychological perspectives on the self* (Vol. 1, pp. 151–181). Hillsdale, NJ: Erlbaum.

Greenwald, A. G., & Banaji, M. R. (1989). The self as a memory system: Powerful, but ordinary. *Journal of Personality and Social Psychology, 57,* 41–54.

Hamilton, D. L., & Gifford, R. K. (1976). Illusory correlation in interpersonal perception: A cognitive basis of stereotypic judgments. *Journal of Experimental Social Psychology, 12,* 392–407.

Hastie, R., & Kumar, P. A. (1979). Person memory: Personality traits as organizing principles in memory for behaviors. *Journal of Personality and Social Psychology, 37,* 25–38.

Heider, F. (1927). Ding und Medium. *Symposium, 1,* 109–157.

Heider, F. (1958). *The psychology of interpersonal relations.* New York: Wiley.

Herek, G. M. (1987). Can functions be measured? A new perspective on the functional approach to attitudes. *Social Psychology Quarterly, 50,* 285–303.

Higgins, E. T., Rholes, W. S., & Jones, C. R. (1977). Category accessibility and impression formation. *Journal of Experimental Social Psychology, 13,* 141–154.

Hilgard, E. R. (1977). *Divided consciousness: Multiple controls in human thought and action.* New York: Wiley.

Hovland, C. I. (1952). A "communication analysis" of concept learning. *Psychological Review, 59,* 461–472.

Hovland, C. I., Janis, I. L., & Kelley, H. H. (1952). *Communication and persuasion.* New Haven: Yale University Press.

Jones, E. E. (1985). Major developments in social psychology during the past five decades. In G. Lindzey & E. Aronson (Eds.), *Handbook of social psychology* (3rd ed.) (pp. 47–108). New York: Random House.

Jones, E. E., & McGillis, D. (1976). Correspondent inferences and the attribution cube: A comparative reappraisal. In J. H. Harvey, W. J. Ickes, & R. F. Kidd (Eds.), *New directions in attribution research* (Vol. 1). Hillsdale, NJ: Erlbaum.

Kass, A. (1990). Developing creative hypotheses by adapting explanations. Ph.D. dissertation, Yale University. Reprinted as Technical Report #6, Institute for the Learning Sciences, Northwestern University.

Katz, D. (1960). The functional approach to the study of attitudes. *Public Opinion Quarterly, 24,* 163–204.

Kinder, D. R., & Sears, D. O. (1985). Public opinion and political action. In G. Lindzey & E. Aronson (Eds.), *Handbook of social psychology* (3rd. ed.) (pp. 659–741). New York: Random House.

Kuklinski, J. H., Luskin, R. C., & Bolland, J. (1991). Where is the schema? Going beyond the "S" word in political psychology. *American Political Science Review, 85*(4), 1341–1356.

Langer, E. J. (1989). *Mindfulness.* Reading, MA: Addison-Wesley.

LaPiere, R. T. (1934). Attitude vs. actions. *Social Forces, 13,* 230–237.

Lehnert, W. G. (1981). Plot units and narrative summarization. *Cognitive Science, 4,* 293–331.

Lewin, K. (1938). The conceptual representation and the measurement of psychological forces. *Contributions to psychological theory* (Vol. 1, No. 4). Durham, NC: Duke University Press.

McGuire, W. J. (1960). A syllogistic analysis of cognitive relationships. In M. J. Rosenberg, C. I. Hovland, W. J. McGuire, R. P. Abelson, & J. W. Brehm, *Attitude organization and change.* New Haven: Yale University Press.

McGuire, W. J. (1968). Personality and attitude change: An information processing theory. In A. G. Greenwald, T. C. Brock, & T. M. Ostrom (Eds.), *Psychological foundations of attitude* (pp. 171–196). New York: Academic Press.

McGuire, W. J. (1985). Attitudes and attitude change. In G. Lindzey & E. Aronson (Eds.), *Handbook of social psychology* (3rd ed.) (Vol. 2, pp. 233–346). New York: Random House.

Minsky, M. (1975). A framework for representing knowledge. In P. H. Winston (Ed.), *The psychology of computer vision.* New York: McGraw Hill.

Minsky, M. (1985). *The society of mind.* New York: Simon & Schuster.

Nemeroff, C., & Rozin, P. (1991). The contagion concept in adult thinking in the United States: Transmission of germs and of interpersonal influence. Unpublished paper, Arizona State University.

Newell, A., & Simon, H. (1972). *Human problem solving.* New York: Prentice Hall.

Norman, D., & Rumelhart, D. (1975). *Explorations in cognition.* San Francisco: Freeman.

Nowak, A., Szamrej, J., & Latane, B. (1990). From private attitude to public opinion: A dynamic theory of social impact. *Psychological Review, 97,* 362–376.

Nunn, C. Z., Crockett, H. J., Jr., & Williams, J. A. (1978). *Tolerance for nonconformity.* San Francisco: Jossey-Bass.

Osgood, C. E., Suci, G. J., & Tannenbaum, P. H. (1957). *The measurement of meaning.* Urbana, IL: University of Illinois Press.

Ostrom, T. M. (1988). Computer simulation: The third symbol system. *Journal of Experimental Social Psychology, 24,* 381–392.

Patnoe, S. (1988). *A narrative history of experimental social psychology: The Lewin tradition.* Berlin: Springer-Verlag.

Petty, R. E., & Cacioppo, J. T. (1986). The elaboration likelihood model of persuasion. In L. Berkowitz (Ed.), *Advances in experimental social psychology, 19,* (pp. 123–205). San Diego, CA: Academic Press.

Pratkanis, A. R., Breckler, S. J., & Greenwald, A. G. (1989). *Attitude structure and function.* Hillsdale, NJ: Erlbaum.

Rainio, K. (1986). *Stochastic field theory of behavior.* Helsinki, Finland: Finnish Society of Sciences and Letters.

Riesbeck, C., & Schank, R. C. (1989). *Inside case-based reasoning.* Hillsdale, NJ: Erlbaum.

Rosenberg, M. J., & Abelson, R. P. (1960). An analysis of cognitive balancing. In M. J. Rosenberg, C. I. Hovland, W. J. McGuire, R. P. Abelson, & J. W. Brehm, *Attitude organization and change* (pp. 112–163). New Haven: Yale University Press.

Rosenberg, S., Nelson, C., & Vivekananthan, P. S. (1968). A multidimensional approach to the study of personality impressions. *Journal of Personality and Social Psychology, 9,* 283–294.

Ross, L., & Nisbett, R. E. (1991). *The person and the situation: Perspectives of social psychology.* New York: McGraw Hill.

Rothbart, M., & John, O. P. (1985). Social categorization and behavioral episodes: A cognitive analysis of the effects of intergroup contact. *Journal of Social Issues, 41,* 81–104.

Rumelhart, D. E., McClelland, J. L., & the PDP Research Group (1986). *Parallel distributed processing: Explorations in the microstructure of cognition.* Cambridge, MA: MIT Press.
Schank, R. C. (1972). Conceptual dependency: A theory of natural language understanding. *Cognitive Psychology, 3,* 552–631.
Schank, R. C. (1982). *Dynamic memory: A theory of reminding and learning in computers and people.* New York: Cambridge University Press.
Schank, R. C. (1986). *Explanation patterns: Understanding mechanically and creatively.* Hillsdale, NJ: Erlbaum.
Schank, R. C. (1990). *That reminds me of a story: A new look at real and artificial intelligence:* New York: Cambridge University Press.
Schank, R. C., & Abelson, R. P. (1977). *Scripts, plans, goals, and understanding.* Hillsdale, NJ: Erlbaum.
Schelling, T. (1984). Self command in practice, in policy, and in a theory of rational choice. *American Economic Review, 74,* 1–11.
Schneider, W., & Shiffrin, R. (1977). Controlled and automatic human information processing: I. Detection, search, and attention. *Psychological Review, 84,* 1–66.
Sears, D. O. (1983). The person positivity bias. *Journal of Personality and Social Psychology, 44,* 233–250.
Sears, D. O., & Lau, R. R. (1983). Inducing apparently self-interested political preferences. *American Journal of Political Science, 27,* 223–252.
Sears, D. O., Huddy, L., & Schaffer, L. G. (1986). A schematic variant of symbolic politics theory, as applied to racial and gender equality. In R. R. Lau & D. O. Sears (Eds.), *Political cognition: 19th Annual Carnegie Symposium on Cognition.* Hillsdale, NJ: Erlbaum.
Seifert, C. M. (1987). Mental representation of social knowledge: A computational approach to reasoning about relationships. Unpublished Ph.D. dissertation, Yale University.
Seifert, C. M., McKoon, G., Abelson, R. P., & Ratcliff, R. (1986). Memory connections between thematically similar episodes. *Journal of Experimental Psychology: Learning, Memory, and Cognition, 12,* 220–231.
Sharkey, N. (1985). Script activation and deactivation. In J. A. Galambos, R. P. Abelson, & J. B. Black (Eds.), *Knowledge structures.* Hillsdale, NJ: Erlbaum.
Shavitt, S. (1989). Operationalizing functional theories of attitude. In A. R. Pratkanis, S. J. Breckler, & A. G. Greenwald (Eds.), *Attitude structure and function* (pp. 311–337). Hillsdale, NJ: Erlbaum.
Shefrin, H. M., & Thaler, R. H. (1992). Mental accounting, saving, and self-control. In G. Loewenstein & J. Elster (Eds.), *Choice over time.* New York: Russell Sage.
Sherif, M., & Sherif, C. (1953). *Groups in harmony and tension.* New York: Harper.
Smith, E. R. (1991). Illusory correlation in a simulated exemplar-based memory. *Journal of Experimental Social Psychology, 27,* 107–113.
Thaler, R. (1980). Toward a positive theory of consumer choice. *Journal of Economic Behavior and Organizations, 1,* 39–60.
Tomkins, S. S. (1992). *Affect Imagery Consciousness* (Vol. 3). New York: Springer.
Uleman, J. S., & Bargh, J. A. (1989). *Unintended thought.* New York: Guilford Press.
Weber, R., & Crocker, J. (1983). Cognitive processes in the revision of stereotypic beliefs. *Journal of Personality and Social Psychology, 45,* 961–977.
White, R. K. (1969). Three not-so-obvious contributions of psychology to peace. *Journal of Social Issues, 25*(4), 23–39.
Wilder, D. A. (1986). Social categorization: Implications for creation and reduction of intergroup bias. *Advances in experimental social psychology* (Vol. 19, pp. 291–355). New York: Academic Press.
Wilson, T. D., Dunn, D. S., Kraft, D., & Lisle, D. J. (1989). Introspection, attitude change, and attitude-behavior consistency: The disruptive effects of explaining why we feel the way we do. In L. Berkowitz (Ed.), *Advances in experimental social psychology* (Vol. 22, pp. 287–343). Orlando, FL: Academic Press.

Wyer, R. S., Jr., & Srull, T. K. (Eds.). (1984). *Handbook of social cognition* (Vol. 3). Hillsdale, NJ: Erlbaum.

Zajonc, R. (1980). Feeling and thinking: Preferences need no inferences. *American Psychologist, 35,* 151–175.

3

Impression Formation: From Recitals to Symphonie Fantastique

Jacques-Philippe Leyens
Susan T. Fiske

One well-known social psychologist charting the history of the field has referred to the "social cognition interlude," in the past tense, as the field returns to its presumably more major themes. The implication is that social cognition research is a mere diversion on the intellectual scene. What difference would it make if the social cognition "interlude" had never occurred? Is it a mere divertimento or rather a magnum opus? In this chapter, we will focus on the study of person perception and impression formation. The study of impression formation should be an area of research par excellence in which to evaluate the progress of social cognition research. Although there is no one consensual definition of social cognition (for reviews, see Fiske & Taylor, 1984, 1991; Leyens, 1983; Markus & Zajonc, 1985; McGuire, 1986; Ostrom, 1984), people talk as if there is a shared melody, played on various instruments, to create a symphony of intellectual endeavor. Whether social cognition is a field in itself, as is sometimes suggested (Ostrom, 1984; Wyer & Srull, 1984), or is, more modestly, "an approach or set of assumptions guiding research in a variety of traditional substantive domains" (Sherman, Judd, & Park, 1989, p. 281) hardly matters. Ordinary people's perception of other people is central to the enterprise, whatever it is.

On one hand, current researchers are still addressing many of the concerns originally raised by the first students of person perception; there is continuity in the concerns, theories, and even some methods. A traditionalist could find comfort there. On the other hand, many things have profoundly changed; the methods, precision, diversity, and enthusiasm of the impression formation field have exploded as a result of the social cognition variations. An innovator could find comfort there. In this chapter, we will illustrate both continuity and change. We find no evidence for a passing interlude, a distracting aberration, a temporary detour.

Indeed, rather than "interlude," a more fitting metaphor for the evolution of the impression formation research might be the classical sonata form of a symphony's first movement: the standard sequence involves the statement of two opposing themes, followed by their development in a free-form fantasy, with a recapitulation of the first two themes at the end of the movement. Playing with a similar structure, this chapter illustrates the contributions of impression formation and person perception research in four phases: statement of the theme, counter theme, fantasia, and return to the opening theme with some synthesis.

ASCH'S THEME

When Solomon Asch started his research on the formation of impressions, he apparently had several goals in mind. Most broadly, is Gestalt theory capable of explaining impression formation? More specifically, "How do we come to know persons as distinctive psychological entities?" (Asch, 1952, p. 205). Operationally, he asked, how do we come to know them when the only basis is a string of trait adjectives? In his studies, Asch clearly wanted to emphasize an aspect of interpersonal relations that had been neglected up to then, namely "the cognitive side of the impressions we form of persons. It should be obvious that we must observe and understand something of a person if we are to form a relation of affection or distrust" (Asch, 1952, p. 205).

Asch's (1946) experiments constituted a breakthrough in person perception. Before then, social psychologists had always been embarrassed in their quest to discover whether or not human beings are accurate perceivers of others. Indeed, the conclusion of any such research could be criticized by disputing the so-called objective criteria of accuracy. With Asch's studies of impression formation, these criteria became irrelevant, the focus turning to the perceiver's own process of making sense of the other person, whether accurate or not, and regardless of whether that other was existing or fictitious.

More important for our present purpose is the fact that Asch's early (1946) and later (Asch & Zukier, 1984) work showed that, without too much difficulty, subjects could "organize the various data of observation into a single, relatively unified impression" (Asch, 1952, p. 207), consistent with the Gestalt view. Within person perception research, this has been a recurring theme, with variations: People continuously build impression theories and use them in their commerce with other people.

To show that the Gestalt approach was superior to an elemental, summative approach, Asch focused his attention on the importance of several kinds of traits: central versus peripheral traits and the first versus last terms in a sequence. According to Asch, central traits were those that colored the big picture, that served as guidelines for the configural interpretation of the complete series of traits. At that time, the discovery of a central trait in a given set essentially was based on empirically verified intuition. Later, Wishner (1960) showed that the centrality of stimulus traits could be predicted from their high positive or negative correlations with the response traits. Moreover, others (Brown, 1986; Rosenberg, Nelson, & Vivekananthan, 1968; Zanna & Hamilton, 1972) defended the idea that central traits are those that are extreme on a different dimension from the rest of the stimulus traits and which, therefore, carry a lot of information weight.

The preponderant impact of the first terms in the sequence—the primacy effect—was also important in showing the appropriateness of a configural explanation of the phenomenon (see Jones & Goethals, 1972, for a review):

> The accounts of the subjects indicate that the first terms set up a direction that exerts a continuous effect on the latter terms. When one hears the first term, a broad, uncrystallized, but directed impression is born. The next characteristic is related to the established direction. The view formed quickly acquires a certain stability; later characteristics are fitted to the prevailing direction when conditions permit. (Asch, 1952, p. 213, original italics omitted)

Several subsequent studies (e.g., Hamilton & Zanna, 1974; Higgins, Rholes, & Jones, 1977; Zanna & Hamilton, 1977) have provided examples of meaning change as a result of the direction provided by the preceding context.

The briefest conclusion of research directly inspired by Asch is that, when forming an impression of persons, perceivers are both theory and data driven, in that they use all the adjectives provided, at least to some extent, but they also organize and interpret them in light of their relations to each other within a larger cognitive structure. Operationally, people were able to use various trait adjectives to form a single general impression that allowed inferences about other attributes and assimilation of still other characteristics. Later, Bruner and Tagiuri (1954) hypothesized that this was possible because of the implicit theories of personality entertained by the individuals. We will take up that refrain next.

IMPLICIT PERSONALITY THEORY: A MAJOR VARIATION ON ASCH'S THEME

According to Asch, the integration of traits produced a general impression that led to personality inferences. But what is responsible for the general impression? Bruner and Tagiuri (1954) suggested that both general impression and inferences were possible because of the prior existence of implicit personality theories (IPT).

These prior theories refer to lay people's naive theories about personality. More precisely, they consist of general beliefs about the frequency and the variability of personality traits in a given population and about the correlations between these traits. The expression was coined by Bruner and Tagiuri (1954); these authors had noticed that the many errors made in person perception were generally consensual; they assumed that these errors were due to shared beliefs or "theories" that guide our perception of others (Leyens, 1983, 1991; Schneider, 1973; Trzebinski, 1985).

Given their personal experiences, individuals can have an idiosyncratic IPT (Beck, McCauley, Segal, & Hershey, 1988; Rosenberg & Sedlak, 1972). Nevertheless, people largely share a common theory, characterized by two almost, but not completely, orthogonal evaluative dimensions: (1) Intellectual Good versus Bad; and (2) Social Good versus Bad (Rosenberg et al., 1968). Notably, in this representation, the central traits warm and cold, used in Asch's paradigm, are on a separate (i.e., social) dimension from the other (i.e., intellectual) dimension, which comprises the other traits on the list. As mentioned earlier, this is one reason why their importance is so crucial in the lists and why they have been called central (Zanna & Hamilton, 1972).

Except to show that personality profiles exist perhaps more in the heads of the observers than in the behavior of the actors (see Leyens, 1983, for a review), the concept of implicit theories of personality did not have much heuristic value; it explained past research more than it produced new studies. Being centered only on personality, its scope was too narrow; there are many things other than traits to which we react when we see someone: behaviors, appearance, roles, ethnicity, and so on (Fiske & Cox, 1979; Park, 1986). Moreover, the concept mirrors a static view of life; except through a long history of past experiences, one does not see how an implicit theory of personality can be changed. By common sense, however, we know that we can have different impressions of people depending on our goals, our mood, and the like. These various limitations probably explain why this concept for the most part has been overpowered by more recent developments (but also see Anderson & Sedikides, 1991; Leyens, 1991).

From a metatheoretical perspective, the IPT research (although not the theory itself) reflects an elemental rather than a Gestalt approach to inferences. That is, the relationships of the elements are described with more and more precision (Van der Kloot & Willemsen, 1991; Van Mechelen, 1991). However, the Gestalt perspective held that the meanings of the trait elements changed as a function of context. IPT research has ignored this Gestalt tenet in practice if not in theory. As such, the IPT research itself is a major variation on the Asch opening theme, which provides a bridge to the explicitly elemental countertheme of Anderson.

ANDERSON'S OPPOSING THEME

Not everyone agreed with Asch's explanation in Gestalt terms. His most vocal opponent was Norman Anderson (e.g., 1966, 1981), who developed an algebraic information integration theory to show that subjects took into account every piece of information and thus worked at a molecular level. Moreover, Anderson asserted that each piece of information could be viewed as an autonomous unit, its meaning (chiefly, its evaluative value) unchanged by the context of the other elements. This led to a hot controversy. Everyone working in the field of impression formation felt obliged to take a position. "The futility of the adversarial approach," in that neither the molar nor the molecular models were stated in falsifiable terms, was denounced by Ostrom (1977) who called for a cease-fire. Some might say that he may as well have preached in the desert; the molar–molecular debate continues in other forms (Fiske & Taylor, 1991, Chapter 1).

The issues raised by Asch and Anderson are fundamental. Current social cognition researchers should have no difficulty recognizing some of their own preoccupations in the specific program set forth by Asch nearly fifty years ago. Yet his original work seems sometimes to receive only lip service in important books on social cognition (e.g., the three volumes of the *Handbook of Social Cognition,* edited by Wyer & Srull, 1984). Why?

Modern social cognition researchers would claim to be interested more in processes than descriptive outcomes. Is that claim justified in regard to the Asch–Anderson debate? First, it does not seem fair to say that neither Asch nor Anderson were interested in processes but only in outcomes. In fact, the object of the controversy was precisely processes, and not outcomes, which were usually predicted to be the same in both cases. Of course, the crux of the matter is that the processes were only assumed, or verified only at a phenomenal level, in the case of Asch, and that they were not phenomenologically convincing, in the case of Anderson. Although it is not fair to say that these authors were not interested in processes but only in outcomes, it is fair to say that they did not have the methods or the theories to approach processes as pointedly as in recent work. This, then, is the core theme developed in a free-form (that is to say, unconstrained) fantasia in the next phase of the social cognition movement. Let us see therefore how current research has approached the problem of processes.

SOCIAL COGNITION AND PROCESS: FANTASIA

In music, a fantasy is not an unnatural, wild, or bizarre mental image but rather a fantasia, "a musical composition of no fixed form, with a structure determined by the composer's fancy" (*New World Dictionary,* 1976). Similarly, "social cognition" is more a label to create a sense of coherence among a group of researchers working on problems determined by their own proclivities, within structures governed by certain conventions, most importantly: unabashed mentalism, cross-fertilization between cognitive and social psychology, process orientation, and commitment to social settings (Fiske & Taylor, 1991; Hastie & Carlston, 1980; Ostrom, 1984; Taylor, 1981). In likening social cognition research to a fantasia on themes stated by Asch and Anderson, we do not intend the second meaning of fantasia, namely "a medley of familiar tunes." Rather, the developments reflect the innovation and enthusiasm of turning old themes upside down and inside out, with new instruments. The fantasia phase can be expressed in three parts: encoding, person memory, and mental representation.

Encoding of Data

Much of social cognition has been devoted to the characteristics of the data provided, to examine the relative importance of theory and data, that is, to verify if people do indeed care about the information given (Higgins & Bargh, 1987). The salience of various traits has especially attracted the interest of researchers, but because salience can be operationalized in many different ways (Taylor & Fiske, 1978), we have chosen to illustrate separately some different ways a trait can be salient. Salience is a property of a stimulus in context, which makes it attract attention. The central finding, of course, is that whatever attracts attention carries more weight in impressions, polarizing evaluations, attracting attributional activity, and increasing perceived causal importance (for a recent review, see Fiske & Taylor, 1991, Chapter 7). In impression formation, the main charge of this chapter, salience at encoding has been reflected in work on data that are vivid, statistically rare or negative, diagnostic, disconfirmatory, and distinctive. Each of these concerns represents an innovation on the older Asch and Anderson themes, using new cognitive theories and methods to explore processes. Because their effects were already noted by Asch, we will not discuss trait centrality and primacy, which are, of course, two ways of being salient.

Vividness

"Whereas salience is determined by the relation of an object to its context, vividness is inherent in the stimulus itself" (Fiske & Taylor, 1984, p. 190). In some of the first work under the new rubric of social cognition, Nisbett, Ross, and their colleagues (Anderson, Lepper, & Ross, 1980; Borgida & Nisbett, 1977; Hamill, Wilson, & Nisbett, 1980; Nisbett & Borgida, 1975) assumed that vividness has the same effects as salience. Several experiments suggested that vivid information attracts more attention, is more persuasive, elicits more cognitive work, is more memorable, and resists counterarguments more than abstract, pallid, information. As Fiske and

Taylor (1991, Chapter 7) suggest, it is not clear whether these effects are really due to vividness per se (see also Taylor & Thompson, 1982); according to these authors, vividness comprises and confounds a lot of variables, which makes the information strictly noncomparable. Vivid information is entertaining, memorable, and believed to be persuasive for people in general, but it is not necessarily persuasive to us as individuals. This much, then, provided new insights.

Statistical Rarity and Negativity

Evaluatively bad events or personal attributes being rarer than good ones, Fiske (1980) hypothesized and found that negative ones would attract more attention and carry more weight. Using a different paradigm, Yzerbyt and Leyens (1991) similarly found that subjects needed more positive items than negative ones to make a decision. Negative information therefore had more weight in the decisions. Within the same paradigm, Leyens and Yzerbyt (1992) showed that negative stereotypes were more informative than positive ones for people deciding whether or not a person belonged to an ingroup. (For reviews of the negativity literature, see Kanouse & Hanson, 1972; Peeters & Czapinski, 1990; Skowronski & Carlston, 1989; Taylor, 1991.) This kind of work explains one reason why, in cognitive terms, negative information is so important in impressions. Asch and Anderson had identified negativity but not explained why. The recent social cognitive approaches thus analyze the phenomenology of Asch and psychologize the algebra of Anderson.

Diagnosticity

Negative information is especially important also because it is unexpected. The same additional weight could then apply to extremely positive evidence because it also is rare (Kanouse & Hanson, 1972); this has been verified by Fiske (1980) in the study already mentioned. Recently, Skowronski and Carlston (1989) have attempted to explain negativity, positivity, and extremity by a single factor: diagnosticity. Their reasoning is similar to that of Reeder (1985), who also concentrates on the domains of ability and morality. For most people, it is not surprising to be moral most of the time and to be only moderately competent in many areas; it is much more surprising to commit an immoral act, such as to kill someone, or to be a genius and win the Nobel prize. These unusual acts are therefore more diagnostic than customary ones and, as such, are more informative.

Disconfirming Evidence

If some newly encoded evidence is diagnostic of a category, other (disconfirming) information may be diagnostic of not belonging to the category. Sometimes we form an impression not for itself or to predict future behavior, but to verify a hypothesis; that is, there is a criterion to which our impression has to be compared. It is relative to that hypothesis or criterion that the information can be confirming, disconfirming, or irrelevant. One is here reminded of the classic warm–cold experiment conducted by Kelley (1950). As the reader knows, this author warned students that their instructor was generally considered a warm or cold person. Apparently students found enough cues in the instructor's behavior to confirm their hypothesis; indeed, not only did they rate the warm instructor more favorably than the cold one, but they initiated more discussion in the former case than in the latter. This type of problem subsequently reappeared in studies by Snyder and colleagues (e.g., Snyder & Swann, 1978b; Snyder & Gangestad, 1981; for a review, see Leyens, 1990).

Because disconfirming information is capable of falsifying a hypothesis, it should have greater weight than confirming information. This was verified in the already-cited studies by Yzerbyt and Leyens (1991; Leyens & Yzerbyt, 1992). In their experiments, subjects needed fewer items to decide whether a candidate was suitable to a specific role or belonged to a particular cultural group when these items disconfirmed the hypothesis. Moreover, when the evidence was mixed, the presentation of disconfirming characteristics almost immediately overrode the confirming information that had preceded it.

Given that positive and negative information has, as we have seen, different weights, what happens when the hypothesis is explicitly evaluative? In a correlational study, Rothbart and Park (1986) showed that positive traits are easier to disconfirm and harder to confirm than negative traits. In other words, one is never sure that an honest person is completely honest, but one can be certain that a dishonest person is not honest. Yzerbyt and Leyens (1991; Leyens & Yzerbyt, 1992) have supported the Rothbart–Park hypothesis experimentally. Work on disconfirmability examines the cognitive dynamics implicit in the Asch studies and ignored in the Anderson studies.

Illusory Correlation

Another encoding phenomenon occurs when information is combined as it is received. In a now-classic series of experiments, Hamilton and his colleagues (Hamilton, Dugan, & Trolier, 1985; Hamilton & Gifford, 1976) have shown that people exaggerate the frequency of infrequent traits supposed to characterize a minority group, therefore perceiving that minority group mostly in terms of these infrequent traits.[1] Because negative information is perceived to be rare, infrequent traits will often be undesirable ones. Paired distinctiveness illusory correlation is highly consistent and generalizable across studies (Mullen & Johnson, 1990; for critiques, see Fiedler,

[1]Sanbonmatsu, Sherman, and Hamilton (1987), however, have suggested that what is salient in the case of a group is not what is salient in the case of an individual. In the individual cases, perhaps it is the more numerous traits that are more important and determine the perception or evaluation. Resolution of this issue awaits further research.

1991; Smith, 1991). The illusory correlation between group membership and behavior valence, reflecting an overestimation of the most distinctive combination, occurs at encoding and at judgment, due to a selective recall process (Fiedler, Hemmeter, & Hofmann, 1984). The detailed cognitive analysis of information pairs has moved the field closer to understanding the joint influence of separate pieces of information that would not have the same impact individually. As such, it speaks to Gestalt ideas about context and goes beyond Andersonian ideas to specify what might determine the weight of information pairs.

Relations between the Traits

Other relationships between traits, besides paired distinctiveness, also influence encoding. Judd and Lusk (1984) have hypothesized that the more correlated the dimensions used to describe a target, the more extremely this target is judged, and that the more orthogonal the dimensions, the less extreme is the judgment. Their reasoning is an attempt to reconcile research by Tesser (1978) and Linville (1982). "Tesser's work suggests that more polarized or extreme evaluative judgments follow from greater thought about a domain of objects, especially when one is relatively familiar with those objects. The mediating process is one of thought inducing perceived evaluative consistency of attributes" (Judd & Lusk, 1984, p. 1194). For Linville, on the other hand, moderate evaluations are caused by complex knowledge structures, which themselves result from familiarity with the relevant domain. The results obtained by Judd and Lusk (1984), in both an experimental study and a correlational one, are intriguing and worth pursuing (also see Marques, Yzerbyt, & Leyens, 1988; Marques & Yzerbyt, 1988). It certainly is in accordance with Gestalt-like notions, to the extent that correlated dimensions would form a good Gestalt, leading to more confident judgment.

Summary

A variety of work on the encoding of data thus examines the impact of stimulus features: vividness, negativity and rarity, diagnosticity, disconfirming evidence, illusory correlation, and correlated dimensions. This work is an exuberant, free-form collection, taking off on various topics severally interesting to their creators, as in a fantasia. We turn next to a more cohesive line of research, memory.

Memory for Data

Person memory research has focused on memory for incongruent information, that is, information descriptively or evaluatively discrepant from previous characteristics of the same target or from a general expectation, such as a stereotype. One could say that incongruent information is unexpected, but we prefer to distinguish the two because unexpected information is not necessarily incongruent (e.g., it could be more extreme but in the same direction as an expectancy). The first person memory researchers emerged from those imprinted on the Asch–Anderson debates; perhaps then it is not surprising that the question of incongruency loomed so large. A good Gestalt requires coherence among its parts, so incongruency is central to this theme. Interestingly, person memory researchers have only recently supported the Gestalt principle that individuals are the basic unit of organization in memory (Mullen & Cooper, 1989; Sedikides & Ostrom, 1988, 1990). With regard to the Andersonian countertheme, the weights in an algebraic combination depend on information value, which follows from nonredundancy, so incongruency matters in this regard as well.

The (in)congruency of the stimulus traits had already been studied by both Asch and Anderson; it was part of the operationalization of the paradigm invented to show the primacy effect. While Asch defended the idea that incongruent traits following congruent ones had less importance because their meaning was influenced in the direction of the preceding items, Anderson argued that it was due to an attention decrement. Recently, Belmore (1987) tested three hypotheses about the link between attention and incongruency. The first is Anderson's *attention decrement* hypothesis, whereby one expects a decrease in looking time regardless of the congruency or incongruency of the information. According to the second hypothesis, the *distinctiveness hypothesis,* the items incongruent with the impression or expectancy receive special attention during encoding in the form of semantic elaboration. The third hypothesis, called *impression sensitivity,* makes different predictions according to the place of incongruency in the sequence of information and depending on whether or not subjects do or do not have a specific expectancy; when there is an expectancy, incongruent material should receive more attention irrespective of the serial position. (For our purposes, this part of the hypothesis is formally identical with the preceding one.) When the impression is formed on-line or bottom-up, on the other hand, the incongruency should be distinctive only later in the sequence. The results support the last part of the third hypothesis (Belmore, 1987, Experiment 2). The distinctiveness hypothesis is only partially supported: longer inspection times for incongruent items are observed only when they are numerically fewer than congruent ones, and when they are compared to the times of those congruent items just preceding. In agreement with the attention-decrement hypothesis, there is always a steady decrease of attention through the sequence; in the studies conducted by Belmore (1987), however, this finding cannot explain the primacy effect, as the incongruent information attracts more attention than the preceding congruent information.

The distinctiveness hypothesis, which received only partial support in Belmore's (1987) experiments, has actually been the focus of much research by social cognition investigators, and the role of information distinctive with regard to an impression created some contradictions in the literature (Higgins & Bargh, 1987). Social cognition researchers brought into fashion concepts such as frame, script, and schema. From that perspective, it was reasonable to assume that people were preferentially theory driven, and, consequently, that they would remember better those items that were congruent with their expectancy. For example, Rothbart, Evans, and Fulero (1979) provided evidence that seemed to support this view. Their subjects expected to read about members of a group that was considered friendly or intelligent. They then read 17 items showing intelligence, 3 unintelligence, 17 friendliness, 3 unfriendliness, and 10 unrelated to personality. Recall was better for the traits congruent with the expectancy.

In a somewhat similar paradigm, Hastie and Kumar (1979) tested the same problem. The expectancy was created by a series of traits that were followed by a certain number of behaviors, the majority of which were congruent with the expectation and the others incongruent (actually opposed to the expectancy) or irrelevant. This time, recall was best for the incongruent information and worst for the irrelevant material. According to Hastie (1981), the two sets of results are not really contradictory because the so-called incongruent items in the Rothbart et al. (1979) study should actually be considered irrelevant to the expectancy. Hastie (1980) explained his results in terms of an associative network model: in order to integrate the incongruent information, subjects have to form a greater number of associative links between the incongruent items and all the other terms than is necessary for items congruent with the expectancy. In subsequent experiments, Hastie (1984) has shown that subjects remember best those behaviors that they have to explain, be they congruent or incongruent with the expectancy. Further support and refinements of this model were made by Srull (1981), Wyer, Bodenhausen, and Srull (1984), and most recently Srull and Wyer (1989). (For reviews of this literature, see Fiske & Taylor, 1991, Chapter 8; Higgins & Bargh, 1987; Rojahn & Pettigrew, 1992; Stangor & McMillan, 1992.)

Higgins and Bargh (1987) noted that there is a confound in the Hastie and Kumar study (1979); in the terminology adopted in this chapter, the items best recalled are salient on two grounds: not only are they incongruent, but they are contextually rare (small "set size"), which is sometimes sufficient to improve recall whether or not in agreement with the expectancy. Also important, they suggest that the subjects in the Hastie–Kumar research were forming an impression rather than testing it. In other words, the induction of an initial impression by a few traits was not strong enough to create a real expectancy. Presumably, when there is a strong belief, people maintain it (Nisbett & Ross, 1980; Ross, Lepper, & Hubbard, 1975), evidently by ignoring or discounting any discordant evidence. In a similar vein, Fiske and Neuberg (1990) have suggested that studies showing greater impact of expectancy-incongruent information have typically used weak (i.e., less developed) stereotypes (also see Ruble & Stangor, 1986).

What has the social cognitive context provided beyond the original insights into these issues? Asch (1946) originally noted the importance of first impressions for the integration of subsequent discrepant information. When Asch and Zukier (1984) asked their subjects to describe in a few sentences a person who was, for instance, cheerful and gloomy, they found that the task was no more difficult (but more interesting) than when the person was intelligent and ambitious. The perceived difficulty was quite different when Asch (1946) asked his subjects to form an impression of both person A, who was intelligent, industrious, and impulsive, and person B, who was critical, stubborn, and envious. Next, he told them that, in fact A and B were the same person, whom they were now to describe. This last task was experienced as extremely difficult, and some subjects, unable to reconcile the contradictions, ended up with the profile of a split personality.

Nevertheless, person memory research has made significant progress on issues related to memory for incongruent information, at least under a certain paradigm (for a recent meta-analysis, see Stangor & McMillan, 1992). It is important to note that, as the procedure becomes more complicated, the incongruency advantage can be eliminated. For example, multiple expectancies eliminate the effect (Hamilton, Driscoll, & Worth, 1989). In addition, the effect seems to require "free recall and experimentally induced expectancies . . . ; evaluative plus descriptive inconsistency (not just descriptive), individual (not group) targets, an explicit impression formation goal (rather than memorizing or evaluating), no interpolated tasks [i.e., no time to reconsider], and location of the whole process within a single experimental session (Stangor & McMillan, 1992)" (Fiske, 1993, p. 160). To be fair, the incongruency effect has been obtained in the real world (Skowronski, Betz, Thompson, & Shannon, 1991). Nevertheless, both its boundaries and its significance directly result from social cognition researchers originally interested in the Asch phenomena (Hamilton, 1989).

Representations of Data

So far, we have pursued themes concerning the encoding of data and memory for data, with references back to enduring issues in impression formation. What kind of representation is formed when subjects have finished reading the series of personality traits proposed by Asch or Anderson to describe a fictitious person? Moreover, what kinds of representations did the subjects have before reading the lists of traits? Extensive social cognition work has examined people's representations that predate the laboratory encounter and that endure beyond the laboratory's interventions.

Schemas

"A schema is a cognitive structure that represents organized knowledge about a given concept or type of stimulus. A schema contains both the attributes of the concept and the relationships among the attributes. . . . The schema concept specifically maintains that information is stored in an abstract form, not simply as a collection of all the original encounters with examples of the general case" (Fiske & Taylor, 1984, p. 140). Like an implicit theory of personality, thus, a schema intervenes after a process of categorization, but it does so with more flexibility; once a person, for instance, has been classified in a particular category of personality, profession, race, and so on, the knowledge accumulated "in" the schema will guide subsequent perception, thinking, and action. The notion is similar to that of prototype and is often used interchangeably (for differences, see Fiske & Taylor, 1991, Chapter 4). According to their generic content, schemas are sometimes distinguished into self-schemas, person schemas, role schemas, event schemas, and content-free schemas. Here, we will mostly treat the first three as a whole (for much more detailed reviews of the recent literature, see Fiske & Taylor, 1991, Chapters 4 & 5; Markus & Zajonc, 1985).

Much research addresses the effects of schemas on perception, memory, and inferences. Essentially, the message is that (1) schemas guide perceivers toward relevant information, and (2) people try to resolve inconsistencies, in order to maintain a coherent impression, just as Asch thought. Rather than dwell on the many studies documenting these phenomena, it may be more interesting to examine two ways in which schema research has evolved over the last decade or so of enthusiastic research activity. Both concern levels of abstraction in schematic organization, but one addresses between-schema relationships, and the other addresses within-schema organization.

Between-schema organization. When we receive information about others, what kinds of schemas are favored; which characteristics are dominant, at what level of abstraction? It has been assumed, first, that social schemas are organized hierarchically. Second, the most useful schemas are assumed to be those that occupy an intermediate level in the hierarchy because they are sufficiently abstract not to be overwhelmed by unnecessary details and sufficiently specific not to be lost in overall generality. Often, this intermediate level corresponds to well-established personality traits (Cantor & Mischel, 1979).

This conclusion has been recently challenged by Andersen and Klatzky (1987). These authors contrast traits and stereotypes. For them, traits relate only to personality and are usually transmitted through adjectives. Stereotypes, on the other hand, relate not only to personality but also to behaviors (e.g., professions) and attitudes (e.g., belief systems); they represent a group of people sharing these attributes and are communicated by nouns. According to these researchers, stereotypes are associatively richer, linked to more visible attributes, and thus more predictive than traits. Moreover, traits would share virtually all their associates with related stereotypes, whereas the social stereotypes would maintain unique associates. To test these hypotheses, Andersen and Klatzky (1987) conducted sorting tasks, free-association tasks, and similarity judgments around two traits (extroverted and introverted) and six stereotypes (comedian, politician, bully, brain, neurotic, and guru). The data indeed show that the stereotypes are richer, more concrete, and more specific than the traits; this supports the idea that "extraverted" and "introverted" occupy a superordinate position relative to the selected stereotypes.

Within-schema organization. Like prototypes, schemas represent the abstract form of the best examples of a category; they inform one about the central tendency of the category. This view, however, is not unanimous. Some authors (Barsalou, 1985; Chapin, John, & Goldberg, 1988) have defended the idea that categories are sometimes better represented by ideal or extreme forms than by average ones. It is true that we prefer to eat in an extremely ideal restaurant rather than in an average one, so in this case the best example is guided by our activity rather than by our average representation of restaurants. It is also true that for many of us, the "real" nun is overhung by a huge white headdress, wears a long, black habit, and always contemplates her hidden toes. Although an almost extinct species, this "real" nun is one representation of "nuns in general" and not linked to any particular function. It is not an extreme (not to mention ideal!) exemplar; it is an illustration of the persistence of schemas in spite of the flux of more recent and contradictory data. Even if the earth was suddenly submerged by the oceans with a little bit of China still floating, the few pandas would still and for a long time be better representatives of mammals than the more numerous whales. For many purposes, the more ideal may be a better representation than the average.

Unlike implicit theories of personality, which were thought to contain knowledge about measures of central tendency, dispersion, and covariation, schemas were thought to represent only the central tendency, and even to overrepresent it (Mayer & Bower, 1986; Rothbart & Lewis, 1988). However, if we have any idea of variability or correlation within a given category, this knowledge has to come from something other than pure schemas. Schematic views have therefore come under severe attack, and some authors have proposed to supplement them by instance or exemplar models (e.g., Smith & Zárate, 1992). According to that perspective, we encode exemplars (specific instances), and when asked to make a global judgment, this is based on the exemplars we can retrieve (Zárate & Smith, 1990).

In several experiments, Park and her colleagues (Judd & Park, 1988; Park & Hastie, 1987; Park & Judd, 1990) have contrasted a nuanced schematic model to a "prototypical" exemplar model:

> According to prototype models, as individual instances of a category are encountered, the perceiver abstracts and stores a unitary prototype of these in memory and may or may not store information about the instances themselves. . . . Proponents of instance storage models argue that the representation of a category is a set of stored exemplars learned at presentation, rather than category-level information that has been abstracted from the exemplars. (Park & Hastie, 1987, p. 621)

When receiving information about a group of individuals that is either very homogeneously intelligent and sociable, or weakly homogeneous on the same dimensions, subjects are sensitive to variability, as predicted by an exemplar model. However, it appears that the variability estimates are calculated on-line rather than at retrieval because manipulating the memorability of the exemplars does not show the effects predicted by an instance storage model (Park & Hastie, 1987). The controversy between the two conceptions (see also Linville, Fischer, & Salovey, 1989) has implications for several phenomena: the generalization of attributes from one person to other members of the category (Nisbett & Borgida, 1975), the effects of individuating information on stereotypes (Locksley, Borgida, Brekke, & Hepburn, 1980; Locksley, Hepburn, & Ortiz, 1982; etc.), illusory correlation (Smith, 1991), and the explanation of out-group homogeneity (Mullen & Hu, 1989).

The growing consensus is that people do not use only schemas or only exemplars; they are able to use both, and they do. Psychologists have to guard against resembling designers of haute couture, who ignore nuances and from one year to the next completely change styles. People on the street, however, do not wear haute couture clothes; they accommodate last-year's purchases to present-day fashion. Likewise, the people psychologists try to study use both schemas and exemplars to varying degrees (Zuroff, 1989).

Social Representations

This concept is a social psychological adaptation (by Moscovici, 1961) of a sociological concept: collective representation (Durkheim, 1898). It refers to an explanatory model categorizing relationships between various objects of the environment, which filters perception and guides action. These models have the function of transforming the strange and the unfamiliar into the familiar so that people sharing a representation about a given object can communicate about it without being experts. Contrary to an IPT and a schema, its objects are almost without limits, including "ideas, thoughts, images, and knowledge which members of a collectivity share: consensual universes of thought which are socially created and socially communicated to form part of a 'common consciousness'" (Augoustinos & Innes, 1990, p. 215). The major difference between a schema and a social representation is that the former can be idiosyncratic, but the latter is by definition a social-cultural creation. Schema research emphasizes individual-level information processing, whereas social representation research emphasizes the content of the representations. However, as social schema research becomes more social (Fiske, 1993), the distinction may evaporate, except in terms of whom authors choose to cite as authorities. Moreover, similarly to schemas, social representations do have a structure (Di Giacomo, 1980), although the structure is quite flexible and will vary with the content of the representations (Farr & Moscovici, 1984; Jodelet, 1989).

The classic example is the study of social representations of psychoanalysis conducted in the fifties by Moscovici (1961) among Parisians. For those people, psychoanalysis was the science about the fight between the conscious and the unconscious; this conflict leads to repression, which engenders complexes; it follows that psychoanalysis is a treatment for those individuals who suffer from complexes. In this representation, one can see the dimension of categorization as well as the resulting simplification: for example, to make the unfamiliar familiar, the persons interrogated by Moscovici completely discarded the central notion of libido. This representation of a given concept is said to be social because it is built and shared by groups of people. Different groups will have different representations; for instance, in the fifties, Catholics were opposed to psychoanalysis because it was related to sexual matters, which were best left unconscious. Marxists, on the other hand, also were opposed to it because psychoanalysis was considered by them to be a luxurious treatment focusing on the individual rather than on social classes. These various reactions to psychoanalysis show how its social representations may guide action. Other work on social representations examines stereotypes, health beliefs, and popular science. Some would argue that a schema and a social representation are identical, but that the latter is a broader theory because it is explicitly social (Augoustinos & Innes, 1990).

Another close equivalent in the American literature may be the concept of construal proposed by Ross and Nisbett (1991). Although, according to these authors, this latter concept fundamentally refers to an individual process, it may have social and cultural significance; given that people share backgrounds, values, environments, priorities, and so on, it is likely that they will construe reality in the same manner. (The same of course is true for a schema.)

Another American equivalent comes from the cognitive literature. In a most cogent paper, Murphy and Medin (1985) try to answer what makes a category, or concept, coherent. According to them, accounts based on similarity and feature correlations provide inadequate answers because none provides enough constraints on possible concepts or categories. They "propose that concepts are coherent to the extent that they fit people's background knowledge or *naive theories about the world*," "people's theories of the world embody conceptual knowledge," and "their conceptual organization is partly represented in their theories" (Murphy & Medin, 1985, pp. 289–290; italics ours). In many ways, people's theories about the world correspond to what is implied by social representations, if one adds the assumption that the naive theories have a social origin. Of course, many social schema theorists also subscribe to the idea of a schema as a coherent theory. In the end, the social representation concept has provided a vehicle for a more sociological level of analysis of people's shared everyday concepts. To the extent that it encourages an examination of the expressly social (as opposed to cognitive) uses of representations, it may address anew part of Asch's original, uncompleted theme in person perception, expressing how our understandings of each other shape our interactions.

SYNTHESIS OF THE OPENING THEMES

The final part of the opening movement in a classical sonata-form symphony is a recapitulation of the opening themes. After Beethoven, however, the two opposing themes commonly would be combined into a third theme. We will follow this genius of the Romantic tradition, with its emphasis on creative synthesis. In this closing section, we will examine several efforts, especially our own, to bring together elements of the opening themes, all of which incorporate the major developments afforded by social cognition approaches.

Continuum Model

One approach explicitly builds both on early work by Asch and on subsequent work in person perception and social cognition, emphasizing the interplay between theory-driven processing and data-driven processing (Fiske & Neuberg, 1990; Fiske & Pavelchak, 1986).[2]

The continuum model's first premise is that impression formation constitutes a *continuum* from fully category-based processes to fully attribute-oriented processes, a distinction parallel to the broader notion of theory-driven and data-driven processes. The model proposes to integrate these two types of process that previously were studied separately: the theory-driven processes were studied in the stereotyping and categorization literatures, and the data-driven processes were studied in the elemental impression formation and attitudes literatures. Examples of the more theory-driven processes include Asch's work on configural impression formation, as well as Allport's (1954) and Tajfel's (1978, 1981) work on categorization and stereotyping. Examples of the more data-driven processes include Anderson's information

[2]There is a related model, the dual process model proposed by Brewer (1988a). Although there are important differences between the models (Brewer, 1988b; Fiske, 1988), they both serve to integrate previous approaches. Lacking all modesty, we will concentrate on Fiske's version here.

integration theory (e.g., 1974, 1981) and Fishbein and Ajzen's (e.g., 1974; Ajzen, 1985) expectancy-value theory of attitudes.

The second premise is that people are lazy: category-based processes have priority, in several respects. People automatically categorize each other on the basis of salient physical cues, and this process appears to be fairly inescapable. If a target person is not trivial to the perceiver, the perceiver will attend further to the other person's attributes. People attempt to confirm this initial category whenever possible, and if successfully confirmed, they do not look any farther. If they cannot reconfirm the category, then they grudgingly examine the person's attributes in hopes of finding a variant on the initial category, one that modifies the category in light of the attributes, resulting in an interaction of the two. For example, they might generate a subcategory such as a seductive woman or a middle-class black; an exemplar, such as great aunt Nancy; or perhaps even a self-reference, such as "this person's independence reminds me of my own." Sometimes they will also generate a new category, for example, reformulating Andre Watts from a black performer to a classical musician. This interactive, Asch-like recategorization process apparently is the most frequent type of impression formation. If this recategorization process fails, people will revert to Andersonian piecemeal, attribute-by-attribute impressions of the other person, as when one is forced to combine qualities without forming an overall, organized impression. The data would suggest that this last process is relatively rare in its pure form. Evidence of all these processes comes from think-aloud data in several studies, which develop one's appreciation for the complexity and agility of people's efforts to make sense of another person, in the Asch tradition (for empirical work, see Erber & Fiske, 1984; Fiske, Neuberg, Beattie, & Milberg, 1987; Fiske, Neuberg, Pratto, & Allman, 1986; Ruscher & Fiske, 1990; Ruscher, Fiske, Miki, & Van Manen, 1991; for methodological discussions, see Fiske & Ruscher, 1989; Taylor & Fiske, 1981).

The continuum model's third premise is that getting people to pay attention to each other is the key to data-driven processing. More formally, attention to the other person's attributes mediates use of the continuum. Unless people attend to another person, they cannot move from category-based or stereotypic impressions to more attribute-based or individuating impressions. Then, as people attend to the attributes of the target person, they may interpret them as contradicting the initial category, and so individuate, or they may interpret them as confirming the category, and so stereotype. Thus, it might seem obvious that attention to another person's attributes would mediate the degree to which one stereotypes or not. However, part of what is important here is that it is increased attention to attributes, not decreased attention to the other person's category. That is, as one individuates another person, one does not forget that the person is a member of category X; one merely learns enough additional information about the person to round out one's impression. This is important because it means that one does not pretend to ignore someone's race or sex, but one does work to go beyond the category to notice other individuating attributes (Fiske et al., 1987; Fiske et al., 1986; Neuberg & Fiske, 1987).

The fourth premise of this model is that information configurations influence the amount of attention and kinds of interpretations that people make about other people's attributes. The influence of information configurations is well documented: people's difficulty in fitting attributes to a given category causes them to move down the continuum. For example, not surprisingly, stereotype-consistent plus mixed information leads people to confirm their stereotypes. Accumulating evidence also indicates that nondiagnostic information leads people to confirm their stereotypes when the category is well established, but not otherwise. On the other hand, dramatically inconsistent information leads people to individuate, as does information that simply cannot be adequately categorized (see Fiske & Neuberg, 1990, for a review). Thus, we can predict fairly well from an information configuration to people's most likely impression formation responses. Putting this together with the idea of initial automatic categorization, it might at first seem that stereotyping and expectancy-driven processing is an inevitable by-product of our cognitive system reacting to the environment, that it is in effect not under intentional control. This idea has come up a number of times, for example, in reviews of the cognitive approaches to stereotyping. But some would argue that it is not quite so (Bargh, 1989; Fiske, 1987, 1989; Uleman, 1989).

This issue of intentional control brings us to the fifth and final premise: motivation also influences people's attention to and interpretation of other people's stereotype-relevant attributes. The model has focused on motivations invoked by interdependence in particular; that is, to the extent a person's own outcomes depend on the other person or on the impression formed of the other person, then the perceiver will pay more attention. In other words, when it is important to people, they can control the processes by which they form impressions of others. This is a fairly radical idea: People's use of the category-based versus attribute-oriented continuum is under their own intentional control. This means that either they can make the easy choice and stay at the beginning of the continuum, or to the extent they are motivated, they can make the hard choice and move down toward individuation of the other person (Erber & Fiske, 1984; Fiske & Von Hendy, 1992; Neuberg & Fiske, 1987; Ruscher & Fiske, 1990; Ruscher et al., 1991; see Fiske & Neuberg, 1990, for a review).

The core of this theory is the balance between categories and data, between the Gestalts of Asch and the attribute-oriented processes of Anderson. As such, it synthesizes some of the opening themes in research on person perception. It also addresses the importance of pragmatic goals, a theme addressed by many other current researchers.

Observation Goals

Early work in social psychology drew on the ideas of set, attitude (in the sense of organizing action), and motivation, but these notions were abandoned during the heyday of the information processing metaphor. As the field returns afresh to early themes, the importance of set, goals, and motivation again becomes clear (Fiske, 1992, 1993). The continuum model expresses some of this theme, but considerable research directly takes up the idea of goals, addressing the classic problems with new vigor.

According to Ebbesen (1980), we generally observe others for one of the following three reasons: learning, impression formation, or evaluation. Subsequent researchers have added other goals: memory, empathy, accuracy, prediction, good structure, and so on. Usually, these goals have been manipulated in order to test global judgment, inferences, or memory, sometimes also processing times.

Often, the goal of impression formation has been contrasted with a memory set and frequently also, the goal of memorizing has been used to block an impression formation set. There is ample evidence (e.g., Hamilton, Katz, & Leirer, 1980; Lichtenstein & Srull, 1987; Wyer & Gordon, 1982) that an impression set facilitates the organizing role of accessible mental categories in information processing, relative to a memory set. The consequence is not obvious; on one hand, better organization could lead to a better memory and, indeed, as just one example, Stangor and Ruble (1989) have shown that memory for material consistent with an expectancy was greater under an impression set than under a memory set (see also Hamilton et al., 1980; Lichtenstein & Srull, 1987; Wyer & Gordon, 1982). On the other hand, the literature on intentional versus incidental learning (de Montpellier, 1985) would suggest better recall when it is made explicit that subjects have to memorize; in agreement with this literature, subjects in one study (Cohen & Ebbesen, 1979) remembered behavioral details better under a memory set than under an impression set. Overall, it seems that when the information is directly related to the personality of individuals (via behaviors as well as traits), an impression set leads to better organized and greater memory than a memory set because the latter favors only rote learning (Srull, Lichtenstein, & Rothbart, 1985), whereas the former creates person-attributes links. Thus, although the number of memorized chunks sometimes may be greater with a memory set, the content of the chunks is likely to be much larger in an impression set, and their links are likely to be more numerous.

More important for our purpose is the way people use and categorize information when they have different goals. In the Cohen–Ebbesen study just mentioned, subjects made inferences about the personality of the actors; when the subjects' task was to form an impression, their inferences were closer to general implicit theories of personality than were those of the subjects who anticipated a memory test. Hoffman, Mischel, and Mazze

(1981) tested another hypothesis; they looked at the way people categorized the information under goals (1) to memorize the behaviors of a target, (2) to empathize with the target, (3) to form an impression of the target, or (4) to predict the target's future behavior. A fifth group received no special goal. The categorization could be made in terms of physical setting (the most obvious criterion), implicit psychological traits, explicit action-goals, or hidden action-goals. Traits were used by those subjects who had to form an impression or to predict future behaviors, and action-goals were used by those who had to memorize or empathize. The same authors showed subsequently that an organization in terms of traits actually led to worse memory than one based on action-goals. According to the authors, action-goals more than traits elicit a coherent temporal sequence, easy to memorize.

Recently, Devine, Sedikides, and Fuhrman (1989) compared the effects of different instruction sets (anticipated interaction, impression formation, self-comparison, best-friend comparison, and memory) on different measures of memory. Only when subjects anticipated an interaction or had to form an impression did they remember the target better than the other individuals. Total recall was not different for the instruction sets. The same results were obtained when subjects had to recall to which individual each bit of information belonged (that is, a measure of name–attribute association). The organization of memory around individuals (i.e., attribute–attribute associations for the same person) was worse for the memory set than for any other, but only under anticipated interaction was memory organization better for the target than for the other persons. If these results prove reliable, one should expect people to make easier inferences about the persons with whom they expect to interact; it would also be interesting to vary the content (e.g., consistent, inconsistent, irrelevant) of the information given the anticipated interaction.

Accuracy has been another goal to be manipulated. Neuberg (1989) has shown that such a goal can overcome a negative expectancy. For half the subjects, the instructions stressed accuracy, while no special goal was given to the rest of the subjects. The negative expectancy for the interviewers with no specific goal led to an unfavorable impression of the applicant at the end of the interview; in other words, the interview had confirmed the hypothesis created by the experimenter. This was not the case, however, for those questioners who had been induced to be accurate; moreover, an analysis of their behavior during the interview showed that they encouraged the applicants and asked questions that allowed them to present themselves in a positive manner.

Another version of the goal of accuracy was proposed by Kruglanski and his colleagues in the framework of his theory of lay epistemology (Kruglanski, 1980; Kruglanski & Ajzen, 1983; Kruglanski & Klar, 1987). According to that theory, people may freeze the generation of new hypotheses because of their need for structure, and the opposite occurs under fear of invalidity (Kruglanski & Freund, 1983; Freund, Kruglanski & Shpitzajzen, 1985); these may actually be the two poles of a single dimension (Kruglanski & Mayseless, 1988). Thus, for example, when people are under time pressure and fear of invalidity is not a main concern, they will be more prone to primacy effects, stereotyping, and neglect of alternative hypotheses than if they know their judgment has to be valid and they have plenty of time to decide. This conjunction of the two needs—structure and validity—leading to freezing or unfreezing does not necessarily correspond to inaccuracy or accuracy (the same is true of accountability: Tetlock & Boettger, 1989). It may be perfectly possible that unfreezing induces inaccuracy, as in the case when "first impressions do count."

In a perspective not alien to Kruglanski's, Zukier (1986) has proposed to distinguish two modes of thinking that correspond more or less to two different goals: paradigmatic (scientific) and narrative (coherent). "The paradigmatic mode is extensive; it sacrifices a specific and comprehensive description for wide applicability of its propositions and trades richness for rigor. By contrast, the narrative mode is intensive; it focuses as much on differences as on similarities and trades generality for singular comprehensiveness, rigor for richness" (Zukier, 1986, p. 476). Adopting one mode or the other leads to different impressions; the narrative mode, for instance, neglects base-rate information (Zukier & Pepitone, 1984) and dilutes stereotypes (Zukier, 1982). This difference in modes of thinking also corresponds to different roles (e.g., the statistician vs. the clinical psychologist), and maybe to various expertises.

The effects of goals on memory organization may be summarized by the level of psychological engagement (from memory to impressions to empathy to interaction); greater engagement facilitates memory. The effects of goals on impression accuracy may be grouped by increasing the costs of being wrong (accuracy, interdependence, accountability in general) versus increasing the costs of being indecisive (e.g., time pressure, narrative mode) (see Fiske & Taylor, 1991, Chapter 4; Fiske, 1992, for reviews). Similar distinctions have been made by Bruner (1957), Festinger (1964), Gollwitzer (1990), Hilton and Darley (1991), Jones and Gerard (1967), Ruble (1993), Snyder (1992), and Stangor and Ford (1992). The efficiency–accuracy trade-off is central to social cognitive goals. All subsequent processes depend on the perceiver's goals.

Priming

Where do the goals come from? Bargh (1990) proposes that motives may be primed by certain contextual cues, just as concepts are primed. Current work on sexual harassment, for example, indicates that sexually explicit or suggestive visual media prime harassing behavior in some men (Borgida & Rudman, 1992; McKenzie-Mohr & Zanna, 1990). Power-related primes can have the same effect (Bargh & Raymond, 1992). This promising line of work may help us to predict people's goals, on which all else rests. The goal-priming work itself builds on Bruner's classic work in construct accessibility.

Research on construct accessibility has documented the wide-ranging impact of priming a particular category on subsequent perceptions, judgments, and memory (see Higgins & Bargh, 1987, for a review). Constructs that are chronically active for particular judges, or, alternatively, constructs that have recently or frequently been activated for that judge, influence the interpretation of ambiguous stimuli that follow. For example, a person primed with positive constructs will interpret the subsequent sensation-seeking behavior of another person as adventurous rather than reckless. These effects operate when judges are not aware of the connection between the stimulus and the prime; they also operate when the priming stimulus is presented subliminally (Bargh & Pietromonaco, 1982). In particular, for example, Devine (1989) has found that subliminally presented words related to blacks cause whites to interpret the behavior of an ambiguous person as hostile (also see Gilbert & Hixon, 1991).

When a specific schema has been activated in judges, they may be particularly sensitive to some kinds of information. This occurs for chronic, long-term activation as well as temporary activation (Bargh, Bond, Lombardi, & Tota, 1986; Higgins, King, & Mavin, 1982). In the case of self-schemas, similarly, Markus (1977) has shown that people process schema-relevant information more sensitively and that this applies to the perception of others as well (e.g., Markus, Smith, & Moreland, 1985). Carpenter (1988) notes that schematics recall and weight schema-relevant information, at least under impression formation conditions.

Experience of the Judge

Of course, there are individual differences in impression formation processes. Early person perception researchers attempted to discover who was a more or less accurate perceiver of other people. When the pursuit of accuracy per se was abandoned, ironically, so was the exploration of individual differences, with a few exceptions. Self-schema research, as just noted, formed one exception (for reviews, see Fiske & Taylor, 1991, Chapter 6; Markus & Wurf, 1987).

It is all the more curious, for a field that considers the judge as an active processor of information, that not many studies have been devoted to this judge's characteristics, which undoubtedly influence the formation of impressions. This becomes curiouser and curiouser, in that the New Look in perception and thinking (Bruner, Goodnow, & Austin, 1956) and almost all theories of person perception have assumed that the processing of information represents a combined influence of stimulus factors and individual differences in social experiences. Observational goals and accessible constructs, just discussed, illustrate this point, but even more so does the social experience and expertise of the judge, which we consider here, and the social rules held by the judge, which we will consider next.

Given the emphasis put on the direction (bottom-up or top-down) and timing (on-line or memory based) of cognitive processes, their controlled or automatic character, as well as the role of memory, it comes as no surprise that authors have investigated the impact of the judge's expertise. What is more surprising is that this characteristic has not been studied more. One source of inspiration for this work is the chess grand master who can memorize all the positions of the pieces during a regular game but is unable to memorize the positions if the pieces are placed at random (Chase & Simon, 1973). The difference between that research and social cognition research is that the social material is not highly specialized, but represents knowledge accessible in common to both experts and novices.

Who, then, should be considered expert at social cognition? Among others, Batson (1975; Batson & Marz, 1979) has shown that experienced psychological helpers are *more* prone to the Fundamental Attribution Error (Ross, 1977) than novices. Reviewing this domain, Leyens (1983) suggested several reasons for that finding. Clinical psychologists are more in a position of observer than actor, they work in a constant environment, and they always entertain the same relationship with their clients. The rich vocabulary of traits is both available and easily accessible to them, and their task is usually to predict future behaviors through stable explanations. Finally, their role is to evaluate others, and this asymmetry in power may also explain why they resort more to personal explanations than do subordinate individuals (Beauvois & Dubois, 1988). Similarly, powerful or dominating people, given no particular incentives, pay less attention to subordinates than do less powerful or dominating people (S. Goodwin & S. Fiske, unpublished data, 1992).

Obviously, the kind of theory entertained by the powerful experts will influence their judgments (e.g., Langer & Abelson, 1974). But will any theory lead its holders to be more influenced by confirming data, or will it lead them to be especially sensitive to odd but confirming data? This question has been tested by Wright and Murphy (1984); in one of their experiments (Experiment 2) they show that novices, who know what the data mean but do not have a theory, are somewhat less influenced by the direction of the data than experts, who have a theory or an expectancy. What is most significant is the idea that knowing what the information means, with or without theory, in some ways protects one from giving importance to deviant data, even when the deviance goes in the direction of the theory. As the authors conclude, ". . . results suggest that the best condition to be in is to know what the data represent but to have no expectancy about the specific results" (Wright & Murphy, 1984, p. 320). This is certainly a condition easier to find inside than outside the laboratory!

Compared to novices, experts tend to encode and classify relevant material efficiently, to think in a focused fashion, to cluster recalled material, and to judge quickly (Dawson, Zeitz, & Wright, 1989; Fiske, Kinder, & Larter, 1983; Fiske, Lau, & Smith, 1990; Hamill, Lodge, & Blake, 1985), but their recall can show a schema-consistent bias (Lodge & Hamill, 1986) and their representations may be more evaluatively organized and extreme than those of novices (Lusk & Judd, 1988); all these findings are compatible with the idea that experts have less differentiated categories than novices do (Murphy & Wright, 1984).

Experts may have some control over their strategies, however. In one data set (Fiske et al., 1983), this time it was the novices who made inferences especially in line with the expectancy, while experts made inferences more in terms of inconsistencies and thus slightly reversed the set. More importantly, memory organization correlated, only for the experts, with the inferences. The authors suggest that novices may use a confirmatory strategy, whereas experts would more often use a disconfirmatory strategy.

This very problem was investigated by Borgida and DeBono (1989), who used still another paradigm to study the effects of expertise. Their question was whether experts would remember better than nonexperts facts confirming a hypothesis relative to disconfirming ones. The experts indeed remembered more disconfirming facts than confirming ones. The difference was due to a greater number of recalled disconfirming facts, as the confirming facts were equally remembered in all the conditions. Thus, experts seemed able to use their knowledge in a more disconfirmatory manner, in agreement with the previous results. Both in Fiske et al. and in Borgida and DeBono, the difference is due to the fact that novices in one of the conditions (the most difficult for them) recall less inconsistent material than experts do.

It also may all depend on degree of expertise. Stangor and Ruble (1989) hypothesized and found that experienced subjects would recall more consistent information than nonexperts. But their theory concerned the development of experience over time, with early stages emphasizing memory for inconsistent information (e.g., the standard person memory effect for newly formed impressions), intermediate stages emphasizing theory-consistent information (as in their experienced subjects), and later stages allowing more flexibility (e.g., Fiske et al.'s and Borgida & DeBono's experts). This theory (Ruble & Stangor, 1986; Ruble, 1994) suggests going beyond Noah's Ark (2×2) designs to examine several levels of experience, at various stages from complete novice to well-practiced expert.

Earlier, we noted that individual experiences have been curiously neglected, except for the promising work on observational goals, accessible constructs, and the experience or expertise of the judge. Next, we consider the social and cultural rules held by the judge.

Social Judgeability Theory

The image emerging from work on impression formation is of perceivers having to resolve the intellectual problem of balancing theory and data. But this image cannot account for the confusion of the obtained results. If categorization rests on social interactions, then social judgment also must respond to certain social norms. Schadron and Yzerbyt (1991) hypothesized that people take account not only of data and theories about data, but also of theories about judgment. Certain of these theories depend importantly on sociocultural context; thus, when Katz and Braly (1933) invented the first measure of stereotypes, it was more socially acceptable to express antiethnic prejudices than to withhold judgment. Just as plausibly, it can be acceptable that perceivers avoid judgment, or judge without much confidence, when they think they have not fulfilled the appropriate conditions for judgment, for example, when they do not have enough information. According to Schadron and Yzerbyt (1991), for example, the dilution of stereotypes through irrelevant information does not occur by reducing perceived similarity to a prototype; instead, it reflects an absence of judgment, when one has been given limited information about the particular target (for a review, see Leyens, Yzerbyt, & Schadron, 1992).

The social judgeability hypothesis fits the interpretation given by Darley and Gross (1983) for the absence of stereotyping by their subjects who knew only the socioeconomic status of a videotaped target. From the social judgeability perspective, the appearance of stereotypes, only after mixed evidence from an intelligence test, did not reflect hypothesis confirmation but the judges' feeling that they were in a position to make a judgment.

Yzerbyt, Schadron, Leyens, & Rocher (1994) directly tested the social judgeability hypothesis by activating an extraversion stereotype and then leading half their subjects to believe that they had subliminally received additional information about the target; only the "informed" subjects allowed themselves to make a judgment, a judgment that in fact had to be stereotypic (because that was all the information they actually had), but the subjects thought their judgment was not stereotypic and pertained specifically to the individual target. In another study, some subjects were led to believe that they had received information about an extroverted category (i.e., comedians). As expected, these subjects did not feel entitled to judge a specific target. This result clarifies that judgeability is due neither to a greater accessibility of the stereotype nor to a demand characteristic. Debriefing also revealed that some of the subjects had misunderstood the instructions and thought they had received individuating rather than categorical information. In line with the continuum model, this finding illustrates that the shift from individualized target to category is an easy one. (For other relevant work, see Leyens, Yzerbyt, & Schadron, 1992.)

The shift is also smooth between feeling entitled to judge and deeming the target judgeable. There is thus no surprise that people also can feel in a position to judge other people because they have been given power (Caetano & Vala, 1993), as noted earlier. Defining power as control over another person's outcomes (Dépret & Fiske, 1993) means that the powerful person is not directly contingent on the subordinate and feels justified in using the easiest categorical judgment. Consistent with this perspective, powerful people, given no other incentives, may well feel justified in relying on their prior categories, even stereotypes (Beauvois & Dubois, 1988; Fiske, 1993; Leyens, 1983).

FINIS

Opening themes in impression formation research reflected Asch's Gestalt thesis and Anderson's algebraic antithesis, with implicit personality theory making a transition in between. The exuberant fantasia of the middle period emphasized the encoding of data (in terms of its isolated and correlational characteristics), memory for data (especially incongruent data), and social theories (e.g., schemas and social representations). Having displayed its virtuosic talents, the social cognition movement has gone on to recapture a synthesis of its opening themes, nevertheless building on the variations of the fantasia period; one sees the culmination of the movement in work incorporating both theory and data, illustrated by work on the continuum model, observational goals, priming of constructs and goals, variations in the experience of the judge, and social judgeability theory. All of these reflect a recent acknowledgment of the pragmatics of social cognition (Fiske, 1992).

Is the current pragmatic era a recapitulation of the opening Asch theme and Anderson countertheme, or is it, as in Beethoven's awesome innovation, rather a synthesis of the two opposing themes, resolving them into a new theme that combines contrasting forces into a new creation? It is this interpretation we prefer.

We have referred throughout to the social cognition movement, not just in the sense of collective action. We also mean the musical reference. This is after all only the opening movement of a multipart work, and we await the ensuing movements that build on the opening one. In this context, it is well to recall the definition of the Romantic tradition as a revolt against principles associated with neoclassism, characterized by freedom of form and spirit, emphasis on originality, and a sympathetic interest in the experiences of the common people.

ACKNOWLEDGMENTS

The writing of this chapter was facilitated by NIMH Grant MH 41801 to S. T. Fiske and by USIA Grant IA-AEGH-G6192688, facilitating a university affiliation program between our two universities.

REFERENCES

Ajzen, I. (1985). From intentions to actions: A theory of planned behavior. In J. Kuhl & J. Beckmann (Eds.), *Action control: From cognition to behavior* (pp. 11–39). New York: Springer-Verlag.

Allport, G. W. (1954). *The nature of prejudice.* Reading, MA: Addison-Wesley.

Andersen, S. M., & Klatzky, R. L. (1987). Traits and social stereotypes: Levels of categorization in person perception. *Journal of Personality and Social Psychology, 53,* 235–246.

Anderson, C. A., & Sedikides, C. (1991). Thinking about people: Contributions of a typological alternative to associationistic and dimensional models of person perception. *Journal of Personality and Social Psychology, 60,* 203–217.

Anderson, C. A., Lepper, M. R., & Ross, L. (1980). Perseverance of social theories: The role of explanation in the persistence of discredited information. *Journal of Personality and Social Psychology, 39,* 1037–1049.

Anderson, N. H. (1966). Component ratings in impression formation. *Psychonomic Science, 6,* 179–180.

Anderson, N. H. (1974). Information integration: A brief survey. In D. H. Krantz, R. C. Atkinson, R. D. Luce, & P. Suppes (Eds.), *Contemporary developments in mathematical psychology.* San Francisco: Freeman.

Anderson, N. H. (1981). *Foundations of information integration theory.* New York: Academic Press.

Asch, S. E. (1946). Forming impressions of personality. *Journal of Abnormal and Social Psychology, 41,* 1230–1240.

Asch, S. E. (1952). *Social psychology.* Englewood Cliffs, NJ: Prentice-Hall.

Asch, S. E., & Zukier, H. (1984). Thinking about persons. *Journal of Personality and Social Psychology, 46,* 1230–1240.

Augoustinos, M., & Innes, J. M. (1990). Towards an integration of social representations and social schema theory. *British Journal of Social Psychology, 29,* 213–321.

Bargh, J. A. (1989). Conditional automaticity: Varieties of automatic influence in social perception and cognition. In J. S. Uleman & J. A. Bargh (Eds.), *Unintended thought* (pp. 3–51). New York: Guilford.

Bargh, J. A. (1990). Auto-motives: Preconscious determinants of social interaction. In E. T. Higgins & R. M. Sorrentino (Eds.), *Handbook of motivation and cognition: Foundations of social behavior* (Vol. 2, pp. 93–130). New York: Guilford Press.

Bargh, J. A., & Pietromonaco, P. (1982). Automatic information processing and social perception: The influence of trait information presented outside of conscious awareness on impression formation. *Journal of Personality and Social Psychology, 43,* 437–449.

Bargh, J. A., & Raymond, P. (1992, October). An automatic power: Sex association in men likely to be sexual harassers. In J. Pryor (Chair), *Social psychological perspectives on sexual harassment.* Symposium conducted at the meeting of the Society of Experimental Social Psychology, San Antonio, Texas.

Bargh, J. A., Bond, R. N., Lombardi, W. L., & Tota, M. E. (1986). The additive nature of chronic and temporary sources of construct accessibility. *Journal of Personality and Social Psychology, 50,* 869–879.

Barsalou, L. W. (1985). Ideals, central tendency, and frequency of instantiation as determinants of graded structure in categories. *Journal of Experimental Psychology: Learning, Memory, and Cognition, 11,* 629–654.

Batson, C. D. (1975). Attribution as a mediator of bias in helping. *Journal of Personality and Social Psychology, 72,* 455–466.

Batson, C. D., & Marz, B. (1979). Dispositional bias in trained therapists' diagnoses: Does it exist? *Journal of Applied Social Psychology, 9,* 476–489.

Beauvois, J. L., & Dubois, N. (1988). The norm of internality in the explanation of psychological events. *European Journal of Social Psychology, 18,* 299–316.

Beck, L., McCauley, C., Segal, M., & Hershey, L. (1988). Individual differences in prototypicality judgments about trait categories. *Journal of Personality and Social Psychology, 55*, 286–292.

Belmore, S. M. (1987). Determinants of attention during impression formation. *Journal of Experimental Psychology: Learning, Memory, and Cognition, 13*, 480–489.

Borgida, E., & DeBono, K. G. (1989). Social hypothesis-testing and the role of expertise. *Personality and Social Psychology Bulletin, 15*, 212–221.

Borgida, E., & Nisbett, R. E. (1977). The differential impact of abstract vs. concrete information on decisions. *Journal of Applied Social Psychology, 7*, 258–271.

Borgida, E., & Rudman, L. (1992, October). Master status and the Swedish Bikini Team: Out of the courtroom and into the laboratory. In J. Pryor (Chair), *Social psychological perspectives on sexual harassment*. Symposium conducted at the meeting of the Society for Experimental Social Psychology, San Antonio, Texas.

Brewer, M. B. (1988a). A dual process model of impression formation. In T. K. Srull & R. S. Wyer, Jr. (Eds.), *Advances in social cognition* (Vol. 1, pp. 1–36). Hillsdale, NJ: Erlbaum.

Brewer, M. B. (1988b). Reply to commentaries. In T. K. Srull & R. S. Wyer, Jr. (Eds.), *Advances in social cognition* (Vol. 1, pp. 1–36). Hillsdale, NJ: Erlbaum.

Brown, R. (1986). *Social psychology: The second edition*. New York: The Free Press.

Bruner, J. S. (1957). On perceptual readiness. *Psychological Review, 64*, 123–152.

Bruner, J. S., & Tagiuri, R. (1954). The perception of people. In G. Lindzey (Ed.), *Handbook of social psychology* (Vol. 2). Reading, MA: Addison-Wesley.

Bruner, J. S., Goodnow, J. J., & Austin, G. A. (1956). *A study of thinking*. New York: Wiley.

Caetano, A., & Vala, J. (1993, September). *Effects of the social interaction context on social judgeability*. Paper presented at the Xth General Meeting of the European Association of Experimental Social Psychology, Lisbon.

Cantor, N., & Mischel, W. (1979). Prototypes in person perception. In L. Berkowitz (Ed.), *Advances in experimental social psychology* (Vol. 12). New York: Academic Press.

Carpenter, S. L. (1988). Self-relevance and goal-directed processing in the recall and weighting of information about others. *Journal of Experimental Social Psychology, 24*, 310–332.

Chapin, W. F., John, O. P., & Goldberg, L. R. (1988). Conceptions of states and traits: Dimensional attributes with ideals as prototypes. *Journal of Personality and Social Psychology, 54*, 541–557.

Chase, W. G., & Simon, H. A. (1973). The mind's eye in chess. In W. G. Chase (Ed.), *Visual information processing*. New York: Academic Press.

Cohen, C. E., & Ebbesen, E. B. (1979). Observational goals and schema activation: A theoretical framework for behavior perception. *Journal of Experimental Psychology, 15*, 305–329.

Darley, J. M., & Gross, P. H. (1983). A hypothesis-confirming bias in labeling effects. *Journal of Personality and Social Psychology, 44*, 20–33.

Dawson, V. L., Zeitz, C. M., & Wright, J. C. (1989). Expert-novice differences in person perception: Evidence of experts' sensitivities to the organization of behavior. *Social Cognition, 7*, 1–30.

de Montpellier, G. (1985). Le rôle de l'intention dans l'apprentissage et la mémoire. *Revue des Questions Scientifiques, 156*, 417–428.

Dépret, E. F., & Fiske, S. T. (1993). Social cognition and power: Some cognitive consequences of social structure as a source of control deprivation. In G. Weary, F. Gleicher, & K. Marsh (Eds.), *Control motivation and social cognition*. (pp. 176–202). New York: Springer-Verlag.

Devine, P. G. (1989). Stereotypes and prejudice: Their automatic and controlled components. *Journal of Personality and Social Psychology, 56*, 5–18.

Devine, P. G., Sedikides, C., & Fuhrman, R. W. (1989). Goals in social information processing: A case of anticipated interaction. *Journal of Personality and Social Psychology, 56*, 680–690.

Di Giacomo, J. P. (1980). Intergroup alliances and rejections within a protest movement. Analysis of the social representations. *European Journal of Social Psychology, 10*, 329–344.

Durkheim, E. (1898). Représentations individuelles et représentations collectives. *Revue de Métaphysique, 6*, 275–302.

Ebbesen, E. B. (1980). Cognitive processes in understanding ongoing behavior. In R. Hastie, T. M. Ostrom, E. B. Ebbesen, R. S. Wyer, D. L. Hamilton, & D. E. Carlston (Eds.), *Person memory: The cognitive basis of social perception*. Hillsdale, NJ: Erlbaum.

Erber, R., & Fiske, S. T. (1984). Outcome dependency and attention to inconsistent information. *Journal of Personality and Social Psychology, 47*, 709–726.

Farr, R. M., & Moscovici, S. (1984). *Social representations*. Cambridge: Cambridge University Press.

Festinger, L. (1964). *Conflict, decision, and dissonance*. Palo Alto, CA: Stanford University Press.

Fiedler, K. (1991). The tricky nature of skewed frequency tables: An information loss account of distinctiveness-based illusory correlations. *Journal of Personality and Social Psychology, 60*, 24–36.

Fiedler, K., Hemmeter, U., & Hofmann, C. (1984). On the origin of illusory correlations. *European Journal of Social Psychology, 14*, 191–202.

Fishbein, M., & Ajzen, I. (1974). Attitudes toward objects as predictors of single and multiple behavioral criteria. *Psychological Review, 81*, 59–74.

Fiske, S. T. (1980). Attention and weight in person perception: The impact of negative and extreme behavior. *Journal of Personality and Social Psychology, 38*. 889–906.

Fiske, S. T. (1987). On the road: comment on the cognitive stereotyping literature in Pettigrew and Martin. *Journal of Social Issues, 43*, 113–118.

Fiske, S. T. (1988). Compare and contrast: Brewer's dual process model and Fiske et al.'s continuum model. In T. K. Srull & R. S. Wyer, Jr. (Eds.), *Advances in social cognition* (Vol. 1, pp. 65–76). Hillsdale, NJ: Erlbaum.

Fiske, S. T. (1989). Examining the role of intent, toward understanding its role in stereotyping and prejudice. In J. S. Uleman & J. A. Bargh (Eds.), *Unintended thought: The limits of awareness, intention, and control* (pp. 253–283). New York: Guilford.

Fiske, S. T. (1992). Thinking is for doing: Portraits of social cognition from daguerreotype to laserphoto. *Journal of Personality and Social Psychology, 63*, 877–889.

Fiske, S. T. (1993). Social cognition and social perception. In M. R. Rosenzweig & L. W. Porter (Eds.), *Annual Review of Psychology* (Vol. 44, pp. 155–194). Palo Alto, CA: Annual Reviews.

Fiske, S. T., & Cox, M. G. (1979). Person concepts: The effects of target familiarity and descriptive purpose on the process of describing others. *Journal of Personality, 47*, 136–161.

Fiske, S. T., & Neuberg, S. L. (1990). A continuum of impression formation, from category-based to individuating processes: Influences of information and motivation on attention and interpretation. In M. P. Zanna (Ed.), *Advances in experimental social psychology* (Vol. 23, pp. 1–74). New York: Academic Press.

Fiske, S. T., & Pavelchak, M. A. (1986). Category-based versus piecemeal-based affective responses: Developments in schema-triggered affect. In R. M. Sorrentino & E. T. Higgins (Eds.), *Handbook of motivation and cognition: Foundations of social behavior* (pp. 167–203). New York: Guilford Press.

Fiske, S. T., & Ruscher, J. B. (1989). On-line processes in category-based and individuating impressions: Some basic principles and methodological reflections. In J. N. Bassili (Ed.), *On-line cognition in person perception* (pp. 141–174). Hillsdale, NJ: Erlbaum.

Fiske, S. T., & Taylor, S. E. (1984). *Social cognition*. New York: Random House.

Fiske, S. T., & Taylor, S. E. (1991). *Social cognition* (2nd ed.). New York: McGraw-Hill.

Fiske, S. T., & Von Hendy, H. M. (1992). Personality feedback and situational norms can control stereotyping processes. *Journal of Personality and Social Psychology, 62*, 577–596.

Fiske, S. T., Kinder, D. R., & Larter, W. M. (1983). The novice and the expert: Knowledge based strategies in political cognition. *Journal of Experimental Social Psychology, 19*, 381–400.

Fiske, S. T., Lau, R. R., & Smith, R. A. (1990). On the varieties and utilities of political expertise. *Social Cognition, 8*, 31–48.

Fiske, S. T., Neuberg, S. L. Pratto, F., & Allman, C. (1986). *Stereotyping and individuation: The effects of information inconsistency and set size on attribute-oriented processing*. Unpublished manuscript, University of Massachusetts at Amherst.

Fiske, S. T., Neuberg, S. L., Beattie, A. E., & Milberg, S. J. (1987). Category-based and attribute-based reactions to others: Some informational conditions of stereotyping and individuating processes. *Journal of Experimental Social Psychology, 23,* 399–427.

Freund, T., Kruglanski, A. W., & Shpitizajzen, A. (1985). The freezing and unfreezing of impression primacy: Effects of the need for structure and the fear of invalidity. *Personality and Social Psychology Bulletin, 11,* 479–487.

Gilbert, D. T., & Hixon, J. G. (1991). The trouble of thinking: Activation and application of stereotypic beliefs. *Journal of Personality and Social Psychology, 60,* 509–517.

Gollwitzer, P. M. (1990). Action phases and mind-sets. In E. T. Higgins & R. M. Sorrentino (Eds.), *Handbook of motivation and cognition: Foundations of social behavior* (Vol. 2, pp. 53–92). New York: Guilford.

Hamill, R., Lodge, M., & Blake, F. (1985). The breadth, depth, and utility of class, partisan, and ideological schemata. *American Journal of Political Science, 29,* 850–870.

Hamill, R., Wilson, T. D., & Nisbett, R. E. (1980). Insensitivity to sample bias: Generalizing from atypical cases. *Journal of Personality and Social Psychology, 39,* 578–589.

Hamilton, D. L. (1989). Understanding impression formation: What has memory research contributed? In P. R. Solomon, G. R. Goethals, C. M. Kelley, & B. R. Stephens (Eds.), *Memory: Interdisciplinary approaches* (pp. 221–242). New York: Springer-Verlag.

Hamilton, D. L., & Gifford, R. K. (1976). Illusory correlation in interpersonal perception: A cognitive basis of stereotypic judgments. *Journal of Experimental Social Psychology, 12,* 392–407.

Hamilton, D. L., & Zanna, M. P. (1974). Context effects in impression formation: Changes in connotative meaning. *Journal of Personality and Social Psychology, 29,* 649–654.

Hamilton, D. L., Katz, L. B., & Leirer, V. O. (1980). Cognitive representation of personality impressions: Organizational processes in first impression formation. *Journal of Personality and Social Psychology, 39,* 1050–1063.

Hamilton, D. L., Dugan, P. M., & Trolier, T. K. (1985). The formation of stereotypic beliefs: Further evidence for distinctiveness-based illusory correlations. *Journal of Personality and Social Psychology, 48,* 5–17.

Hamilton, D. L., Driscoll, D. M., & Worth, L. T. (1989). Cognitive organization of impressions: Effects of incongruency in complex representations. *Journal of Personality and Social Psychology, 57,* 925–939.

Hastie, R. (1980). Memory for behavioral information that confirms or contradicts a personality impression. In R. Hastie, T. M. Ostrom, E. B. Ebbesen, R. S. Wyer, D. L. Hamilton, & D. E. Carlston (Eds.), *Person memory: The cognitive basis of social perception*. Hillsdale, NJ: Erlbaum.

Hastie, R. (1981). Schematic principles in human memory. In E. T. Higgins, C. P. Herman, & M. P. Zanna (Eds.), *Social cognition: The Ontario Symposium* (Vol. 1, pp. 39–88). Hillsdale, NJ: Erlbaum.

Hastie, R. (1984). Causes and effects of causal attribution. *Journal of Personality and Social Psychology, 46,* 44–56.

Hastie, R., & Carlston, D. (1980). Theoretical issues in person memory. In R. Hastie, T. M. Ostrom, E. B. Ebbesen, R. S. Wyer, D. L. Hamilton, & D. E. Carlston (Eds.), *Person memory: The cognitive basis of social perception* (pp. 1–53). Hillsdale, NJ: Erlbaum.

Hastie, R., & Kumar, P. A. (1979). Person memory: Personality traits as organizing principles in memory for behavior. *Journal of Personality and Social Psychology, 37,* 25–38.

Higgins, E. T., & Bargh, J. A. (1987). Social cognition and social perception. In M. R. Rosenzweig & L. W. Porter (Eds.), *Annual review of psychology* (Vol. 38). Palo Alto, CA: Annual Review.

Higgins, E. T., Rholes, W. S., & Jones, C. R. (1977). Category accessibility and impression formation. *Journal of Experimental Social Psychology, 13,* 141–154.

Higgins, E. T., King, G. A., & Mavin, G. H. (1982). Individual construct accessibility and subjective impressions and recall. *Journal of Personality and Social Psychology, 43,* 35–47.
Hilton, J. L., & Darley, J. M. (1991). The effects of interaction goals on person perception. *Advances in Experimental Social Psychology, 24,* 235–267.
Hoffman, C., Mischel, W., & Mazze, K. (1981). The role of purpose in the organization of information about behavior: Trait-based versus goal-based categories in person cognition. *Journal of Personality and Social Psychology, 40,* 211–225.
Jodelet, D. (1989). *Les representations sociales.* Paris: PUF.
Jones, E. E., & Gerard, H. B. (1967). *Foundations of social psychology.* New York: Wiley.
Jones, E. E., & Goethals, G. R. (1972). Order effects in impression formation: Attribution context and the nature of the entity. In E. E. Jones, D. E. Kanouse, H. H. Kelley, R. E. Nisbett, S. Valins, & B. Weiner (Eds.), *Attribution: Perceiving the causes of behavior* (pp. 27–46). Morristown, NJ: General Learning Press
Judd, C. M., & Lusk, C. M. (1984). Knowledge structures and evaluative judgments: Effects of structural variables on judgmental extremity. *Journal of Personality and Social Psychology, 46,* 1193–1207.
Judd, C. M., & Park, B. (1988). Out-group homogeneity: Judgments of variability at the individual and group levels. *Journal of Personality and Social Psychology, 54,* 778–788.
Kanouse, D. E., & Hanson, L. R., Jr. (1972). Negativity in evaluations. In E. E. Jones, D. E. Kanouse, H. H. Kelley, R. E. Nisbett, S. Valins, & B. Weiner (Eds.), *Attribution: Perceiving the causes of behavior* (pp. 47–62). Morristown, NJ: General Learning Press.
Katz, D., & Braly, K. W. (1933). Racial stereotypes of 100 college students. *Journal of Abnormal and Social Psychology, 28,* 280–290.
Kelley, H. H. (1950). The warm-cold variable in first impressions of persons. *Journal of Personality, 18,* 431–439.
Kruglanski, A. W. (1980). Lay epistemo-logic—Process and contents: Another look at attribution theory. *Psychological Review, 87,* 70–87.
Kruglanski, A. W. (1989). The psychology of being "right": On the problem of accuracy in social perception and cognition. *Psychological Bulletin, 106,* 395–409.
Kruglanski, A. W., & Ajzen, I. (1983). Bias and error in human judgment. *European Journal of Social Psychology, 13,* 1–44.
Kruglanski, A. W., & Freund, T. (1983). The freezing and unfreezing of lay-inferences: Effects of impressional primacy, ethnic stereotyping, and numerical anchoring. *Journal of Experimental Social Psychology, 19,* 448–468.
Kruglanski, A. W., & Klar, Y. (1987). A view from a bridge: Synthesizing the consistency and attribution paradigms from a lay epistemic perspective. *European Journal of Social Psychology, 17,* 211–241.
Kruglanski, A. W., & Mayseless, O. (1988). Contextual effects in hypothesis testing: The role of competing alternatives and epistemic motivations. *Social Cognition, 6,* 1–20.
Langer, E. J., & Abelson, R. P. (1974). A patient by any other name. . . . Clinician group difference in labeling bias. *Journal of consulting and Clinical Psychology, 42,* 4–9.
Leyens, J.-Ph. (1983). *Sommes-nous tous des psychologues? Approche psychosociale des théories implicites de la personnalité.* Bruxelles: Mardaga.
Leyens, J.-Ph. (1990). Intuitive personality testing: A social approach. The Jos Jaspars Lecture. In J. Extra, A. van Knippenberg, J. van der Pligt, & M. Poppe (Eds.), *Fundementele Sociale Psychologie* (Vol 4). Tilburg: Tilburg University Press.
Leyens, J.-Ph. (1991). Prolegomena for the concept of implicit theories of personality. *European Bulletin of Cognitive Psychology, 11* 131–136.
Leyens, J.-Ph., & Yzerbyt, V. Y. (1992). The ingroup overexclusion effect: Impact of valence and confirmation on stereotypical information search. *European Journal of Social Psychology, 22,* 549–569.
Leyens, J.-Ph., Yzerbyt, V. Y., & Schadron, G. (1992). The social judgeability approach to stereotypes. In W. Stroebe & M. Hewstone (Eds.), *European review of social psychology,* (Vol. 3, pp. 91–120).

Lichtenstein, M., & Srull, T. K. (1987). Processing objectives as a determinant of the relationship between recall and judgment. *Journal of Experimental Social Psychology, 23,* 93–118.

Linville, P. W. (1982). The complexity-extremity effect and age-based stereotyping. *Journal of Personality and Social Psychology, 42,* 193–211.

Linville, P. W., Fischer, G. W., & Salovey, P. (1989). Perceived distributions of the characteristics of ingroup and outgroup members: Empirical evidence and a computer simulation. *Journal of Personality and Social Psychology, 57,* 165–188.

Locksley, A., Borgida, E., Brekke, N., & Hepburn, C. (1980). Sex stereotypes and social judgment. *Journal of Personality and Social Psychology, 39,* 821–831.

Locksley, A., Hepburn, C., & Ortiz, V. (1982). Social stereotypes and judgments of individuals: An instance of the base rate fallacy. *Journal of Experimental Social Psychology, 18,* 23–42.

Lodge, M., & Hamill, R. (1986). A partisan schema for political information processing. *American Political Science Review, 80,* 505–519.

Lusk, C. M., & Judd, C. M. (1988). Political expertise and the structural mediators of candidate evaluations. *Journal of Experimental Social Psychology, 24,* 105–126.

McGuire, W. J. (1986). The vicissitudes of attitudes and similar representational constructs in twentieth century psychology. *European Journal of Social Psychology, 16,* 89–130.

McKenzie-Mohr, D., & Zanna, M. P. (1990). Treating women as sexual objects: Look to the (gender schematic) male who have viewed pornography. *Personality and Social Psychology Bulletin, 16,* 296–308.

Markus, H. (1977). Self-schemata and processing information about the self. *Journal of Personality and Social Psychology, 35,* 63–78.

Markus, H., & Wurf, E. (1987). The dynamic self-concept: A social psychological perspective. In M. R. Rosenzweig & L. W. Porter (Eds.), *Annual review of psychology* (Vol. 38, pp. 299–337). Palo Alto, CA: Annual Reviews.

Markus, H., & Zajonc, R. B. (1985). The cognitive perspective in social psychology. In G. Lindzey & E. Aronson (Eds.), *The handbook of social psychology,* Vol. 1 (3rd ed.) (pp. 137–230). New York: Random House.

Markus, H., Smith, J., & Moreland, R. L. (1985). Role of the self-concept in the social perception of others. *Journal of Personality and Social Psychology, 49,* 1494–1512.

Marques, J. M., & Yzerbyt, V. Y. (1988). The black sheep effect: Judgmental extremity towards ingroup members in later- and intra-group situations. *European Journal of Social Psychology, 18,* 287–292.

Marques, J. M., Yzerbyt, V. Y., & Leyens, J.-Ph. (1988). The black sheep effect: Extremity of judgments towards ingroup members as a function of group identification. *European Journal of Social Psychology, 18,* 1–16.

Mayer, J. D., & Bower, G. H. (1986). Learning and memory for personality prototypes. *Journal of Personality and Social Psychology, 51,* 473–492.

Moscovici, S. (1961). *La Psychanalyse: Son image et son public.* (2nd ed. 1976.) Paris: Presses Universitaires de France.

Mullen, B., & Cooper, C. (1989). The privileged position of person categories: A comment on Sedikides and Ostrom. *Social Cognition, 7,* 373–388.

Mullen, B., & Hu, L. (1989). Perceptions of ingroup and outgroup variability: A meta-analytic integration. *Basic and Applied Social Psychology, 10,* 233–252.

Mullen, B., & Johnson, C. (1990). Distinctiveness-based illusory correlations and stereotyping: A meta-analytic integration. *British Journal of Social Psychology, 29,* 11–28.

Murphy, G. L., & Medin, D. L. (1985). The role of theories in conceptual coherence. *Psychological Review, 92,* 289–316.

Murphy, G. L., & Wright, J. C. (1984). Changes in conceptual structure with expertise: Differences between real-world experts and novices. *Journal of Experimental Psychology: Learning, Memory and Cognition, 10,* 144–155.

Neuberg, S. L. (1989). The goal of forming accurate impressions during social interactions: Attenuating the impact of negative expectancies. *Journal of Personality and Social Psychology, 6,* 374–386.

Neuberg, S. L., & Fiske, S. T. (1987). Motivational influences on impression formation: Outcome dependency, accuracy-driven attention, and individuating processes. *Journal of Personality and Social Psychology, 53,* 431–444.

Nisbett, R. E., & Borgida, E. (1975). Attribution and the psychology of prediction. *Journal of Personality and Social Psychology, 32,* 932–943.

Nisbett, R. E., & Ross, L. (1980). *Human inference: Strategies and shortcomings of social judgment.* Englewood Cliffs, NJ: Prentice-Hall.

Ostrom, T. M. (1977). Between-theory and within-theory conflict in explaining context effects in impression formation. *Journal of Experimental Social Psychology, 13,* 492–503.

Ostrom, T. M. (1984). The sovereignty of social cognition. In R. S. Wyer, Jr. & T. K. Srull (Eds.), *Handbook of social cognition* (Vol. 1, pp. 1–38). Hillsdale, NJ: Erlbaum.

Park, B. (1986). A method for studying the development of impressions of real people. *Journal of Personality and Social Psychology, 51,* 907–917.

Park, B., & Hastie, R. (1987). Perception of variability in category development: Instance- versus abstraction-based stereotypes. *Journal of Personality and Social Psychology, 53,* 621–635.

Park, B., & Judd, C. M. (1990). Measures and models of perceived group variability. *Journal of Personality and Social Psychology, 59,* 173–191.

Peeters, G., & Czapinski, J. (1990). Positive–negative asymmetry in evaluations: The distinction between affective and informational negativity effects. *European Review of Social Psychology, 1,* 33–60.

Reeder, G. D. (1985). Implicit relations between dispositions and behaviors: Effects on dispositional attribution. In J. H. Harvey & G. Weary (Eds.), *Attribution: Basic issues and applications* (pp. 87–116). Orlando, FL: Academic Press.

Rojahn, K., & Pettigrew, T. F. (1992). Memory for schema-relevant information: A meta-analytic resolution. *British Journal of Social Psychology, 31,* 81–109.

Rosenberg, S., & Sedlak, A. (1972). Structural representations of implicit personality theory. In L. Berkowitz (Ed.), *Advances in Experimental Social Psychology* (Vol. 6, pp. 235–297). New York: Academic Press.

Rosenberg, S., Nelson, C., & Vivekanathan, P. S. (1968). A multidimensional approach to the structure of personality impressions. *Journal of Personality and Social Psychology, 9,* 283–294.

Ross, L. (1977). The intuitive psychologist and his shortcomings: Distortions in the attribution process. In L. Berkowitz (Ed.), *Advances in experimental social psychology* (Vol. 10). New York: Academic Press.

Ross, L., & Nisbett, R. E. (1991). *The person and the situation: Perspectives of social psychology.* New York: McGraw-Hill.

Ross, L., Lepper, M. R., & Hubbard, M. (1975). Perseverance in self-perception and social perception: Biased attribution processes in the debriefing paradigm. *Journal of Personality and Social Psychology, 32,* 880–892.

Rothbart, M., & Lewis, S. (1988). Inferring category attributes from exemplar attributes: Geometric shapes and social categories. *Journal of Personality and Social Psychology, 55,* 861–872.

Rothbart, M., & Park, B. (1986). On the confirmability and disconfirmability of trait concepts. *Journal of Personality and Social Psychology, 50,* 131–142.

Rothbart, M., Evans, M., & Fulero, S. (1979). Recall for confirming events: Memory processes and the maintenance of social stereotyping. *Journal of Experimental Social Psychology, 15,* 343–355.

Ruble, D. N. (1994). Motivational consequences of social-cognitive transitions. In M. P. Zanna (Ed.), *Advances in experimental social psychology* (Vol. 26, pp. 163–214). San Diego, CA: Academic Press.

Ruble, D. N., & Stangor, C. (1986). Stalking the elusive schema: Insights from developmental and social-psychological analyses of gender schemas. *Social Cognition, 4,* 227–261.

Ruscher, J. B., & Fiske, S. T. (1990). Interpersonal competition can cause individuating processes. *Journal of Personality and Social Psychology, 58,* 832–843.
Ruscher, J. B., Fiske, S. T., Miki, H., & Van Manen, S. (1991). Individuating processes in competition: Interpersonal versus intergroup. *Personality and Social Psychology Bulletin, 17,* 595–605.
Sanbonmatsu, D. M., Sherman, S. J., & Hamilton, D. L. (1987). Illusory correlation in the perception of individuals and groups. *Social Cognition, 5,* 1–25.
Schadron, G., & Yzerbyt, V. Y. (1991). Social judgeability: Another perspective in the study of social inference. *European Bulletin of Cognitive Psychology, 11,* 229–258.
Schneider, D. J. (1973). Implicit personality theory: A review. *Psychological Bulletin, 79,* 294–309.
Sedikides, C., & Ostrom, T. M. (1988). Are person categories used when organizing information about unfamiliar sets of persons? *Social Cognition, 6,* 252–267.
Sedikides, C., & Ostrom, T. M. (1990). Persons as privileged categories: A rejoinder to Mullen and Cooper. *Social Cognition, 8,* 229–240.
Sherman, S. J., Judd, C. M., & Park, B. (1989). Social cognition. *Annual Review of Psychology, 40,* 281–326.
Skowronski, J. J., & Carlston, D. E. (1989). Negativity and extremity biases in impression formation: A review of explanations. *Psychological Bulletin, 105,* 131–142.
Skowronski, J. J., Betz, A. L., Thompson, C. P., & Shannon, L. (1991). Social memory in everyday life: Recall of self-events and other-events. *Journal of Personality and Social Psychology, 60,* 831–843.
Smith, E. R. (1991). Illusory correlation in a simulated exemplar-based memory. *Journal of Experimental Social Psychology, 27,* 107–123.
Smith, E. R., & Zárate, M. A. (1992). Exemplar-based model of social judgement. *Psychological Review, 99,* 3–21.
Snyder, M. (1992). Motivational foundations of behavioral confirmation. *Advances in Experimental Social Psychology, 25,* 67–114.
Snyder, M., & Gangestad, S. (1981). Hypothesis-testing processes. In J. H. Harvey, W. Ickes, & R. F. Kidd (Eds.), *New directions in attribution research* (Vol. 3). Hillsdale, NJ: Erlbaum.
Snyder, M., & Swann, W. B. (1978). Hypothesis-testing processes in social interaction. *Journal of Personality and Social Psychology, 36,* 1202–1212.
Snyder, M., & Swann, W. B., Jr. (1978). Hypothesis-testing processes in social interaction. *Journal of Personality and Social Psychology, 36,* 1202–1212.
Srull, T. K. (1981). Person memory: Some tests of associative storage and retrieval models. *Journal of Experimental Psychology: Human Learning and Memory, 7,* 440–462.
Srull, T. K., & Wyer, R. S., Jr. (1989). Person memory and judgment. *Psychological Review, 96,* 58–83.
Srull, T. K., Lichtenstein, M. & Rothbart, M. (1985). Associative storage and retrieval processes in person memory. *Journal of Experimental Psychology: Learning, Memory, and Cognition, 11,* 316–345.
Stangor, C., & Ford, T. E. (1992). Accuracy and expectancy-confirming processing orientations and the development of stereotypes and prejudice. In W. Stroebe & M. Hewstone (Eds.), *European Review of Social Psychology* (Vol. 3, pp. 57–89).
Stangor, C., & McMillan, D. (1992). Memory for expectancy-congruent and expectancy-incongruent information: A review of the social and social developmental literatures. *Psychological Bulletin, 111,* 42–61.
Stangor, C., & Ruble, D. N. (1989). Strength of expectancies and memory for social information: What we remember depends on how much we know. *Journal of Experimental Social Psychology, 25,* 18–35.
Tajfel, H. (Ed.). (1978). *Differentiation between social groups.* London: Academic Press.
Tajfel, H. (1981). *Human groups and social categories: Studies in social psychology.* Cambridge, MA: Cambridge University Press.

Tajfel, H., & Wilkes, A. L. (1963). Classification and quantitative judgment. *British Journal of Psychology, 54,* 101–114.

Taylor, S. E. (1981). A categorization approach to stereotyping. In D. L. Hamilton (Ed.), *Cognitive processes in stereotyping and intergroup behavior* (pp. 88–114). Hillsdale, NJ: Erlbaum.

Taylor, S. E. (1991). Asymmetrical effects of positive and negative events: The mobilization–minimization hypothesis. *Psychological Bulletin, 110,* 67–85.

Taylor, S. E., & Fiske, S. T. (1978). Salience, attention and attribution: Top of the head phenomena. *Advances in Experimental and Social Psychology, 11,* 249–288.

Taylor, S. E., & Fiske, S. T. (1981). Getting inside the head: Methodologies for process analysis in attribution and social cognition. In J. H. Harvey, W. Ickes, & R. F. Kidd (Eds.), *New directions in attribution research.* Hillsdale, NJ: Erlbaum.

Taylor, S. E., & Thompson, S. C. (1982). Stalking the elusive "vividness" effect. *Psychological Review, 89,* 155–181.

Tesser, A. (1978). Self-generated attitude change. In L. Berkowitz (Ed.), *Advances in experimental social psychology* (Vol. 11). New York: Academic Press.

Tetlock, P. E., & Boettger, R. (1989). Accountability: A social magnifier of the dilution effect. *Journal of Personality and Social Psychology, 57,* 388–398.

Trzebinski, J. (1985). Action-oriented representations of implicit personality theories. *Journal of Personality and Social Psychology, 48,* 1266–1278.

Uleman, J. S. (1989). A framework for thinking intentionally about unintended thoughts. In J. S. Uleman & J. A. Bargh (Eds.), *The direction of thought: Limits of awareness, intention, and control* (pp. 425–449). New York: Guilford.

Van der Kloot, W. A., & Willemsen, T. M. (1991). The measurement, representation and predictive use of implicit personality theory. *European Bulletin of Cognitive Psychology, 11,* 137–154.

Van Mechelen, I. (1991). Symptom and diagnosis inference based on implicit theories of psychopathology: A review. *European Bulletin of Cognitive Psychology, 11,* 155–171.

Webster's new world dictionary of the American language (2nd College Ed.). New York: W. M. Collins & World Publishing Co.

Wishner, J. (1960). Reanalysis of "impressions of personality." *Psychological Review, 67,* 96–112.

Wright, J. C., & Murphy, G. L. (1984). The utility of theories and intuitive statistics: The robustness of theory-based judgments. *Journal of Experimental Psychology: General, 113,* 301–332.

Wyer, R. S., Jr., & Gordon, S. E. (1982). The recall of information about persons and groups. *Journal of Experimental Social Psychology, 18,* 128–164.

Wyer, R. S., Jr., & Srull, T. K. (Eds.). (1984). *Handbook of social cognition* (Vols. 1–3). Hillsdale, NJ: Erlbaum.

Wyer, R. S., Jr., Bodenhausen, G. V., & Srull, T. K. (1984). The cognitive representation of persons and groups and its effect on recall and recognition memory. *Journal of Experimental Social Psychology, 20,* 445–469.

Yzerbyt, V. Y., & Leyens, J.-Ph. (1991). Requesting information to form an impression: The influence of valence and confirmatory status. *Journal of Experimental Social Psychology, 27,* 337–356.

Yzerbyt, V., Schadron, G., Leyens, J.-Ph., Rocher, S. (1994). Social judgeability: The impact of meta-informational cues on the use of stereotypes. *Journal of Personality and Social Psychology, 66,* 48–55.

Zanna, M. P., & Hamilton, D. L. (1972). Attribute dimensions and patterns of trait inferences. *Psychonomic Science, 27,* 353–354.

Zanna, M. P., & Hamilton, D. L. (1977). Further evidence for meaning change in impression formation. *Journal of Experimental Social Psychology, 13,* 224–238.

Zárate, M. A., & Smith, E. R. (1990). Person categorization and stereotyping. *Social Cognition, 8,* 161–185.

Zukier, H. (1982). The role of the correlation and the dispersion of predictor variables in the use of nondiagnostic information. *Journal of Personality and Social Psychology, 43*, 1163–1175.

Zukier, H. (1986). The paradigmatic and narrative modes in goal guided inference. In R. M. Sorrentino & E. T. Higgins (Eds.), *Handbook of motivation and cognition* (pp. 465–502). New York: The Guilford Press.

Zukier, H., & Pepitone, A. (1984). Social roles and strategies in prediction: Some determinants of the use of base information. *Journal of Personality and Social Psychology, 47*, 349–360.

Zuroff, D. C. (1989). Judgments of frequency of social stimuli: How schematic is person memory? *Journal of Personality and Social Psychology, 56*, 890–898.

4

Social Cognition Contributions to Attribution Theory and Research

Eliot R. Smith

Attribution is often cited as *the* major research topic within social psychology in the 1970s, just as dissonance held that role in the 1960s. Though this statement suggests that attribution long since began to wane in popularity as a research issue, perhaps with the rise of social cognition circa 1980, in fact, there is still no evidence that the number of attribution articles published annually has peaked (as I shall discuss below). It seems that an attributional analysis has been developed for virtually every social-psychological phenomenon, ranging from achievement motivation (Weiner, 1974) through various social problems (Frieze, Bar-Tal, & Carroll, 1979) to depression (Abramson, Seligman, & Teasdale, 1978), to dissonance itself (Bem, 1967). Has social cognition had a notable impact on this huge body of literature, which is still accumulating at a rate of over 300 articles per year?

Before beginning to answer this question I will draw a distinction, pointing out an ambiguity that has been present since the beginnings of research interest in attribution. In effect, the term *attribution* itself has two meanings. Its primary usage in the social-psychological literature refers to *inferences about the causes of a target person's behavior, with a special focus on the possibility of learning about that person's traits or other dispositions*. This is clearly the focus in the seminal theoretical works by Jones and Davis (1965) and Kelley (1967). Similarly, the famous "orange book" (Jones et al., 1972), which contained a number of classic chapters, was entitled *Attribution: Perceiving the Causes of Behavior*. Research on the trait attributions or correspondent inferences that can be made from observed behaviors, and on the determinants of internal versus external (dispositional vs. situational) attributions, exemplifies this perspective on the issue.

Attribution also refers to another, broader question. This perspective is more characteristic of Heider's writings in his classic 1958 *Psychology of Interpersonal Relations* than of the upsurge of attribution theory in the late 1960s and 1970s. In this perspective the goal of the attributor is to *infer the stable properties of the world in general from observable cues.* Heider's definition of "dispositional properties" is not limited to personality traits, nor to properties of people. He draws a strong analogy between the perception of social and nonsocial dispositional properties (pp. 80–82). In his example, the appearance of some sand on his desk has no meaning in itself, but may motivate a search for the underlying cause—perhaps a dangerous crack in the room's ceiling. Similarly, a person's behavior has little meaning except as an indicator of that person's more stable underlying motives, traits, and other qualities. Summarizing this viewpoint, Heider writes,

> We note first, that man is usually not content simply to register the observables that surround him; he needs to refer them as far as possible to the invariances of his environment. Second, the underlying causes of events, especially the motives of other persons, are the invariances of the environment that are relevant to him; they give meaning to what he experiences and it is these meanings that are recorded in his life space, and are precipitated as the reality of the environment to which he then reacts. (p. 81)

Put in more modern terms, Heider's "life space" might be called the perceiver's "mental model" (cf. Johnson-Laird, 1983) of the world, and attribution —in this second, broader perspective—is the process of interpreting perceptual input for the purpose of constructing such a model.

Of course, the behavior of most people most of the time is oriented toward the social, rather than the nonsocial (physical) environment. Hence, inferring traits and other personal qualities on the basis of a target person's behavior is an important subset of this broader definition of "attribution." Under either definition, it is clear that the dispositions that are constructed or inferred by the perceiver, rather than the observable evidence on which they were based, should be primary determinants of the perceiver's reactions and behaviors. This insight has been followed up extensively in research relating perceived causes as independent variables to such consequences as interpersonal attraction, motivation, affective reactions, learned helplessness, and the like (Kelley & Michela, 1980). In this chapter, I take the inference of causes as the main topic, and so will have little to say about the consequences of attributions.

TRENDS IN ATTRIBUTION RESEARCH

To begin to analyze the impact of social cognition on attribution theory and research, it is worthwhile to look at some trends in the attribution field over time. After all, this research area has a respectably long history, during

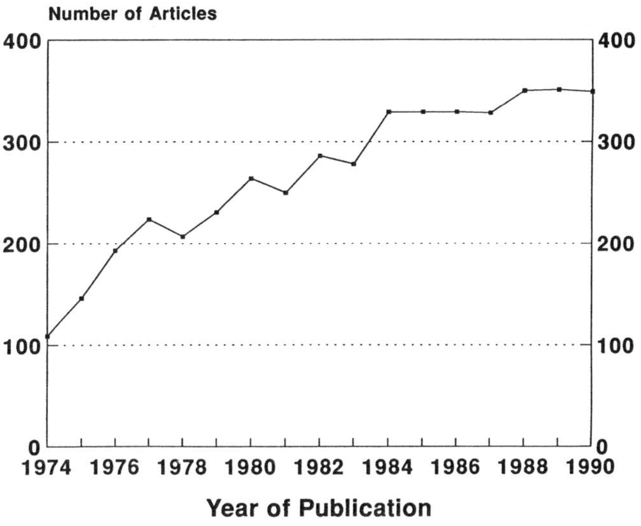

FIGURE 1.
Number of articles published on attribution research from 1974 to 1990.

which changes in research emphasis may be visible. Figure 1 gives a picture of the overall literature over time, showing the number of journal articles published in each year since 1974 indexed with "attribution" as a descriptor in the PsycINFO database (American Psychological Association, 1988). The number of attribution articles climbed steadily and steeply through the 1970s, tripling between 1974 and 1984. No falloff of publication activity is yet evident even in 1990.

Several interrelated trends appear to characterize the development of this field from the earlier years to more recent times. I shall argue that each of these trends reflects the influence of social cognition on attribution research.

From a Narrower to a Broader Definition of Attribution

First, the field has shifted over time from the narrower to the broader definition described in the introduction to this chapter. The early attribution theories focused on the attribution of traits to actors in the context of person perception. Researchers analyzed internal versus external (or dispositional vs. situational, or person vs. stimulus or circumstances) attributions, with the ultimate goal of understanding when people would attribute traits to actors based on observed behaviors.

In contrast, recent approaches to attribution emphasize the continuity between the attribution of traits to actors and the perception and comprehension of the perceiver's environment in general. For example, attribution papers such as Smith and Miller (1979b), Read (1987), and Leddo and Abelson (1986) explicitly cite the cognitive literature on text comprehension. As Hewstone (1989) notes, "it makes . . . sense to think of explanation as part of the general process of understanding. From this perspective, explanation should be based on, not divorced from, world-knowledge, the kind of knowledge . . . necessary . . . to understand stories or even to explain events" (pp. 109–110). Jones's historical discussion (1985) makes a similar point: attribution research "has become practically synonymous with research based on the premise that people act with reference to their conception of causal forces in the environment. Such a premise covers a very large terrain" (p. 92). Thus, from the earlier focus on actors' behaviors and traits, we have seen something of a return to the Heiderian conception of attribution as the perceiver's construction of a "life space" or mental model of the enduring causal structure of the social and nonsocial environment. This shift is consistent with the general emphasis within social cognition on the continuities between social cognition and nonsocial cognition (e.g., Ostrom, 1984; Jones, 1985, pp. 82–83).

From Content-Free to Content-Specific Inference Rules

Jones's and Kelley's early attribution theories postulated that people infer causes using rules that are general and content free, rather than being limited to specific types of behaviors or traits. For example, Kelley's (1967) covariation principle specifies "an information processing rule but is open ended with respect to the types of causes and effects involved" (Kelley & Michela, 1980, p. 462), though most applications assumed persons, stimuli, and circumstances were the dimensions of interest. Later elaborations of Kelley's covariation-based approach including Kelley (1972) and Orvis, Cunningham, and Kelley (1975) maintained the assumption that attributional inference rules did not incorporate the content of specific behaviors. Likewise, Jones and Davis's model (1965; Jones & McGillis, 1976) held that analyses of desirability and noncommon effects would suffice to indicate when a correspondent inference should be made, regardless of the type of behavior in question.

More recently, however, attribution researchers have begun to emphasize that content-specific knowledge structures are often used to make attributional inferences. Reeder and Brewer (1979) in an influential paper argued that different types of behaviors (e.g., in achievement vs. moral domains) were processed with systematically different attributional principles. Smith and Miller (1979a) suggested that scripts (stored knowledge about expected sequences of events and their causal interrelationships) could furnish a list of candidate causes for the attributor to consider. Read (1987) and Abelson and Lalljee (1988) elaborated a "knowledge structure" approach to attribution, which draws explicit links with the literature on the use of specific knowledge in text comprehension (e.g., Schank & Abelson, 1977; Trabasso & Van den Broek, 1985). Hilton and Knibbs (1988) directly contrasted covariation-based and knowledge-based strategies for making attributions. All of these papers assume that when given an event, instead of seeking covariation information or even retrieving "assumed" covariation information from memory, subjects analyze the meaning of the event and ascribe traits or goals to the actors based on their specific world knowledge regarding scripts, plans, and goals.

This shift in the attribution field parallels similar changes in emphasis in cognitive psychology, cognitive science, and social cognition (Allport, 1980; Jacoby & Kelley, 1987; Smith, 1990). Early cognitive researchers like Newell and Simon (1972) assumed that a few, content-general inference rules would suffice to produce generally "intelligent" or adaptive behavior. More recently the trend is toward the representation and application of extensive domain-specific knowledge as a basis for problem solving and adaptive behavior (e.g., in "expert systems"). Social cognition has fully participated in this trend, as researchers generally assume that people possess a vast library of specific knowledge organized in scripts, schemas, prototypes, exemplars, inference rules, and the like, on which they draw to make judgments and enact behaviors.

From Normative Models to "Errors and Biases" to a New Synthesis

An oft-noted shift in emphasis over time in the attribution field is from a picture of the attributor as rational to one that emphasizes error and bias in attributional inferences. The early attribution theories (Kelley, 1967; Jones & Davis, 1965) were developed on the basis of logical analysis of when person attributions (or correspondent inferences) would be reasonably justified. In a sense they constitute normative models of how attributors *should* proceed as well as proposals about how they actually *do* perform. Of course, the early empirical studies designed to test these models produced evidence that the predicted effects did account for significant amounts of variance in attribution responses (e.g., McArthur, 1972).

However, systematic departures from the predictions of the normative models were quickly noted. These were summarized in terms of a host of errors and biases ranging from the fundamental attribution error (Ross, 1977) to the underuse of consensus information (Nisbett & Borgida, 1975) to various self-serving biases (Miller & Ross, 1975). An overall portrayal of attribution processes as understood in the mid- to late 1970s might have involved two types of process: normatively appropriate reasoning processes (such as the analysis of covariation) plus a handful of motivational biases. Under conditions that did not trigger the biases, people would apply normative processes and derive correct answers to attributional questions. Under other conditions, biases would influence their responses, leading, for instance, to overly internal attributions for personal successes and external attributions for failures. Thus, fundamentally different sorts of processes were thought to be responsible for normatively correct judgments and for biased judgments—a conception reflected in the repeated debates, which became intense at times, over the "cognitive" versus "motivational" nature of various phenomena.

Attribution researchers today—reflecting the trend in social cognition—are likely to reject this dual-process view. Instead, current accounts depict attributions (as well as other judgments) as affected by limited processing capacity and the use of shortcut heuristic strategies, effects of salience and accessibility on what information is used, and the application of schematic "default assumptions." The *same* processes are assumed to lead sometimes to correct and pragmatically useful results, and at other times to invalid and biased results—depending on the amount of information available, the cognitive resources available to the perceiver, his or her motivation to think hard about the judgment, and other factors (Smith, in press). Researchers today understand that cognitive activity always serves specific processing goals—which can involve motives to self-enhance or to self-present as well as to comprehend the world accurately (Chaiken, Liberman, & Eagly, 1989). Thus, cognition and motivation are inseparable, both necessarily being involved in the generation of any overt judgment or behavior. The old debates between cognition and motivation appear superfluous once the old, misleading identification of "cognitive" processes with normative outcomes and "motivational" processes with biased outcomes is discarded.

From Rules or Algorithms to Process

Psychologists and cognitive scientists have often distinguished different levels of analysis of cognitive processes. The key distinction is between the *algorithm,* the program or set of rules that guide the processing of information and the generation of output, and the *implementation,* the properties of the underlying "hardware" that actually carry out the computation. This distinction has been drawn in cognitive science by Pylyshyn (1984) as "representational" versus "functional architecture" levels, in psychology by Anderson (1983) and Wyer and Srull (1986) as the specific contents of declarative and procedural representations versus the basic architecture of the cognitive system, and in social cognition by Ostrom (1981, p. 420) as the rules that people use to interpret behavior versus the psychological processes or "generative mechanisms" that underlie those rules. The same distinction has been made specifically in the attribution context. Hewstone (1989) distinguishes the logic of attribution (the level of rules or algorithms, such as the use of covariation) from process and content (the detailed specification of cognitive processes and knowledge structures as they interact in making attributions). Gilbert (1989, p. 191) distinguishes a set of rules by which an intelligent system might determine causes from the processes by which those rules are carried out.

The importance of this distinction rests on the fact that the algorithm and implementation levels are independent in a fundamental sense, as can be illustrated in the context of computer programs. The same algorithm (e.g., to calculate mortgage payments given the principal amount, interest rate, and term of the loan) can be performed by a variety of computers whose implementations may differ (e.g., based on integrated circuits, vacuum tubes, mechanical relays, or even a human clerk carrying out the elementary logical and arithmetic operations specified by the program). By the definition of an algorithm (the rules for generating output given a set of input values), the same results will be obtained by every implementation—although, of course, they may be obtained with different degrees of speed and reliability. Conversely, many different programs (i.e., algorithms) can be carried out by a single implementation (e.g., a single physical computer).

The fact that the output of a process depends only on the algorithm and not on the implementation has implications—not always clearly recognized—for both theory and research strategy.

1. Theories at the algorithm level, such as theories that attributions depend in specified ways on covariation information, can be framed without any concern for the details of implementation. Neither the exact functional architecture (the nature of the "basic" cognitive processes that are available inside the skull) nor a choice among different ways of representing, accessing, and combining the input information (e.g., different sequences of operations) need be specified by the theorist. Obviously, this simplifies the theorist's task and permits a deeper focus on the issues of concern at the algorithm level.

2. To the extent that people's responses follow the predictions of a theory stated at the algorithmic level, that fact is *not informative* about properties of the implementation level. This follows from the fact that any (correctly functioning) implementation that uses the same algorithm will produce the same output—by the definition of what an algorithm is.

3. As a consequence, researchers interested in implementation-level issues, such as the nature of limitations in cognitive capacity, or the particular ways in which covariation information is represented in memory and the sequence in which different types of information are combined, cannot limit themselves to looking at the content of people's responses. They must look either for *errors* or departures from the predictions of the algorithm (which might be caused by representations being lost from memory because of inadequate short-term store capacity, for instance) or for patterns of *response times* or other indicators of processing load. Implementation-level theories can be empirically tested if they support hypotheses concerning such types of dependent variables.

4. Finally, properties of the implementation level, such as capacity limita-

tions or preferred modes of information representation, will hold across a variety of algorithms (cf. Cheng & Novick, 1990), although their effects might appear different depending on the program the subject is carrying out. This fact suggests that as facts about the implementation level of human psychology become well established, such as severe limitations on reliably holding information in short-term memory, they can be used to constrain theories at the algorithm level. For example, an interpretation of Kelley's ANOVA model of attribution that says people process covariation information by mentally calculating *F* ratios and the like would not be plausible, for it would require the reliable storage of too many intermediate results.

The trend I wish to point out is now surely obvious to the reader. Early theories of attribution were directed at the algorithm or logic level: they specified rules relating attributional judgments to various types of input information, and were generally tested by examining the content of subjects' responses to explicit attributional question. More recent theories have been more concerned with implementation-level issues: the way information is represented and retrieved from memory, and the processes by which various inputs are combined to calculate a response. Empirical tests have involved process-oriented measures such as error rates and RTs, as I shall discuss later. Among the first papers aimed at these issues were Ferguson and Wells (1980), Fiske, Kenny, and Taylor (1982), Pryor and Kriss (1977), and Smith and Miller (1979b). In a specific illustration of the trend toward process-oriented research questions, attribution researchers have followed social cognition researchers in general in employment the measurement of response times to make inferences about cognitive processes (see Fazio, 1990). Studies in this category include Smith and Miller (1979a), Ferguson and Wells (1980), Smith and Miller (1983), Smith (1984a), Zuckerman and Evans (1984), Graham and Brown (1988), Hamilton (1988), Hilton and Knibbs (1988), Bassili and Racine (1990), Newman (1991), and Macrae and Shepherd (1991).

Theoretical Integration

Besides a concern with the implementation-level details of cognitive process and structure, another hallmark of the social cognition approach is a preference for broadly integrative theory. Table 1 shows in chronological order several papers that have specifically attempted to place attributions in the context of broader theoretical models. Most of these papers have sought not only to integrate a range of research paradigms and dependent variables, but also to make use of findings and theoretical insights from fields beyond social psychology, including primarily cognitive psychology but also developmental, personality, and clinical.

TABLE 1
Papers Putting Attribution in a More General Theoretical Context

Paper	Framework
Fischoff (1976)	Judgment under uncertainty
Wyer (1981)	Wyer and Srull's person memory model
Ostrom (1981)	Social judgment theory
Shustack and Sternberg (1981)	Multiple-cue judgment model
Smith (1984b)	J. R. Anderson's ACT*
Read (1987)	Schank and Abelson's knowledge structure approach

THREE THREADS OF ATTRIBUTION RESEARCH TODAY

Let me turn from characterizing trends in attribution research to reviewing currently active areas with an eye to characterizing the influence of social cognition on each. Three areas involve intense research interest at present: a resurgence of research inspired by the Kelley (1967) ANOVA model, a focus on linguistic influences on attribution, and (by far the largest area) an elaboration of research on the cognitive processes and memory structures involved in attribution.

The ANOVA Model Revivified

A research tradition dating back to Kelley (1967) is theoretically based on the ANOVA model of attribution and empirically focuses on the effects of covariation information. This approach initially seemed to decline in popularity during the late 1970s as researchers discovered a series of "biases" and wondered just how rational and logical attribution processes were. However, the ANOVA approach has seen renewed interest in the last few years, largely in Europe. Jaspars, Hewstone, and Fincham (1983; Hewstone & Jaspars, 1987) developed a "Logical Model" of attribution. According to this model, subjects given a configuration of consensus, distinctiveness, and consistency covariation information attempt to identify a causal factor (person, stimulus, or circumstances) or conjunction of factors that is *necessary and sufficient* for the target event to occur. That is, they look for factors that are always present when the event occurs, and absent when the event does not occur. Unlike Kelley's original model, which made predictions for only three of the eight ($2 \times 2 \times 2$) possible configurations of these three covariation dimensions, this model makes predictions for all eight. In this regard, an important methodological contribution has been recently advanced by Iacobucci and McGill (1990). They demonstrated how to analyze data to examine specific theoretical predictions rather than simply—and less appropriately—looking for main effects and interactions of the three covariation dimensions.

Another contribution was made by several theorists who noted that the usual three dimensions of covariation information actually do not convey the total pattern of presence or absence of the target event in all regions of the 3-dimensional (person by stimulus by circumstances) ANOVA cube. For example, with the target event "John laughs at the comedian," consensus information tells whether most other people laugh at this comedian and distinctiveness information tells whether John laughs at most comedians. Subjects are not told whether *other people* generally laugh at *other comedians*. (Of course, in this example it is likely that subjects will assume they do.) This lack was first recognized by Pruitt and Insko (1980) and elaborated into a complete attribution model by Hilton and Slugoski (1986). Their "abnormal conditions focus model" holds that subjects possess background knowledge about the presence of the event in all the cells of the ANOVA cube. They use this knowledge as well as information about the usual three covariation dimensions in making attributions. Subjects "treat [covariation] information as contrast cases that define the abnormal conditions facilitating the production of the target event. Abnormal conditions focused in this way are dignified as the causes of the target event" (p. 80). On the other hand, normal conditions will not be identified as causes, just as the presence of oxygen in the air is normally not cited as a cause of a fire even though it is a necessary condition. This model embodies a counterfactual criterion of causation: causes are abnormal events in whose absence the target event would not have occurred. Indeed, under this model, normal, expected events cannot be explained at all! For example, "Sally bought something on her visit to the supermarket" cannot sensibly be explained in terms of anything unusual about Sally, the supermarket, or the specific circumstances (Hilton, 1990).

Försterling (1989) combines aspects of the above two approaches. Like Hilton and Slugoski, he holds that people make assumptions about the occurrence or nonoccurrence of the target event in all cells of the complete ANOVA cube. To this given or assumed information base, Försterling holds that people apply an inference principle that is equivalent to that of Jaspars et al.'s (1983) Logical Model: a factor or conjunction of factors is selected as causal if it is both necessary and sufficient for the event to occur.

The most recent contribution to this currently rapid theoretical development has been offered by Cheng and Novick (1990, 1992). They also hold that people operate from a complete (given or assumed) pattern of information rather than just the three types of covariation information specified by Kelley (1967). Their process model differs from those cited above in two ways. First, it maintains a closer analogy than previous models between people's causal reasoning and the scientist's analytic procedures (specifically, statistical contrasts in an ANOVA). People are assumed to name a factor or conjunction of factors as the cause if it was encoded with the event, and if the *probability of the event occurring when that factor or conjunction is present differs from the probability when the factor or conjunction is absent.* The factor(s) need not be either necessary or sufficient to be identified as causal. Both facilitative and inhibitory causes can be identified, depending on whether the event's probability given the factor in question is greater or less than the probability when the factor is absent. This approach also deals with the issue of causes versus constantly present conditions, for only factors that are encoded with the memory representation of the event are candidate causes. Factors like the presence of oxygen in the air that are invariably present are unlikely to be encoded and hence unlikely to be cited as causes, even if they are logically necessary for the occurrence of the event.

Second, Cheng and Novick hold that people make these comparisons without calculating sums of squares, F ratios, and the like. Their model requires only that people can estimate and compare proportions, which people are known to do reasonably well. The point of this specification is that Cheng and Novick depart from the traditional focus of this literature on the *logic* of attribution by bringing in *process* issues. That is, Kelley (1967) proposed in effect that people make attributions *as if* they were performing an ANOVA, focusing on subjects' overt responses without much attention to the processing mechanisms involved. In contrast, Cheng and Novick are concerned with demonstrating that the details of processing under their model are psychologically plausible and consistent with other models of problem solving, covariation detection, probability estimation, and the like.

The more recent models in the ANOVA tradition illustrate several themes. First, recent models suggest that people use content-specific world knowledge to fill in assumed patterns of covariation, including information outside of the traditional consensus, distinctiveness, and consistency portions of the ANOVA cube. Second, the processing assumptions of more recent models (particularly Cheng & Novick, 1990) are becoming more realistic as theorists attend to research evidence about the types of processes that people may plausibly carry out. Third, recent models (since Hilton & Slugoski, 1986) embody the distinction between normal and abnormal conditions and incorporate the insight that people generally do not cite normal conditions as causes of events.

Two important issues remain in this literature. One is the whole question of biases in attribution. As I noted above, much research through the 1970s and 1980s was devoted to an examination of biases, such as the "fundamental attribution error" or tendency to overattribute events to person causes, and the underuse of consensus information. The discovery of a host of biases was probably one factor that contributed to a decline of interest in the seemingly overly rational ANOVA models. But ANOVA-like models and biases are not basically incompatible; the issue is really one of parsimony. If a single process model can account both for normative outcomes and for biases, specifying the conditions under which each occurs, it should be preferred over an alternative model—like Kelley (1967)—that predicts only normative outcomes and has to be supplemented with a list of biases. Cheng and Novick (1990, 1992) make this claim for their model. It has reasonable claims to be considered as normative by virtue of its close analogy with statistical contrasts in ANOVA. It also predicts the "fundamental attribution error" and the underuse of consensus information, as well as actor–observer differences in attributions. The import of this claim is that these and possibly another known biases are not due to deficiencies in people's processing, but can be explained by the pattern of information subjects assume. The existence and nature of attributional biases have been a frequent battleground—for example, between advocates of motivational versus nonmotivational viewpoints. Thus, it is exciting to contemplate the possibility that a single, reasonable set of processing assumptions like Cheng and Novick's might be able to account for either biased or nonbiased results, depending on the specific assumptions that subjects make.

The second remaining issue is the uneasy coexistence between covariational processing and the use of content-specific knowledge. Most studies in the ANOVA tradition either implicitly or explicitly request subjects to set aside their general knowledge and answer the causal questions based only on the given covariation information. That is, these studies generally either describe events specifically chosen so that prior knowledge is inapplicable (e.g., statements about a warrior performing a strange ritual) or events that are highly abstract and involve individuals about whom nothing else is known (e.g., statements about John laughing at a comedian). The studies also generally employ intensive within-subjects designs—with each subject responding to dozens, perhaps hundreds, of events with different patterns of information. Both of these methodological features probably encourage subjects to formulate special, logical strategies for the experiment (McArthur, 1972; Hilton, 1985).

So are people accurately characterized as "naive scientists" who apply ANOVA-like analyses to infer causes? In everyday life, perceivers probably use covariation information to make attributions much less often than they draw on their rich, detailed world knowledge. Indeed, it is probably true that all types of human reasoning and judgment rest less often on highly general, abstract rules than on content-specific knowledge (e.g., Cheng & Holyoak, 1985). The difference between analyzing covariation and accessing stored knowledge is not simply an efficiency difference (an implementation issue). That is, it is not just the difference between computing a judgment on-line versus retrieving a ready-made judgment. Instead, covariation analysis and the use of stored knowledge to make attributions seem to be basically different tasks (Hilton, 1985; Hilton & Knibbs, 1988; Read, 1987). If everyday attributions are made more often on the basis of stored knowledge, we must question the relevance of studies of the use of covariation information abstracted from context and divorced from any relevant knowledge. That is, even though such studies show that people *can* use experimenter-provided covariation information to make attributions in a sensible way, it does not follow that people *naturally* either notice or use covariation information to explain events in everyday life when they have access to relevant knowledge (Hewstone, 1989, pp. 93–94). Perhaps the scientist metaphor should be supplemented by consideration of the person as "story understander" (Read, 1987).

Linguistic and Conversational Influences

Events and attributional judgments are often encoded verbally in memory or communicated from one person to another. Influences of these processes on attribution have been of interest almost from the beginning. Heider (1958) analyzed a number of verbs such as "can," "try," "love," and "request" in order to draw conclusions about the implicit causal structures underlying them. Schank and Abelson (1977) are responsible for a more recent effort along similar lines. Kanouse (1972) described linguistic effects on the attributions subjects made about events described in sentences. And among McArthur's (1972) findings were clear differences between attributions for different types of verbally described events: actions and emotions. Recent work has begun to systematically investigate linguistic effects on attribution.

The basic assumption is that particular linguistic constructs such as categories of verbs contain implicit information about causality. To demonstrate this, Brown and Fish (1983) gave subjects extremely simple sentences describing events, such as "Ted helps Paul" or "Ted likes Paul," and obtained ratings of causation. Patterns of response revealed differences between two categories of verbs, which could be independently distinguished on linguistic grounds by examining the adjectives derivable from the verbs. Verbs like *help* for which the derived adjective (*helpful*) describes the subject of the sentence (i.e., Ted) gave rise to perceptions that the subject was causal. For *like* and similar verbs for which the adjective *likable* describes the object (Paul), on the other hand, subjects perceived that the object was the primary cause of the event.

The sentences in the Brown and Fish study described fictitious events, and it might be argued that any effects of linguistic factors would be minimized when people make attributions concerning actual events about which they have considerable information. Brown and van Kleeck (1989) had subjects describe and explain an actual interpersonal event that they had experienced. Specifically, subjects were given a sentence frame like "(person 1) *bores* (person 2) *because* ______________________." They filled in names and wrote an explanation for the event. Based on both causal ratings and coding of the open-ended explanation, subjects were found most often to cite the stimulus person rather than the experiencer, as the cause of the events. Brown and van Kleeck used two categories of verbs to unconfound grammatical case (sentence subject versus object) from the underlying roles of stimulus and experiencer. *Bore* is an example of a verb where the stimulus is the subject, whereas *admire* takes the experiencer as subject and stimulus as object. So subjects tended to say that Erika bores Bill because of something about Erika, whereas Sue admires Peg because of something about Peg. Brown and van Kleeck point out that people make these attributions even though we are all familiar with easily bored Bills and easily impressed Sues. This study, then, establishes the existence of at least two categories of verbs denoting interpersonal reactions or experiences; overt action verbs, such as *help* in Brown and Fish (1983), form a third category. The study also shows that the implicit causality in language can have effects even when sentences describe real events and subjects have other information that might suggest causes.

Similar results have been obtained by a variety of other researchers (e.g., Fiedler & Semin, 1988; Au, 1986). The conclusion must be that language does contain implicit information about causality, which can influence people's attributions for both fictitious and real events. It is interesting to reflect that sentences describing an emotion and an action may be essentially interchangeable in meaning (for example, "I like the *New Yorker* magazine" and "I subscribe to the *New Yorker*"). Yet these sentences might give rise to substantially different attributional judgments, with the first leading more readily to inferences about the magazine's characteristics and the second to inferences about the personal attributes of the actor. Though these linguistic effects undoubtedly have boundary conditions, they hold for languages other than English (Afrikaans: Vorster, 1985; German: Fiedler & Semin, 1988) and also when covariation information as well as verb type is manipulated (van Kleeck, Hillger, & Brown, 1988). Explanations of the effects tend to invoke knowledge structures that are cued by the verbs used in linguistic materials (see Brown & Fish, 1983; Fiedler & Semin, 1988; Semin & Fiedler, 1988). Research on linguistic effects on attributions, then, illustrates the trend away from content-free principles such as the analysis of covariation information, and toward theories based on content-specific attribution rules that may differ for different categories of events. In a way, this trend points back toward Heider's original emphasis on the causality implicit in language (Hilton, 1985, p. 76).

Attributional language is often used in an interpersonal context, not just when an individual verbally encodes an event or an attribution for him- or herself. Thus, a speaker's specific goals, such as to convey information to a hearer in unbiased fashion, to ingratiate, or to self-promote, may influence the attributions that the speaker makes and communicates. Perhaps less obviously, goals that are implicit in any conversational interchange (Grice, 1975) may also have an effect. An explanation is always *for someone,* and the individual's conceptions of what knowledge someone possesses or assumes will therefore affect how an explanation is communicated, or indeed what explanation is given in the first place (Hilton, 1990; Turnbull & Slugoski, 1988). For example, a question about why Don went to the basketball game would be answered differently when asked by an acquaintance who didn't know Don is a passionate fan of the game ("He loves to watch basketball") or by someone who knows him well ("He was able to get tickets"). Similarly, we explain things differently to young children and to adults because we take account of differences in what they can be supposed to know.

This impact of Gricean conversational principles on the communication of causal explanations has relevance not only to everyday explanations, but also to social-psychological research. An experiment is a social interaction, and the explanations subjects give to researchers, naturally, depend on what they think the researcher can be expected to know already (Hilton, 1990; Gilovich, Jennings, & Jennings, 1983). People's efforts to adapt the explanations they give to conversational norms may thus serve as a source of "bias"; two people with similar information about an event, and similar perceptions of the causal factors at work, may end up verbalizing different "causes." There is persuasive evidence that the well-known actor–observer difference in attributions is due at least in part to this factor (McGill, 1989; Semin & Fiedler, 1989). Thus language, and the interpersonal and conversational contexts in which it is used to communicate events or explanations, has a pervasive impact on attributions.

Information Processing Models

The major body of research involving attribution currently is focused on processing variables. I will briefly summarize research on four specific issues, though these do not exhaust the range of attributional topics that are currently being addressed from a cognitive-process perspective.

Spontaneity of Attributional Inferences

Perhaps in reaction to the greatly expanding volume of published attribution research around the end of the 1970s, some voices were heard asking a basic question. Do people actually make attributions in everyday life? Certainly (the argument goes) they *can* do so when social psychologists push questionnaires under their noses, but is this complex, cognitively flavored processing something that people typically perform under other circumstances?

Several approaches have been taken in answering this question. Researchers have coded attributional content in written materials (e.g., stories in newspaper sports pages; Lau & Russell, 1980) or verbal communications produced in unconstrained contexts (e.g., Harvey, Yarkin, Lightner, &

Town, 1980). They have performed studies to identify the conditions under which people are more or less likely to make attributions (e.g., Hastie, 1984). However, I shall focus here on research that applies innovative methods in attempts to get at the attribution of traits in the on-line comprehension of written stimulus materials describing events or behaviors. This line of research owes much theoretically to the literature on text comprehension (e.g., Kintsch & van Dijk, 1978; Schank & Abelson, 1977) with its general emphasis on the necessity of inferences during comprehension.

Smith and Miller (1983) and Smith (1984a) used a response-time methodology. Subjects read sentences describing events (e.g., "Larry steps on his girlfriend's feet as they foxtrot") and then were timed as they answered a yes/no question about the vent. A number of question types were used, including a trait that pretesting showed was often inferred from the event (e.g., clumsy), questions about person or situational causation of the event, whether the event was intended, and so on. Results showed that trait questions could be answered quickly—nearly as fast as control questions about the gender of the actor in the sentence. The researchers concluded that trait inferences were probably made "automatically" during the comprehension of the sentences. However, response-time measures often face interpretive difficulties (see Hewstone, 1989, pp. 112–113), and support for the conclusion cannot be considered clear-cut.

Uleman and his associates (Winter & Uleman, 1984; Winter, Uleman, & Cunniff, 1985) used a cued-recall method. Subjects read similar sentences without any instructions to make attributions about the events. They were surprised with a cued-recall test, in which the cue for a sentence was either the trait (e.g., clumsy), a gist description of the event (e.g., dancing), or a semantic associate of the actor, who in this experiment was identified by an occupational label. The trait cue was about as effective as a gist cue, and more effective than no cue or a semantic-associate cue, in eliciting retrieval of the sentence. These researchers also concluded that the disposition was inferred when the sentence was originally comprehended. This conclusion rests on Tulving's encoding specificity principle, which states that if the trait was inferred as the sentence was comprehended, and therefore encoded in memory together with the sentence, it should function as a powerful retrieval cue.

The researchers' conclusion was bolstered by the finding (cited in Uleman, 1987, p. 342) that a higher memory load imposed on subjects at the time they initially read the sentences specifically reduced the effectiveness of the trait cue (but not other types of cues). This suggests that the effectiveness of the trait cue does depend on processing that goes on during comprehension, and is not simply due to a retrieval-time search strategy subjects might adopt. It also shows that the inference of a trait is not "automatic" in the strong sense of requiring no cognitive resources (because otherwise it would not be affected by a concurrent memory load). For this reason, this literature has generally addressed the question of "spontaneous" rather than "automatic" trait inferences.

Bassili (1989b) used a third methodological approach. Subjects read short vignettes describing behaviors under instructions either to form an impression of the actor or to allocate causality between person and situation. Some of the vignettes included covariation information suggesting that the behavior was caused either by the person or by the situation. Subjects were later presented with a trait word corresponding to the behavior with several letters deleted (e.g., g-n--u- for generous). They tried to complete the fragmented trait word, and an improvement over the completion rate among control subjects was interpreted as an indicator that the trait concept had been activated. Bassili concluded that the trait concepts were activated when subjects were instructed to form impressions of the actor, even when covariation information suggested situational causation. In contrast, when subjects' task was to allocate causality between person and situation, they could not complete the trait words at a higher rate than baseline. In a similar study by Bassili and Smith (1986), completion of fragmented trait words was low when subjects had been instructed simply to memorize the sentences.

These studies, Bassili argued, constitute evidence against much spontaneous trait inference. Only specific subject goals to form impressions led to high rates of trait activation. Even an attributional task (causal allocation between person and situation) showed no evidence of leading to inference of a trait from behavior.

A fourth methodological approach to the issue of spontaneous trait inferences from behaviors is currently being pursued. Newman (1991) applied methods developed by McKoon and and Ratcliff (1986) for the study of text-based inferences in general. Subjects believed that they were participating in a memory study and were not instructed to form impressions. On each trial, the subject heard a sentence that implies a trait, and then saw a trait word visually presented. The subject indicated whether or not the word occurred in the previous sentence, and the RT was measured. The logic is that the correct "no" response will be slower when the sentence implies the trait than when the trait is unrelated to the sentence. Control sentences are constructed to rule out effects due to the simple association of the trait with individual words included in the sentence. With this paradigm, Newman found evidence for spontaneous trait inferences among fifth-grade subjects but not among college students.

Fifth and finally, d'Agostino (1991) applied a related approach. Subjects read behavior sentences that either did or did not explicitly mention a related trait word. Later, they were presented with trait words for a recognition test. Spontaneous trait inferences made as the sentence was studied should reduce recognition accuracy. Results suggested that traits were inferred when the sentences were read under impression formation instructions, but generally were not under memorization instructions.

Taken as a group, these studies lead to several important conclusions. First, spontaneous trait inferences are extremely sensitive to subjects' goals. Good evidence for trait inferences is usually found under impression formation instructions, but little evidence under memorization or other types of instructions. This goal dependence, taken together with the general effects of conversational norms outlined earlier, suggests a hypothesis that Gilbert and Hixon (1991) and others have noted. If subjects expect experimenters' verbal communications (in the form of behavior sentences) to be meaningful and informative (Grice, 1975), perhaps the use of written materials in typical attribution studies implicitly gives subjects a goal of looking for trait inferences or other implications of the materials. This idea would suggest that subjects watching videotaped enactments of behaviors would be less likely to derive trait inferences than those who read sentences. No studies have directly tested this hypothesis, partly because of the near impossibility of equating the information in visual and verbal presentations of the "same" behavior. Carlston and Skowronski (1986), however, in their pioneering study of inferences from visually presented behaviors, found no evidence that subjects spontaneously inferred traits when they observed behaviors. For example, subjects saw a brief vignette in which "Dave" decided to return $20 that he and his friends found in an unused room, but did not infer that Dave was honest unless they had been specifically instructed to form impressions of the actors' honesty.

A second conclusion that may be drawn from these studies is equally important: all types of attributional inferences are not created equal (Hewstone, 1989). Several studies clearly demonstrate that a trait corresponding to a behavior can be activated or inferred without a complete causal analysis being performed (Bassili, 1989a). For example, Smith and Miller (1979b) found that people could infer traits much more rapidly than they could answer questions about causality. Uleman and his associates find that the trait is *not* a particularly effective cue for recall of the sentence actor, suggesting that the trait is not linked to the actor as a dispositional inference. And Bassili (1989b) found that a causal allocation task did not lead to trait activation, while an impression formation task did—even when the available information suggested that the actor's trait characteristics did not cause the behavior. Lupfer, Clark, and Hutcherson (1990) used a cued-recall method related to Uleman's and also obtained results suggesting that trait inference and causal ascription processes operate independently. I shall return to this important insight below, in the discussion of overall models of the attribution process.

Research on spontaneous trait inferences perhaps best exemplifies the impact that social cognition has had on attribution. The questions being addressed are process oriented: *when* do people make attributions—on-line in the process of comprehending an event, or only when they are asked explicit causal questions? The methods being applied are borrowed from nonsocial cognitive psychology: response time measurement, word-fragment completion, cued recall, and errors in recognition. It has been clear to many researchers that traditional pencil-and-paper questions, while they may reveal the patterns of attributions or other inferences that subjects can make given explicit goals, are less useful for getting at what people do as they comprehend events or behaviors on their own. As methods for investigating on-line inferences are further developed and refined in this area, they may prove useful for researchers in other areas as well—for example, in the study of cognitive responses to persuasive messages.

Attributions and Memory

In contrast to the widespread use of memory measures in research in social cognition in general and on attribution in particular (e.g., Winter et al., 1985), there is a remarkably small body of research directly assessing effects of attribution on memory. Wells (1982) found that making an attribution for an event could influence subjects' memory for details of the event, tested a week later. He argued that attributional processing led subjects to later access a reconstructed memory for the event, rather than the original event information. Sherman and Titus (1982) manipulated covariation information to indicate that either the person or stimulus was causal in events described in sentences. Later, subjects were given probe words in a recognition test, and their latency to respond "yes" to words that had been included in the original materials was measured. Persons or objects that were suggested as causal by the covariation information gave rise to *slower* recognition latencies, and the authors argued that they were embedded more deeply in the cognitive representation of the event, which therefore took longer to "decompose."

Two more studies of attribution effects on memory are in the theoretical context of the Hastie and Kumar (1979) effect: under certain circumstances people better recall behaviors that are inconsistent with their expectations about the actor, compared to behaviors that are consistent. Crocker, Hannah, and Weber (1983) discovered that this finding held only when subjects were given a dispositional attribution for the unexpected behavior; if it was attributed to aspects of the situation, it no longer possessed a memory advantage. Hastie (1984) presented a general two-step model for the recall advantage of inconsistent events. People are more likely to make an attribution for unexpected (compared to expected) events. In addition, attributional processing results in a more elaborated memory representation of the event, which is well known to enhance later recall.

Finally, Hamilton, Grubb, Acorn, Trolier, and Carpenter (1990) gave subjects behaviors sentences with several items of additional "context" information, each item implying either person or situational causation. Subjects made attributions to the person or situation, and were later given a recall test. Subjects could better recall the behaviors themselves when the context information was mixed so that the initial judgment was more difficult. In addition, subjects better recalled context information that implied a different causal agent than the majority of the context information. The implicational inconsistency presumably led to more elaborative thought about the information at the time the judgment was made, benefiting recall later.

Given the theoretical importance of memory, the prevalence of memory measures in social cognition research in recent years, and the general assumption that unsolicited attributions are made with some frequency at least for important or unexpected events, it is surprising that there is not more research specifically focused on the effects of attributional processing on memory. Perhaps research efforts that would otherwise have been devoted to these issues have gone into a somewhat broader theme, relations between memory and inferences or judgments in general (e.g., Hastie & Park, 1986).

Effects of Accessibility and Salience on Attributions

Perhaps the prototypical line of research in social cognition demonstrates that perceptual salience or the accessibility of a memory structure can influence people's judgments and inferences (e.g., Higgins, Rholes, & Jones, 1977). If attributions are often made by a process that includes accessing knowledge structures from memory, then accessibility ought to influence attributions. It does, as Rholes and Pryor (1982), Ferguson and Wells (1980), and others have demonstrated. When there are several potential causes for a given event, a factor that is made more accessible by priming manipulations tends to be cited as "the" cause.

Similarly, salience affects attributions in a wide variety of situations, as a deservedly influential article by Taylor and Fiske (1978) pointed out. Their theoretical interpretation held, against the background of the rational ANOVA model that predominated at the time, that salience effects stemmed from perceivers' efforts to economize on cognitive processing, to give attributional responses off the "top of the head" without much thought. That is, it was assumed that perceivers just name as causal whatever object is perceptually salient or highly accessible in memory. However, not all salience effects are based on little or no cognitive processing. Smith and Miller (1979b) tested this idea directly, using a heavy-handed instructional manipulation of the amount of effortful thought subjects gave to an attributional response. They found that increased levels of thought did not weaken the effects of salience (manipulated by the order of presentation of subject and object in a sentence, following Pryor & Kriss, 1977). In addition, the effects of salience were significantly stronger after a delay than on an immediate test. Smith and Miller suggested that salience influenced the way information was encoded and stored in memory, and therefore indirectly influenced later responses based on that stored representation, rather than affecting only low-effort, "top of the head" responses.

In their theoretical treatment of causal inferences, Einhorn and Hogarth (1986) advance still another viewpoint on the mediation of salience effects. They note the distinction (already discussed above) between causes and conditions—for example, the distinction between a carelessly discarded cigarette and the presence of oxygen in the air as causes of a forest fire. Conditions, being normally present, are generally not cited as causes even when they are necessary for the occurrence of the effect. Einhorn and Hogarth further note that what is "cause" and what is "condition" varies easily with context. In their example, if a watch face is hit with a hammer and breaks, the cause is ordinarily given as the hammer blow. But if this same event occurs in the watch factory, where all the watches are struck as part of a testing procedure, the cause is much more likely to be seen as some defect in this particular watch face. Einhorn and Hogarth (1986, pp. 5–6) believe that salience influences attributions by affecting what people consider as conditions (nonsalient factors) versus causes (salient factors). Salient factors are more likely to be nominated as causes, because they stand out from a background of mere conditions that are not considered to be causes.

Kahneman and Miller (1986) make a similar argument, extending the cause-condition distinction to explaining the Jones and Nisbett (1972) actor–observer asymmetry in judging causation. If I am asked why I acted in the way I did toward a particular object, I will tend to treat the identity of the actor (myself) as a condition; this factor is constant across all my behaviors. I will therefore tend to explain my action in terms of the object's properties. In contrast, in explaining someone else's identical behavior, the causal question is more likely to be interpreted as "why did this person (among all people) behave thus?" This invites comparisons among actors and therefore explanations in terms of the actor's own characteristics. McGill (1989) provides strong evidence consistent with this argument.

Overall, the conclusion must be that salience and accessibility can have multiple effects. Clearly, these factors can influence causal judgments that are given with little thought, but their effects are also evident when people take much time and effort to make their judgments. This observation is consistent with the suggestion (Smith & Miller, 1979b; Einhorn & Hogarth, 1986) that salience influences the way potential causal factors are interpreted and encoded in a mental representation of the event. Similar themes are evident in some of the recent ANOVA-based models treated above. Hilton and Slugoski (1986) hold that only abnormal (i.e., unusual, salient) conditions are candidates for being considered as causes. And Cheng and Novick (1990) state that only factors encoded as part of the target event are analyzed as potential causes; clearly, salient or unusual factors will be encoded with a higher probability than fixed, unchanging background conditions like the presence of oxygen in the air.

Recent theoretical developments in this area therefore hold promise of unifying what had initially seemed almost opposite theoretical approaches (cf. Taylor & Fiske, 1978): the "rational" ANOVA approaches and the "top of the head" effects of salience and accessibility. We can now see the outlines of a model where salience and accessibility influence how events are encoded (e.g., what potential causal factors are noted as abnormal, what memory representations are retrieved and used to interpret events), and then further processing, based on that perceptual or memory representation, arrives at attributional judgments.

Information Processing Models of Attributional Inferences

Over the last decade or so, several overall process models of attribution have been advanced. They divide into two general categories: schematic and sequential-stage models. Many theorists have approached attribution with an emphasis on the role of content-specific schematic knowledge structures. Models focusing on linguistically based causal schemas (Reeder & Brewer, 1979; Brown and Fish, 1983; and others) and knowledge-structure approaches (Leddo & Abelson, 1986; Read, 1987; and others) constitute two subcategories. (Kelley's, 1972, "schematic" approach does not fit this category because his schemas are content-free, abstract patterns of covariational information.) Considered as process models, all these approaches share the basic assumptions of schematic models (Brewer & Nakamura, 1984). With the target event or behavior and its context as cues, including most importantly the specific nature of the event, perceivers retrieve information from memory for use in interpreting and making inferences about the event. In simple cases, the retrieved information might directly suggest a plausible candidate cause, as when "Bill dropped his expensive camera on the pavement" retrieves information suggesting that this event was probably not intended and would most likely be due to Bill's clumsiness. In more complex cases, processing of the sort outlined by Schank and Abelson (1977) might be necessary to use background knowledge and construct a scenario in which a plausible cause for the event can be located. An example (Read, 1987, p. 288) is:

> Anne walks in the front door and is greeted by her husband Dave. "The doctor thinks the operation will be quite expensive," says Anne. "Oh well," replies Dave, "there's always Uncle Henry." Dave then reaches for the telephone book.

Presumably the reader constructs an explanation in which Dave's action is part of a plan of contacting the wealthy Uncle Henry and asking for money for the operation. (Or perhaps Uncle Henry is a cheap doctor!) The point is that this complex but relatively effortless feat of understanding could not be accomplished without extensive use of detailed social and nonsocial world knowledge, which has generally been assumed to be organized in schemas.

While knowledge-structure approaches to attribution generally have not provided explicit models of processing, two recent comprehensive attribution models have postulated sequential processing stages. Trope (1986) advanced a two-stage model of identification and inference. First, the target behavior is identified or categorized by perceptual processes that use not only cues provided by the behavior itself, but also cues drawn from the situation and the perceiver's prior knowledge. For example, the identical ambiguous emotional display might be identified as silent weeping in the situation of a funeral, but suppressed giggles at a comedy film. In a second stage, the identities of the behavior and situation are used to make a dispositional inference about the actor. Here, such familiar processes as discounting and augmentation may come into play. One interesting type of prediction that is closely associated with Trope's perspective is that situational cues can have opposite effects at the identification and dispositional inference stages. For example, for a perceiver seeing an ambiguous emotional display, the context of a funeral may make it both *more* likely that the behavior will be identified as weeping and *less* likely that a sad disposition will be attributed to the actor (because the situation is a plausible cause of the behavior). Trope's theory contains additional complexities beyond the summary sketched above, such as the possibility that an unambiguously perceived behavior may itself influence the identification of crucial situational features. The model has been empirically supported (Trope & Cohen, 1989; Trope, Cohen, & Maoz, 1988) and appears both conceptually sophisticated and cognitively plausible.

Gilbert (e.g., Gilbert, Pelham, & Krull, 1988a; Gilbert, Krull, & Pelham, 1988b) has built on Trope's theory as well as on Quattrone's (1982) suggestion that dispositional inference may be divided into two substages of characterization (assigning the previously identified disposition to the actor) and correction (adjusting that inference for relevant situational characteristics). Gilbert's unique contribution is the claim that correction requires more cognitive effort than characterization; his research is characterized by imaginative tests of versions of the general hypothesis that overly correspondent inferences will be produced by perceivers under cognitive load. For example, Gilbert et al. (1988a) had subjects observe a target behaving anxiously on a video clip without sound, and then rate the target's dispositional level of anxiety. Some subjects were given information that clearly suggested the target's situation was anxiety producing (i.e., that she was discussing personal topics such as sexual fantasies or embarrassing moments), while others were told that she was discussing innocuous topics. Subjects who did not have any extra cognitive load discounted appropriately, rating the target as more dispositionally anxious when the situation was not particularly anxiety provoking. Other subjects were given an added cognitive load, which impaired their ability to discount in making dispositional inferences: they rated her trait anxiety as equally high regardless of the topics. This result cannot be attributed to the cognitively busy subjects' forgetting or ignoring the topic information, for the manipulation of cognitive load was to rehearse the topics themselves!

Other studies by Gilbert and his colleagues have confirmed the generality of this pattern of results, across diverse types of information and diverse manipulations of cognitive load (e.g., effortful regulation of the perceiver's own behavior). The theoretical conclusion is that the identification and characterization stages of the overall attribution process require lower levels of cognitive resources than the correction stage does. Therefore, cognitive loads, arising from whatever source, will predictably lead perceivers to make overly correspondent attributions.

Multiple-stage models of attribution appear highly promising. Trope shows how separating identification and inference stages can clear up certain paradoxes in the literature, clarifying the different logic that applies at each stage. Gilbert adds a breakdown of the inference stage into two substages. His analysis of the cognitive load requirements of each stage give researchers a powerful process-oriented variable to manipulate in pursuing further refinements of stage models, and also suggest that cognitive load (caused, for example, by the perceiver's own role in an ongoing social interaction) may have important effects on attribution in everyday life. Perhaps most important, these stage models capture a distinction that was already noted above in the discussion of evidence concerning spontaneous inferences. Several studies have obtained strong evidence of the relative independence of correspondent trait inferences and more extensive attributional reasoning (Hamilton, 1992). For example, given impression formation goals, people appear to activate traits without regard to the causation suggested by available covariation information (Lupfer et al., 1990; Bassili, 1989b). Clearly, we can hypothesize that these subjects are going through the first stage but lack the motivation or cognitive capacity to go on to the second. Trait inferences based directly on observed behaviors are quickly and easily made (though only under certain processing goals). On the other hand, a fuller consideration of multiple possible causes of behavior requires effort and capacity and will not be performed unless people have some reason to do so.

SUMMARY: WHAT HAS SOCIAL COGNITION DONE FOR ATTRIBUTION?

Social cognition is sometimes seen—by participants as well as observers—as somewhat narrow. Endless investigations look at details of memory structure or question how many processes can dance on the head of a pin. But these are trees. If we step back a bit, we can see that for social cognition, the forest is a focus on issues of cognitive structure, representation, and process. Researchers interested in attribution are coming to understand that investigating these process issues can liberate theoretical development—freeing it, for example, from the constraints on what can be learned from questionnaire studies that implicitly give subjects special processing goals. The research reviewed in this chapter points to several major types of impact of social cognition on attribution theory and research. I shall summarize three relatively specific and two general impacts, and advance some tentative prognostications for the future.

1. Social cognition generally emphasizes the importance of people's goals (e.g., Srull & Wyer, 1989). Correspondingly, we now realize that whether attributions are made at all, the nature of the attributional questions that people seek to answer, and what causal information people communicate to others, also depend on their purposes and goals. Goal dependence is clearest in the research on spontaneous attributional inferences. No doubt, the focus on goals will continue, as researchers seek to develop a taxonomy of social goals, to categorize the strategies that people use to attain various goals, and to learn what goals tend to be activated in various social situations (see Chaiken et al., 1989; Smith, in press; Bargh, 1990).

2. Social cognition stresses that people generally access and use specific knowledge drawn from memory, rather than applying general, content-free reasoning principles (Smith & Zárate, 1992; Wyer & Srull, 1986). More recent attribution approaches that emphasize the use of stored knowledge (e.g., Read, 1987) appear to better match people's everyday reasoning processes than do covariation-based approaches—which people probably use only as a last resort. Further development of models of attribution as story comprehension is sorely needed. One exciting possibility is that this development may draw on parallel distributed processing models of knowledge-based explanation (Read & Marcus-Newhall, 1993).

3. Recent research on attributional issues has been strongly influenced by methods borrowed from social cognition, as investigators have sought to determine what knowledge is activated and brought to bear in causal reasoning tasks. I have reviewed research using cued recall, response time measurement, word-fragment completion, and other sophisticated, process-oriented methods. The future presumably holds more of the same, as researchers increasingly recognize the deficiencies of questionnaire methods for getting at what people *do* in everyday life as opposed to what they *can* do when encouraged to sit up straight, pay attention, and think logically.

These three specific impacts are subsumed in two broader trends that also owe much to the general impact of social cognition.

4. Research questions that are process oriented—aimed at implementation rather than algorithmic issues—are predominant in attribution today. Researchers ask *when* people make attributions, how knowledge is organized and represented in memory and accessed for use in judgment, what resources are required and how capacity overload affects judgment, and in what sequence people carry out different types of process. For example, Fletcher and Fincham (1990), addressing the role of attributions in close relationships, found it useful to ask process-oriented questions involving the

distinction between automatic and controlled inferences. All of these represent important applications of the general social-cognition perspective, with its fundamental concern for the cognitive processes and mental representations involved in social inference and judgment.

5. Finally, the most fundamental contribution of social cognition to the attribution field—and perhaps to other classic areas of social psychology as well—is increased theoretical integration. Attribution is becoming incorporated into a broader theoretical framework dealing with how people make conceptual sense of their entire environment, or construct mental models of the world. The content of one's model or interpretation of the world then becomes the key proximal cause both of one's "cold" cognitive judgments and social evaluations, and "hot" responses including emotion, as appraisal theories have postulated. Heider's insights about the important place of attribution within this more general process of the perceiver's construction of a "life space" ring even truer now than they did in 1958, because in the intervening years, advances in cognitive and social psychology mean that notions like interpretation of the environment and construction of mental models are no longer just metaphors, and can be operationalized in terms of concrete, specific cognitive and interpersonal processes.

ACKNOWLEDGMENTS

Preparation of this chapter was supported by the National Science Foundation under Grants BNS-8613584 and BNS-9020807 and by the National Institutes of Mental Health under Grant 1R01-MH46840. I am grateful to John Bassili, Donal Carlston, Dan Gilbert, Miles Hewstone, Denis Hilton, Ned Jones, and Ben Slugoski, as well as the editors of this volume, for thoughtful comments on an earlier version of this chapter.

REFERENCES

Abelson, R. P., & Lalljee, M. (1988). Knowledge structures and causal explanation. In D. J. Hilton (Ed.), *Contemporary science and natural explanation: Commonsense conceptions of causality.* Brighton, England: Harvester Press.

Abramson, L. Y., Seligman, M. E. P., & Teasdale, J. D. (1978). Learned helplessness in humans: Critique and reformulation. *Journal of Abnormal Psychology, 87,* 49–74.

Allport, D. A. (1980). Patterns and actions: Cognitive mechanisms are content-specific. In G. Claxton (Ed.), *Cognitive psychology: New directions* (pp. 26–64). London: Routledge and Kegan Paul.

American Psychological Association. (1988). *Thesaurus of psychological index terms.* Washington, DC.

Anderson, J. R. (1983). *The architecture of cognition.* Cambridge, MA: Harvard University Press.

Au, T. K. (1986). A verb is worth a thousand words: The causes and consequences of interpersonal events implicit in language. *Journal of Memory and Language, 25,* 104–122.

Bargh, J. A. (1990). Auto-motives: Preconscious determinants of social interaction. In E. T.

Higgins & R. M. Sorrentino (Eds.), *Handbook of motivation and cognition* (Vol. 2, pp. 93–130). New York: Guilford.

Bassili, J. N. (1989a). Traits as action categories versus traits as person attributes in social cognition. In J. N. Bassili (Ed.), *On-line cognition in person perception* (pp. 61–89). Hillsdale, NJ: Erlbaum.

Bassili, J. N. (1989b). Trait encoding in behavior identification and dispositional inference. *Personality and Social Psychology Bulletin, 15,* 285–296.

Bassili, J. N., & Racine, J. P. (1990). On the process relationship between person and situation judgments in attribution. *Journal of Personality and Social Psychology, 59,* 881–890.

Bassili, J. N., & Smith, M. C. (1986). On the spontaneity of trait attribution: Converging evidence for the role of cognitive strategy. *Journal of Personality and Social Psychology, 50,* 239–245.

Bem, D. J. (1967). Self-perception: An alternative interpretation of cognitive dissonance phenomena. *Psychological Review, 24,* 183–200.

Brewer, W. F., & Nakamura, G. V. (1984). The nature and functions of schemas. In R. S. Wyer & T. K. Srull (Eds.), *Handbook of social cognition* (Vol. 1, pp. 119–160). Hillsdale, NJ: Erlbaum.

Brown, R., & Fish, D. (1983). The psychological causality implicit in language. *Cognition, 14,* 237–273.

Brown, R., & van Kleeck, M. H. (1989). Enough said: Three principles of explanation. *Journal of Personality and Social Psychology, 57,* 590–604.

Carlston, D. E., & Skowronski, J. J. (1986). Trait memory and behavior memory: The effects of alternative pathways on impression judgment response times. *Journal of Personality and Social Psychology, 50,* 5–13.

Chaiken, S., Liberman, A., & Eagly, A. H. (1989). Heuristic and systematic information processing within and beyond the persuasion context. In J. S. Uleman & J. A. Bargh (Eds.), *Unintended thought* (pp. 212–252). New York: Guilford.

Cheng, P. W., & Holyoak, K. J. (1985). Pragmatic reasoning schemas. *Cognitive Psychology, 17,* 391–416.

Cheng, P. W., & Novick, L. R. (1990). A probabilistic contrast model of causal induction. *Journal of Personality and Social Psychology, 58,* 545–567.

Cheng, P. W., & Novick, L. R. (1992). Covariation in natural causal induction. *Psychological Review, 99,* 365–381.

Crocker, J., Hannah, D. B., & Weber, R. (1983). Person memory and causal attributions. *Journal of Personality and Social Psychology, 15,* 961–977.

d'Agostino, P. R. (1991). Spontaneous trait inferences: Effects of recognition instructions and subliminal priming on recognition performance. *Personality and Social Psychology Bulletin, 17,* 70–77.

Einhorn, H. J., & Hogarth, R. M. (1986). Judging probable cause. *Psychological Bulletin, 99,* 3–19.

Fazio, R. H. (1990). A practical guide to the use of response latency in social psychological research. *Review of Personality and Social Psychology, 11,* 74–97.

Ferguson, T. J., & Wells, G. L. (1980). Priming of mediators in causal attribution. *Journal of Personality and Social Psychology, 38,* 461–470.

Fiedler, K., & Semin, G. R. (1988). On the causal information conveyed by different interpersonal verbs: The role of implicit sentence context. *Social Cognition, 6,* 21–39.

Fischhoff, B. (1976). Attribution theory and judgment under uncertainty. In J. H. Harvey, W. J. Ickes, & R. F. Kidd (Eds.), *New directions in attribution research* (Vol. 1). Hillsdale, NJ: Erlbaum.

Fiske, S. T., Kenny, D. A., & Taylor, S. E. (1982). Structural models for the mediation of salience effects on attribution. *Journal of Experimental Social Psychology, 18,* 105–127.

Fletcher, G.J.O., & Fincham, F. D. (1990). Attribution processes in close relationships. In G.

Fletcher & F. Fincham (Eds.), *Cognition in close relationships* (pp. 7–35). Hillsdale, NJ: Erlbaum.

Försterling, F. (1989). Models of covariation and attribution: How do they relate to the analogy of analysis of variance? *Journal of Personality and Social Psychology, 57,* 615–625.

Frieze, I. H., Bar-Tal, D., & Carroll, J. S. (1979). *New approaches to social problems.* San Francisco: Jossey-Bass.

Gilbert, D. T. (1989). Thinking lightly about others: Automatic components of the social inference process. In J. S. Uleman & J. A. Bargh (Eds.), *Unintended thought* (pp. 189–211). New York: Guilford.

Gilbert, D. T., & Hixon, J. G. (1991). The trouble of thinking: Activation and application of stereotypic beliefs. *Journal of Personality and Social Psychology, 60,* 509–517.

Gilbert, D. T., Pelham, B. W., & Krull, D. S. (1988a). On cognitive busyness: When person perceivers meet persons perceived. *Journal of Personality and Social Psychology, 54,* 733–740.

Gilbert, D. T., Krull, D. S., & Pelham, B. W. (1988b). Of thoughts unspoken: Social inference and the self-regulation of behavior. *Journal of Personality and Social Psychology, 55,* 685–694.

Gilovich, T., Jennings, D. L., & Jennings, S. (1983). Causal focus and estimates of consensus: An examination of the false-consensus effect. *Journal of Personality and Social Psychology, 45,* 550–559.

Graham, S., & Brown, J. D. (1988). Attributional mediators of evaluation, expectancy, and affect: A response time analysis. *Journal of Personality and Social Psychology, 55,* 873–881.

Grice, H. P. (1975). Logic and conversation. In P. Cole & J. L. Morgan (Eds.), *Syntax and semantics 3: Speech acts* (pp. 41–58). New York: Academic Press.

Hamilton, D. L. (1988). Causal attribution viewed from an information-processing perspective. In D. Bar-Tal & A. W. Kruglanski (Eds.), *The social psychology of knowledge* (pp. 359–385). Cambridge, England: Cambridge University Press.

Hamilton, D. L. (1992). *Dispositional and attributional inferences: Similarities and differences.* Paper presented at Joint Meeting of European Association of Experimental Social Psychology and Society for Experimental Social Psychology, Leuven, Belgium, July 1992.

Hamilton, D. L., Grubb, P. D., Acorn, D. A., Trolier, T. K., & Carpenter, S. (1990). Attribution difficulty and memory for attribution-relevant information. *Journal of Personality and Social Psychology, 59,* 891–898.

Harvey, J. H., Yarkin, K. L., Lightner, J. M., & Town, J. P. (1980). Unsolicited interpretation and recall of interpersonal events. *Journal of Personality and Social Psychology, 38,* 551–568.

Hastie, R. (1984). Causes and effects of causal attribution. *Journal of Personality and Social Psychology, 46,* 44–56.

Hastie, R., & Kumar, P. A. (1979). Person memory: Personality traits as organizing principles in memory for behaviors. *Journal of Personality and Social Psychology, 37,* 25–38.

Hastie, R., & Park, B. (1986). The relationship between memory and judgment depends on whether the judgment task is memory-based or on-line. *Psychological Review, 93,* 258–268.

Heider, F. (1958). *The psychology of interpersonal relations.* New York: Wiley.

Hewstone, M. (1989). *Causal attribution: From cognitive processes to collective beliefs.* Oxford: Basil Blackwell.

Hewstone, M., & Jaspars, J. (1987). Covariation and causal attribution: A logical model of the intuitive analysis of variance. *Journal of Personality and Social Psychology, 53,* 663–672.

Higgins, E. T., Rholes, W. S., & Jones, C. R. (1977). Category accessibility and impression formation. *Journal of Experimental Social Psychology, 13,* 141–154.

Hilton, D. J. (1985). Causal beliefs: From attribution theory to cognitive science. In J. Allwood & E. Hjelmquist (Eds.), *Foregrounding background.* Lund, Sweden: Doxa.

Hilton, D. J. (1990). Conversational processes and causal explanation. *Psychological Bulletin, 107,* 65–81.

Hilton, D. J., & Knibbs, C. S. (1988). The knowledge-structure and inductivist strategies in causal attribution: A direct comparison. *European Journal of Social Psychology, 18,* 79–92.

Hilton, D. J., & Slugoski, B. R. (1986). Knowledge-based causal attribution: The abnormal conditions focus model. *Psychological Review, 93,* 75–88.

Iacobucci, D., & McGill, A. L. (1990). Analysis of attribution data: Theory testing and effects estimation. *Journal of Personality and Social Psychology, 59,* 426–441.

Jacoby, L. L., & Kelley, C. M. (1987). Unconscious influences of memory for a prior event. *Personality and Social Psychology Bulletin, 13,* 314–336.

Jaspars, J., Hewstone, M.R.C., & Fincham, F. D. (1983). Attribution theory and research: The state of the art. In J. Jaspars, F. Fincham, & M. Hewstone (Eds.), *Attribution theory: Essays and experiments* (pp. 3–36). London: Academic Press.

Johnson-Laird, P. N. (1983). *Mental models.* Cambridge, MA: Harvard University Press.

Jones, E. E. (1985). Major developments in social psychology during the past five decades. In G. Lindzey & E. Aronson (Eds.), *Handbook of social psychology* (Vol. 1, pp. 47–108). New York: Random House.

Jones, E. E., & Davis, K. E. (1965). From acts to dispositions: The attribution process in person perception. In L. Berkowitz (Ed.), *Advances in experimental social psychology* (Vol. 2). New York: Academic Press.

Jones, E. E., & McGillis, D. (1976). Correspondent inferences and the attribution cube: A comparative reappraisal. In J. H. Harvey, W. J. Ickes, & R. F. Kidd (Eds.), *New directions in attribution research* (Vol. 1). Hillsdale, NJ: Erlbaum.

Jones, E. E., & Nisbett, R. E. (1972). The actor and the observer: Divergent perceptions of the causes of behavior. In E. E. Jones, D. E. Kanouse, H. H. Kelley, R. E. Nisbett, S. Valins, & B. Weiner (Eds.), *Attribution: Perceiving the causes of behavior.* Morristown, NJ: General Learning Press.

Jones, E. E., Kanouse, D. E., Kelley, H. H., Nisbett, R. E., Valins, S., & Weiner, B. (Eds.). (1972). *Attribution: Perceiving the causes of behavior.* Morristown, NJ: General Learning Press.

Kahneman, D., & Miller, D. T. (1986). Norm theory: Comparing reality to its alternatives. *Psychological Review, 93,* 136–153.

Kanouse, D. E. (1972). Language, labeling, and attribution. In E. E. Jones, D. E. Kanouse, H. H. Kelley, R. E. Nisbett, S. Valins, & B. Weiner (Eds.), *Attribution: Perceiving the causes of behavior.* Morristown, NJ: General Learning Press.

Kelley, H. H. (1967). Attribution theory in social psychology. In D. Levine (Ed.), *Nebraska symposium on motivation.* Lincoln, NE: University of Nebraska Press.

Kelley, H. H. (1972). Causal schemata and the attribution process. In E. E. Jones, D. E. Kanouse, H. H. Kelley, R. E. Nisbett, S. Valins, & B. Weiner (Eds.), *Attribution: Perceiving the causes of behavior.* Morristown, NJ: General Learning Press.

Kelley, H. H., & Michela, J. L. (1980). Attribution theory and research. *Annual Review of Psychology, 31,* 457–501.

Kintsch, W., & van Dijk, T. A. (1978). Toward a model of text comprehension and production. *Psychological Review, 82,* 363–394.

Lau, R. R., & Russell, D. (1980). Attributions in the sports pages. *Journal of Personality and Social Psychology, 39,* 29–38.

Leddo, J., & Abelson, R. P. (1986). The nature of explanations. In J. A. Galambos, R. P. Abelson, & J. B. Black (Eds.), *Knowledge structures.* Hillsdale, NJ: Erlbaum.

Lupfer, M. B., Clark, L. F., & Hutcherson, H. W. (1990). Impact of context on spontaneous trait and situational attributions. *Journal of Personality and Social Psychology, 58,* 239–249.

McArthur, L. Z. (1972). The how and what of why: Some determinants and consequences of causal attribution. *Journal of Personality and Social Psychology, 22,* 171–193.

McGill, A. L. (1989). Context effects in judgments of causation. *Journal of Personality and Social Psychology, 57,* 189–200.

McKoon, G., & Ratcliff, R. (1986). Inferences about predictable events. *Journal of Experimental Psychology: Learning, Memory, and Cognition, 12,* 82–91.

Macrae, C. N., & Shepherd, J. W. (1991). Categorical effects on attributional inferences: A response-time analysis. *British Journal of Social Psychology, 30,* 235–245.

Miller, D. T., & Ross, M. (1975). Self-serving biases in the attribution of causality: fact or fiction? *Psychological Bulletin, 82,* 213–225.

Newell, A., & Simon, H. A. (1972). *Human problem solving.* Englewood Cliffs, NJ: Prentice-Hall.

Newman, L. S. (1991). Why are traits inferred spontaneously? A developmental approach. *Social Cognition, 9,* 221–253.

Nisbett, R. E., & Borgida, E. (1975). Attribution and the psychology of prediction. *Journal of Personality and Social Psychology, 32,* 932–943.

Orvis, D., Cunningham, J. D., & Kelley, H. H. (1975). A closer examination of causal inference: The role of consensus, distinctiveness, and consistency information. *Journal of Personality and Social Psychology, 32,* 605–615.

Ostrom, T. M. (1981). Attribution theory: Whence and whither? In J. H. Harvey, W. J. Ickes, & R. F. Kidd (Eds.), *New directions in attribution research* (Vol. 3, pp. 405–424). Hillsdale, NJ: Erlbaum.

Ostrom, T. M. (1984). The sovereignty of social cognition. In R. S. Wyer & T. K. Srull (Eds.), *Handbook of social cognition* (Vol. 1, pp. 1–38). Hillsdale, NJ: Erlbaum.

Pruitt, D. J., & Insko, C. A. (1980). Extension of the Kelley attribution model: The role of comparison-object consensus, target-object consensus, distinctiveness, and consistency. *Journal of Personality and Social Psychology, 39,* 39–58.

Pryor, J. B., & Kriss, M. (1977). The cognitive dynamics of salience in the attribution process. *Journal of Personality and Social Psychology, 35,* 49–55.

Pylyshyn, Z. W. (1984). *Computation and cognition.* Cambridge, MA: MIT Press.

Quattrone, G. A. (1982). Overattribution and unit formation: When behavior engulfs the person. *Journal of Personality and Social Psychology, 42,* 1427–1433.

Read, S. J. (1987). Constructing causal scenarios: A knowledge structure approach to causal reasoning. *Journal of Personality and Social Psychology, 52,* 288–302.

Read, S. J., & Marcus-Newhall, A. (1993). Explanatory coherence in social explanations: A parallel distributed processing account. *Journal of Personality and Social Psychology, 65,* 429–447.

Reeder, G. D., & Brewer, M. B. (1979). A schematic model of dispositional attribution in interpersonal perception. *Psychological Review, 86,* 61–79.

Rholes, W. S., & Pryor, J. B. (1982). Cognitive accessibility and causal attributions. *Personality and Social Psychology Bulletin, 8,* 719–727.

Ross, L. (1977). The intuitive psychologist and his shortcomings. In L. Berkowitz (Ed.), *Advances in experimental social psychology* (Vol. 10). New York: Academic Press.

Schank, R., & Abelson, R. P. (1977). *Scripts, plans, goals, and understanding.* Hillsdale, NJ: Erlbaum.

Semin, G. R., & Fiedler, K. (1988). The cognitive functions of linguistic categories in describing persons: Social cognition and language. *Journal of Personality and Social Psychology, 54,* 558–568.

Semin, G. R., & Fiedler, K. (1989). Relocating attributional phenomena within a language–cognition interface: The case of actors' and observers' perspectives. *European Journal of Social Psychology, 19,* 491–508.

Sherman, R. C., & Titus, W. (1982). Covariation information and cognitive processing: Effects of causal implications on memory. *Journal of Personality and Social Psychology, 42,* 989–1000.

Shustack, M. W., & Sternberg, R. J. (1981). Evaluation of evidence in causal inference. *Journal of Experimental Psychology: General, 110,* 101–120.

Smith, E. R. (1984a). Attributions and other inferences: Processing information about the self versus others. *Journal of Experimental Social Psychology, 20,* 97–115.
Smith, E. R. (1984b). Model of social inference processes. *Psychological Review, 91,* 392–413.
Smith, E. R. (1990). Content and process specificity in the effects of prior experiences. In T. K. Srull & R. S. Wyer (Eds.), *Advances in social cognition* (Vol. 3, pp. 1–59). Hillsdale, NJ: Erlbaum.
Smith, E. R. (in press). Procedural knowledge and processing strategies in social cognition. In R. S. Wyer & T. K. Srull (Eds.), *Handbook of social cognition* (2nd ed.). Hillsdale, NJ: Erlbaum.
Smith, E. R., & Miller, F. D. (1979a). Attributional information processing: A response time measure of causal subtraction. *Journal of Personality and Social Psychology, 37,* 1723–1731.
Smith, E. R., & Miller, F. D. (1979b). Salience and the cognitive mediation of attribution. *Journal of Personality and Social Psychology, 37,* 2240–2252.
Smith, E. R., & Miller, F. D. (1983). Mediation among attributional inferences and comprehension processes: Initial findings and a general method. *Journal of Personality and Social Psychology, 44,* 492–505.
Smith, E. R., & Zárate, M. A. (1992). Exemplar-based model of social judgment. *Psychological Review, 99,* 3–21.
Srull, T. K., & Wyer, R. S. (1989). The role of chronic and temporary goals in social information processing. In R. M. Sorrentino & E. T. Higgins (Eds.), *Handbook of motivation and cognition* (pp. 503–549). New York: Guilford.
Taylor, S. E., & Fiske, S. T. (1978). Salience, attention, and attribution: Top of the head phenomena. In L. Berkowitz (Ed.), *Advances in experimental social psychology* (Vol. 11). New York: Academic Press.
Trabasso, T., & Van den Broek, P. (1985). Causal thinking and the representation of narrative events. *Journal of Memory and Language, 24,* 612–630.
Trope, Y. (1986). Identification and inferential processes in dispositional attribution. *Psychological Review, 93,* 239–257.
Trope, Y., & Cohen, O. (1989). Perceptual and inferential determinants of behavior-correspondent attributions. *Journal of Experimental Social Psychology, 25,* 142–158.
Trope, Y., Cohen, O., & Maoz, Y. (1988). The perceptual and inferential effects of situational inducements on dispositional attribution. *Journal of Personality and Social Psychology, 55,* 165–177.
Turnbull, W., & Slugoski, B. R. (1988). Conversational and linguistic processes in causal attribution. In D. J. Hilton (Ed.), *Contemporary science and natural explanation: Commonsense conceptions of causality* (pp. 66–93). Brighton, England: Harvester Press.
Uleman, J. S. (1987). Consciousness and control: The case of spontaneous trait inferences. *Personality and Social Psychology Bulletin, 13,* 337–354.
van Kleeck, M. H., Hillger, L. A., & Brown, R. (1988). Pitting verbal schemas against information variables in attribution. *Social Cognition, 6,* 89–106.
Voter, J. (1985). Implicit causality in language: Evidence from Afrikaans. *South African Journal of Psychology, 15,* 62–67.
Weiner, B. (1974). *Achievement motivation and attribution theory.* Morristown, NJ: General Learning Press.
Wells, G. L. (1982). Attribution and reconstructive memory. *Journal of Experimental Social Psychology, 18,* 447–463.
Winter, L., & Uleman, J. S. (1984). When are social judgments made? Evidence for the spontaneousness of trait inferences. *Journal of Personality and Social Psychology, 47,* 237–252.
Winter, L., Uleman, J. S., & Cunniff, C. (1985). How automatic are social judgments? *Journal of Personality and Social Psychology, 49,* 904–917.
Wyer, R. S. (1981). An information-processing perspective on social attribution. In J. H.

Harvey, W. J. Ickes, & R. F. Kidd (Eds.), *New directions in attribution research* (Vol. 3, pp. 359–404). Hillsdale, NJ: Erlbaum.

Wyer, R. S., & Srull, T. K. (1986). Human cognition in its social context. *Psychological Review, 93,* 322–359.

Zuckerman, M., & Evans, S. (1984). Schematic approach to the attributional processing of actions and occurrences. *Journal of Personality and Social Psychology, 47,* 469–478.

5

The Role of Trait Constructs in Person Perception: An Historical Perspective

Robert S. Wyer Jr.
Alan J. Lambert

Personality trait adjectives play an important role in the exchange of information about people. As communicators, we often use trait adjectives to describe an acquaintance and, in some cases, ourselves. We also use traits as explanations of a person's behavior. Thus, a man kicks a cat because he is cruel, and a woman avoids parties because she is shy. As recipients of information, we use others' trait adjective descriptions of a person to form an impression of whether we will like this person, or to predict how the person will behave. Certainly, we are more apt to accept a blind date with someone who is described as attractive, friendly, and intelligent than with someone who is described as domineering, humorless, and provincial. Moreover, we are more likely to admit a graduate student whose reference letters portray her as hardworking, bright, and creative rather than one whose letters characterize her as frivolous and dull. In the language of the lay person, therefore, trait terms are used to describe important ingredients of a personality that provide explanations of a person's behavior, influence our evaluation of the person, and guide our decisions about how to interact with this person.

Personality traits have historically played an equally important role in the language of the psychologist. The traditional role of traits in personality theory, for example, is conveyed in Figure 1(A). That is, traits are viewed as fundamental components of an individual's personality (e.g., Allport, 1937, 1954; Cattell, 1965; Eysenck, 1952). These traits, which could be acquired either genetically or through social learning, influence both the individual's behavior in specific situations and, more generally, the person's social adjustment and global sense of well-being.

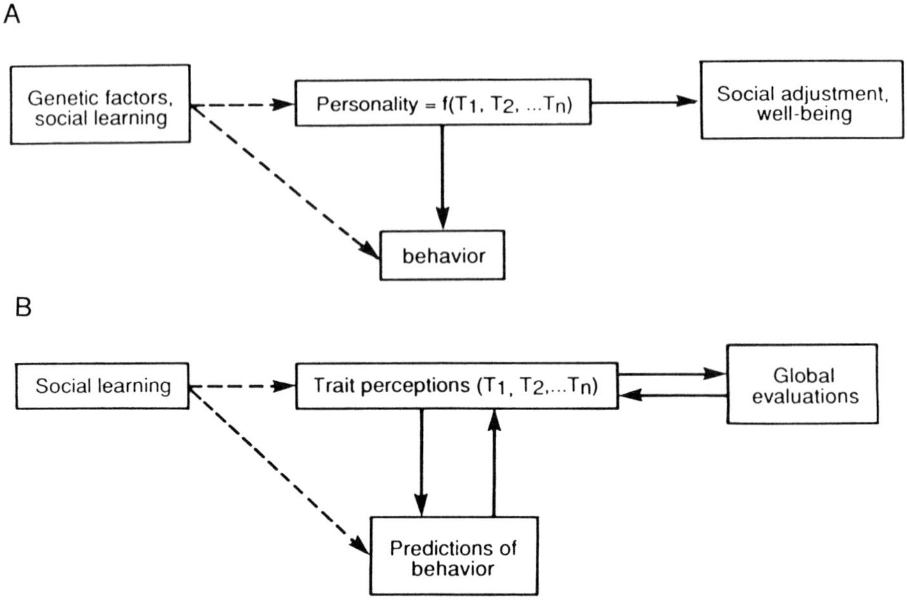

FIGURE 1.

Diagrams conveying the causal relations involving trait constructs that have been historically investigated in research on personality and social perception. (A) Role of traits in personality theory and research; (B) role of traits in social perception theory and research. Solid lines denote the relations of primary empirical and theoretical interest; dashed lines denote assumed relations that have less often been investigated. T_1, T_2, . . . T_n denote traits.

Personality traits have also been the focus of research in social perception (cf. Schneider, Hastorf, & Ellsworth, 1979). Specifically, researchers have assumed that lay people, like personality theorists, regard traits as fundamental to a person's personality, and that they base their evaluations of a person, and decisions about how to behave toward the person, on perceptions of these traits.

The role of traits in social perception research is conveyed in Figure 1(B). This diagram is somewhat analogous to Figure 1(A). In this case, however, the causal relations that involve trait concepts are bidirectional. Specifically, research has investigated the influence of trait adjective descriptions of a person on both general evaluations of a person and predictions of the person's behavior. By the same token, it has examined the effects of both behavioral information about a person and global evaluations of the person (or, alternatively, of a group to which the person belongs) on inferences of the individual's traits. These issues have been examined with respect to inferences about not only other persons but also oneself.

The past decade, however, has witnessed a major change in the role that personality trait constructs play in psychological theory and research. This change has come about primarily as a result of the emergence of interest in social cognition (for reviews, see Sherman, Judd, & Park, 1989; Sorrentino & Higgins, 1986; Wyer & Srull, 1984). Although this area of inquiry is also concerned with the nature of the relations specified in Figure 1(B), its primary objective is to explicate the cognitive processes that mediate these relations. The emphasis on information processing has decreased the tendency to view trait terms to refer to inherent characteristics of an individual's personality. Instead, these terms refer to *concepts* that are used, by both lay persons and psychologists, in much the same way that other semantic concepts are used in the processing of information to which they are applicable.

In personality theory, for example, traits have become less frequently regarded as characteristics of an individual that predict and explain the person's behavior. Often, they are simply treated as conceptual devices for describing the clusters of semantically or functionally related behaviors (e.g., Hogan, DeSoto, & Solano, 1977). In social psychological theory, traits are less often viewed as central components of person impressions than as semantic concepts that influence the way information about a person is interpreted, organized, and stored in memory. Once trait concepts are applied, they can provide a basis for inferences and evaluations. However, their role in these judgmental phenomena is no longer considered to the exclusion of other types of judgment-relevant information. Indeed, a major question of concern in current research is precisely when trait concepts actually influence the formation of impressions and judgments under conditions in which other types of knowledge are available.

Figure 2 provides an oversimplified description of the component processes that can underlie the use of information to make judgments and behavioral decisions (for a more detailed theoretical analyses of these and other processes, and of how the processes interface, see Wyer & Srull, 1986, 1989). This diagram artificially distinguishes between semantic knowledge about people and events in general and referent-specific knowledge about the particular person, object, or event to which stimulus information pertains. In the diagram, overt responses to the stimulus information (trait inferences, behavior predictions, evaluations, etc.) are mediated by (1) the *comprehension* of the information in terms of previously acquired semantic concepts, (2) its *organization* into a mental representation of its referent, (3) the *storage* of this representation in memory, (4) the subsequent *retrieval* of the representation along with other, previously acquired knowledge about its referent, and (5) the *inference* and *integration* of its implications for the overt response to be made. Research and theory in social cognition is concerned with the cognitive operations that are involved at these component stages of information processing, and with the role of previously acquired semantic and referent-specific knowledge in these operations.

Trait concepts could be involved in any or all of the memory and processing components shown in Figure 2. That is, trait concepts compose part of

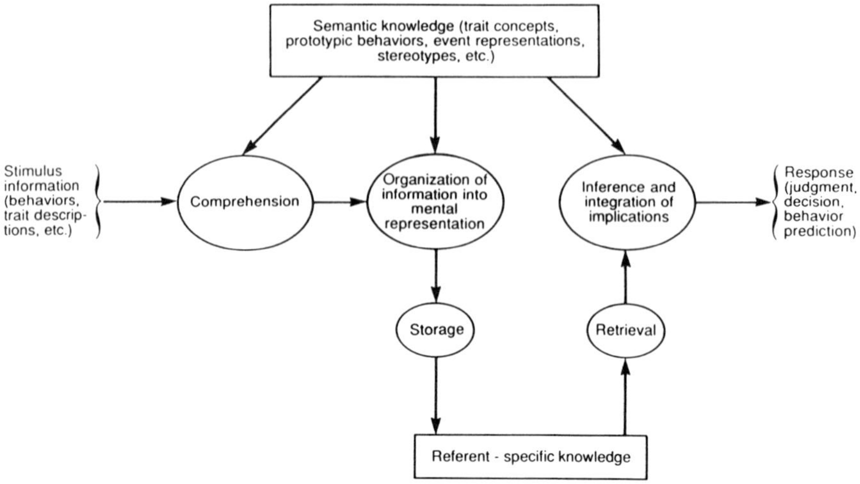

FIGURE 2.

Simplified flow diagram conveying the sequence of cognitive processes postulated to mediate the influence of stimulus information on judgments. Ovals denote component processes, and rectangles denote sources of knowledge, stored in memory, that come into play in these processes.

one's semantic or general world knowledge about people. They could also be contained in one's referent-specific knowledge about the person or object to which the stimulus information refers. The stimulus information itself could, in some instances, include a trait description, and the response to be made could be a trait judgment. At intermediate stages of processing, trait concepts could be used to interpret stimulus information and to organize it into a mental representation of the person it describes. In addition, trait concepts can serve as retrieval cues for previously acquired knowledge about the person. Finally, trait concepts can themselves be used as information that has implications for the judgment or decision to be made. Thus, trait concepts potentially play a role at all stages of information processing. On the other hand, they are hardly the only factors that one must consider.

In this chapter, we provide some specific examples of the shift in the role of trait concepts in person perception. In doing so, we will organize our discussion around each of the four primary types of relations in which trait constructs have traditionally come into play in person perception research (see Figure 1(B)). In each case, we first indicate the role that trait constructs typically played before the advent of social cognition. Then, we discuss the changes in the role that have taken place. Finally, after considering the role of traits in perceptions of other people, we consider briefly their role in self-perceptions and evaluations. Space limitations obviously preclude an exhaustive review of either past or present work in these areas. We therefore restrict ourselves to representative theory and research that exemplify the changes that have taken place.

INFERENCES OF OTHERS' TRAITS FROM THEIR BEHAVIOR

Then

Inferences of traits from behavior have traditionally been investigated within the framework of attribution theory (Heider, 1958; Jones & Davis, 1965; Kelley, 1967, 1971). This research focused on the conditions in which a person's behavior is likely to be attributed to a general disposition of the person (i.e., a trait) rather than to a more transitory state of the person or of the situation in which the behavior occurs. Two general principles dominated this research.

1. Attributions of a behavior to a personality trait of the actor are often mediated by perceptions that the behavior generalizes over situations (Kelley, 1967). Correspondingly, attributions of a behavior to situational factors are mediated by perceptions that the behavior would be performed by other actors in the same situation but would not occur in other situations.

2. A behavior is likely to be attributed to a general trait of the actor if it deviates from normative expectations for behavior in the situation. These expectations, in turn, may be affected by perceptions of external pressure or incentives to engage in the behavior, or by social norms that govern the appropriateness of the behavior in the situation (Jones & Davis, 1965).

The second principle is, of course, subsumed by the first. The perception that there are situational pressures or incentives to perform a particular behavior in a given situation usually increases beliefs that many people would engage in the behavior. Thus, a particular actor who performs the behavior is unlikely to be attributed the trait that the behavior exemplifies. On the other hand, an actor who performs a behavior despite external pressures and incentives to do otherwise may be inferred to behave this way in a variety of situations, regardless of situational constraints. Consequently, as implied by this reasoning, the behavior is likely to be attributed to a trait or disposition of this particular actor.

A decade of research on attribution processes inevitably led to refinements of the original principles (cf. Kelley, 1971) and to qualifications on their applicability (cf. Reeder & Brewer, 1979). Moreover, other factors that affect attributions were identified. For example, subjects appear to attribute the events that occur in a situation to whatever aspects of the situation they happen to be thinking about when they observe or imagine it (e.g., people that are within their real or imagined line of sight; see Fiske, Taylor, Etcoff, & Laufer, 1979; Regan & Totten, 1975; Storms, 1973). Note that the person who performs a behavior is typically more salient to an observer than is the situational context of the behavior. Consequently, the salience bias noted above may lead the observer to overestimate the extent to which the person's behavior is attributable to dispositional (e.g., trait) factors rather than situational ones (Ross, 1977). The specific traits that were responsible for the influence of such a person were not always identified in this research. It nevertheless seems likely that trait attributions implicitly accompanied the causal inferences that were observed.

Several important phenomena were identified in the course of studying social attribution. It is unclear, however, whether the overall gain in our understanding of social inference phenomena has been commensurate with the enormous amount of research performed. As Fiske and Taylor (1984) point out, the area was theoretically fragmented. Very little attempt was made to integrate the numerous theories and empirical findings that emerged, and to specify the role of attribution phenomena within a broader framework of person perception.

In addition, fundamental ambiguities existed in the approach itself. To give but one example, behaviors can in principle exemplify a personality trait even when this trait and, therefore, the behaviors that exemplify it, are widely shared. For reasons that are not clear, attribution theory and research tended to consider only conditions in which a behavior reflected a greater amount of a trait than people in general were likely to possess. This tendency resulted in both conceptual confusion and in potential misinterpretations of the research that was performed.

Consider, for example, the classic study by Jones, Davis, and Gergen (1961). Subjects listened to a person being interviewed for a job that required either extraversion or introversion. During the interview, the candidate described himself in ways that were either consistent or inconsistent with the job requirements. Job candidates were judged to have more of the attribute implied by their self description when this attribute was not required by the job than when it was. Based on these results, the authors concluded that subjects were more likely to attribute a candidate's self-description to an underlying trait of the candidate in the first condition than in the second. Imagine, however, that subjects had not been asked to judge the candidate's extraversion or introversion, but rather, had been asked to judge his materialism, conformity, social dependence, or feelings of insecurity (i.e., traits that might predispose a person to comply with external incentives or social pressure). It seems likely that the candidate would be attributed more extreme amounts of these attributes in the second condition than in the first. The point is that many behaviors can often exemplify more than one trait. Situational factors can certainly influence perceptions of the trait that the behavior is most likely to exemplify. However, the failure for subjects to attribute a behavior to the particular trait of interest to an experimenter does not mean that they believe the behavior to exemplify no trait at all.

Now

Contemporary research on the inference of traits from behaviors has investigated quite different questions than were examined by attribution research. This current work reflects the conceptualization of traits as semantic concepts that are defined in terms of different (e.g., behavioral) features. As noted earlier, these concepts can have an impact on the processing of behavioral information about a person at several different stages. Attribution theory and research implicitly assumed that attributions of traits to an actor were made during the inference stage of processing (see Figure 2), and that they involved a deliberate assessment and integration of the trait implications of an actor's behavior under the conditions in which the behavior occurred. In contrast, the current research on the role of trait concepts in person perception has focused on the impact of these concepts at earlier stages of processing. In particular, it has been concerned with both the initial encoding of behaviors in terms of trait concepts and the role of these concepts in organizing the encoded behaviors into a mental representation of the person they describe.

Three questions have been paramount. First, *which* trait concepts are used to interpret behavior under conditions in which more than one concept is applicable? Second, at what point in the processing of behaviors are these interpretations made (i.e., at the time the behaviors are learned or later, at the time of judgment)? Third, what effects do the encodings of behavior in terms of trait concepts have on both the recall of the behaviors and judgments of the person who performed them?

Which Trait Concepts Are Applied?

When people receive information about someone's behavior for the purpose of forming an impression of the person, they appear to interpret the behavior in terms of the trait concepts it exemplifies. Often, however, a behavior is ambiguous; that is, its features overlap those of two or more different concepts. (Giving someone an answer on an examination, for example, can be either kind or dishonest; crossing the Atlantic in a sailboat can be either adventurous or foolhardy; refusing to pay the rent until the landlord paints one's apartment can be hostile or simply assertive.) Stimulated by the ground-breaking work of Higgins, Rholes, and Jones (1977), a considerable amount of research has been performed on the situational and individual difference factors that lead one or another trait concept to be applied (for reviews of this literature, see Bargh, 1984; Higgins & King, 1981; Wyer & Srull, 1986, 1989). Although there is a theoretical controversy concerning the cognitive processes that underlie the accessibility and use of a trait concept to interpret behavior (cf. Higgins, Bargh, & Lombardi, 1985; Smith, 1990; Wyer & Srull, 1989), several empirical conclusions seem unequivocal.

1. Subjects typically do not attempt to identify all of the alternative concepts that might potentially be used to interpret a behavior. Rather, they apply the first applicable concept that comes to mind and ignore other concepts that are equally appropriate.

2. The likelihood of using a trait concept to interpret a behavior is a function of both the recency and the frequency with which the concept has been used in the past (Higgins et al., 1985; Srull & Wyer, 1979).

3. The concept that is used to interpret a behavior can sometimes be activated by the purpose for which the information is to be used, or by features of the situation in which it is presented (cf. Carlston, 1980; Higgins & Rholes, 1978; Manis, Nelson, & Shedler, 1988). Often, however, quite fortuitous events that have nothing objectively to do with information or the person it describes can activate concepts that are used to interpret this information (Devine, 1989; Higgins et al., 1977; Srull & Wyer, 1979, 1980). These concepts may be applied even though subjects are apparently unaware of the stimuli that initially activated them (Bargh & Pietromonco, 1982). In fact, when subjects *are* aware that the concept that comes to mind most quickly may have been activated as the result of a judgment-irrelevant experience, they may actively avoid using it, leading to a lower probability of applying the concept than would otherwise be the case (Lombardi, Higgins, & Bargh, 1987; Martin, 1986).

4. Transitory, situational factors are obviously not the only thing that affect the accessibility of concepts. Individual differences exist in the "chronic" accessibility of concepts and, therefore, in the likelihood that these concepts are used to interpret behaviors for which they are applicable (Bargh, Bond, Lombardi, & Tota, 1986). Concepts activated by values, or general and specific life goals, can have similar effects (e.g., Anderson, Reynolds, Schallert, & Goetz, 1976; Bruner, 1971; Klinger, 1975).

5. The effect of activated trait concepts on the interpretation of behavioral information typically occurs at the time this information is first received (Srull & Wyer, 1989). Thus, if a behavior has already been interpreted in terms of a trait concept at the time the behavior is first encountered, the behavior is unlikely to be reencoded in terms of a different concept that is accessible at the time a judgment is made. Rather, the initial trait encoding is retrieved and used as a basis for judgment independently of any implications of the original behavior for the judgment (Carlston, 1980). Moreover, the effect of the initial encoding on judgments, relative to that of the original information, increases over time (Carlston, 1980; Higgins, et al., 1977; Srull & Wyer, 1980).

6. Once the trait encodings are made of the behaviors that are described in information about a person, the person is typically inferred to have the traits that these behaviors imply. (For an elaboration of the distinction between the interpretation of behaviors in terms of trait concepts and the

attribution of traits to the actor, see Trope, 1986.) Once these inferences are made, they may affect both global evaluations of the person (Higgins et al., 1977) and beliefs that the person has other attributes that are typically possessed by people with the traits to which the person's behavior was relevant (Srull & Wyer, 1979).

It is important to recognize, however, that the encoding of a particular behavior in terms of a trait concept does not in itself imply that the concept applies to the behavior of the actor in general and, therefore, reflects a general disposition of this actor (see Trope, 1986). A person can sometimes perform a hostile act without being generally hostile. The conditions in which behaviors, once encoded in terms of a trait concept, are inferred to reflect a general disposition of the actor could be governed by the attribution principles noted earlier in this section. To this extent, the conclusions drawn from social cognition research and the implications of attribution theory and research are complementary and not antagonistic.

The Role of Trait Concepts in Organizing Information

When a behavior is encoded in terms of a trait concept, the behavior and the concept presumably become associated in memory. Wyer and Srull (1989; see also Hamilton, Katz, & Leirer, 1980) hypothesized that when several different behaviors are encoded in terms of the same concept, their mutual association with the concept leads the behaviors to be mentally organized into a "trait-behavior cluster" (Srull & Wyer, 1989; Wyer & Srull, 1989). When a person's behaviors exemplify each of several different traits, a number of such trait-behavior clusters are formed as a result of this encoding process. The organization of the behaviors into these mental configurations can facilitate their later recall. Moreover, if the content of one such configuration is reported before that of another configuration, the behaviors that are recalled are likely to be clustered in terms of the trait concepts that they exemplify.

Support for these hypotheses was first reported by Hamilton et al. (1980). Subjects received a randomly ordered set of behaviors that exemplified several different trait and other semantic concepts. Some subjects were told explicitly to remember the behaviors, and others were told to form an impression of the actor. Later, all subjects were asked to recall the behaviors they had read. The surprising outcome (at least, at the time the study was conducted) was that subjects recalled more behaviors overall under impression-objective conditions than they did when they had been told explicitly to try and remember them. Moreover, the recalled behaviors were clustered in terms of the trait concepts they exemplified in the first condition but not in the second. Later research (Gordon & Wyer, 1987; Wyer & Gordon, 1982) provided further evidence that subjects with an impression formation objective encode and organize a person's behaviors in terms of trait concepts and that these concepts, if recalled themselves, serve as retrieval cues for the behaviors that exemplify them. (For a recent challenge to this conceptualization, however, see Klein & Loftus, 1990.)

When Are Behaviors Encoded in Terms of Trait Concepts?

The above results bear on an additional question that was not directly confronted by attribution research; that is, there is no a priori reason to believe that people who encounter a behavior spontaneously engage in the cognitive activity that is required to interpret it in terms of a trait concept: a behavior may often be interpreted in terms of concrete noun and action concepts alone. More abstract (e.g., trait) encodings may be performed only if these encodings are necessary in order to attain some implicit or explicit goal (Wyer & Srull, 1986, 1989).

The above conclusion is not universally accepted. Winter, Uleman, and Cunniff (1985), for example, suggested that subjects spontaneously encode behaviors in terms of trait concepts without any specific objective that requires it. In their study, subjects were exposed to behaviors that exemplified different traits as part of an incidental learning task. These subjects were better able to recall the behaviors later when they were given the traits implied by these behaviors as retrieval cues. The authors argued that cueing with trait concepts would not have had a facilitating effect on recall unless the behaviors had been encoded in terms of these concepts at the time they were first presented.

The weight of the accumulated evidence, however, suggests that trait encoding does not occur unless subjects have an a priori goal that requires it. Bassili and Smith (1986), for example, found that the effects identified by Winter et al. (1985) are much more evident when subjects review the information for the purpose of forming an impression than when they do not. Similar conclusions are drawn from research in other paradigms. Hamilton et al. (1980), for example, found little evidence that recalled behaviors were clustered according to the trait adjectives they exemplified when subjects' objective at the time they read the behaviors was to remember them. This clustering occurred only when subjects had been told to form an impression of the actor.

A later study by Wyer and Gordon (1982) has similar implications. Subjects were given both trait adjective descriptions and behaviors as part of the original information presented and, later, were asked to recall both types of information. When subjects had received the information for the purpose of forming an impression, the recall of a trait adjective spontaneously cued the recall of behaviors that exemplified it. When subjects' goal at the time they received the information was simply to remember it, however, the trait adjectives they recalled did not have this cueing effect. Therefore, both this study and Hamilton et al.'s (1980) suggest that behaviors are only encoded in terms of trait concepts when subjects' processing objective at the time they learn the behaviors is one to which trait encodings are relevant. Thus, they argue against Winter et al.'s (1985) conclusion.[1]

The evidence that people do *not* spontaneously encode behavior in terms of trait concepts unless they have reason to perform these encodings at the time they learn the behaviors has important implications. In particular, it suggests that much of the knowledge we acquire about people's behavior is likely to be represented in memory in its episodic form, and may later be retrieved and used as a basis for judgments and decisions without having first been interpreted in terms of the traits that the behavior exemplifies. This possibility, which was first recognized by Abelson (1976, 1981), will be elaborated presently.

EFFECTS OF TRAIT DESCRIPTIONS ON EVALUATIONS OF OTHERS

Then

The effects of trait descriptions of a person on overall evaluations of the person were first explored by Asch (1946). His research suggested that the impressions of persons formed on the basis of a series of trait adjective descriptions depended substantially on the order in which the information was presented, and also on the presence of certain "central" adjectives ("warm" or "cold") in the stimulus series. In Asch's view, trait descriptions of a person were responded to configurally, and the meaning of any given adjective could not be viewed in isolation from the other adjectives that accompanied it.

Asch's work was provocative, and his conclusions were consistent with intuitions about how impressions were formed. However, studies by Wishner (1960) and Anderson (1962) showed that the effects of trait adjective descriptions of both trait inferences and overall evaluations of a person could be described as a function of the contributions of the individual adjectives considered in isolation, and that the interactive effects identified by Asch may have been illusory. Stimulated by the work of Norman Anderson (1971, 1974; for a summary, see Anderson, 1981), a decade of research in

[1]An alternative interpretation of Winter et al.'s (1985) results is possible. Suppose subjects in their study who had difficulty remembering a behavior were given a trait adjective to use as a retrieval cue. They might never before have considered this trait. However, in an effort to aid their recall, they might intentionally generate prototypic behaviors that exemplify the trait in hopes that one of them would resemble a behavior that was actually presented and, therefore, would help them to remember it. Because the stimulus behaviors used in Winter et al.'s study were, in fact, prototypic, such a strategy would often be successful. To this extent, however, the cueing with trait adjectives did not facilitate the recall of the stimulus behaviors because of encoding operations that were performed at the time the stimulus behaviors were learned. Rather, the facilitation resulted from the adjective's a priori association with prototypic behaviors whose features happened to match those of the actual behaviors that had been presented earlier.

impression formation was devoted almost exclusively to the manner in which different types and numbers of personality trait adjectives were used to infer the likeableness of a person they described. This work was based on several implicit assumptions.

1. The primary component of one's impression of a person is evaluative, and is reflected in one's reported liking for the person.

2. The favorableness of a person's traits, independently of their descriptive implications, provides the primary basis for an impression of this person.

3. The effects of trait adjective descriptions of a person on evaluations of the person are independent and additive. Consequently, the overall evaluation of a person can be expressed as a simple algebraic function (e.g., a weighted average) of the favorableness of each adjective description when considered in isolation.

4. The impression of a person is based on only those trait adjectives that have been used to describe the person. In other words, the impression is formed without considering other attributes of the target that might be indirectly inferred from the trait information presented.

This research was almost invariably conducted within a restricted paradigm; that is, subjects read sets of trait adjectives that varied systematically in their favorableness but were otherwise randomly chosen. (Therefore, the plausibility of a person actually being described by some of these sets was sometimes questionable.) Moreover, over 50 stimuli sets were often presented to a given subject (cf. Anderson, 1962; Birnbaum, 1974). As pointed out elsewhere (Wyer & Carlston, 1979; Wyer & Srull, 1989), these procedures can predispose subjects to respond to the sets of trait adjective descriptions in mechanistic ways that do not correspond to the way they would respond to trait adjective descriptions of a single person that are conveyed in a nonlaboratory context.

Several attempts were made within this paradigm to evaluate the assumptions underlying it. Birnbaum (1974), for example, showed that unfavorable trait adjectives were weighted more heavily than favorable ones, thus qualifying an earlier assumption that the influence of adjectives was independent of either their evaluative or their descriptive implications. Other research (cf. Hamilton & Zanna, 1974; Wyer, 1974; Wyer & Watson, 1969) attempted to demonstrate support for Asch's original hypothesis that the descriptive implications of an individual trait varied with its context. The novelty, semantic redundancy, and inconsistency of adjectives (Wyer, 1968, 1970), and also their grammatical context (Wyer, 1973), determined their influence on liking for the individuals they described. In general, however, the implicit premise that guided most of the impression formation research conducted during this period was that the evaluative component of personality traits had the primary influence on the impressions that were formed.

Now

Current research and theory also recognizes that one's evaluation of a person is sometimes based on a "person impression." However, the evaluation is not *itself* the impression. Rather, it is simply a reflection of a much richer set of cognitive representations of the person that are formed on the basis of the knowledge one has accumulated about this individual. Moreover, trait adjectives per se may not be the central component of the particular representation on which an evaluation of the person is based. Two areas of research and theory in social cognition bear on these matters. One concerns the structure and content of person representations that are typically formed from trait and behavior information about a person and how these representations are used to make judgments. The second focuses more directly on the way that general (e.g., categorical) and specific (e.g., behavioral) information about a person combine to affect evaluative judgments. In neither of these lines of work do traits play as central a role in evaluative judgments as the earlier research on person impression formation implicitly assumed.

The Structure and Use of Person Representations

Impression formation research in the Anderson tradition made no assumptions about the mental representations that are formed of a person from the information acquired about this person. In contrast, current research and theory on impression formation focuses directly on the content and structure of these representations and on how they are used to make both evaluative and nonevaluative judgments of the individual to whom they refer. The need to postulate such representations as mediators of judgments is made salient by the fact that judgments of a person are often unrelated to the implications of the information that people can recall about the person at the time the judgment is made (cf. Anderson & Hubert, 1963; Dreben, Fiske, & Hastie, 1979).

Several conceptualizations of the cognitive representations that are formed of a person have been proposed (Cantor & Mischel, 1979; Carlston & Skowronski, 1986; Hastie, 1980; Wyer & Carlston, 1979). The Person Memory model developed by Srull and Wyer (1989; Wyer & Srull, 1989) provides a convenient illustration. Under conditions in which this model is typically applied, subjects receive a series of behaviors a person has performed. These behaviors usually vary both in favorableness and in the trait concept they exemplify. In some cases, the behaviors are preceded by favorable or unfavorable trait adjective descriptions of the person. Later, subjects are asked to evaluate the person, to infer various traits that the person possesses, and to recall the information presented.

A concrete example helps to convey the model's implications. Suppose subjects with the objective of forming an impression of a target person read a series of kind (favorable) behaviors the target has performed followed by a series of stupid (unfavorable) ones. The subjects theoretically engage in several cognitive activities in the course of forming an impression on the basis of this information. First, as noted earlier, people encode the target's behaviors in terms of trait concepts they exemplify, thereby forming trait-behavior clusters. Second, if the initial information about the target is consistent in its evaluative implications (as in our example), subjects extract an *evaluative* concept of the person as likeable or unlikeable on the basis of this information. Once this concept is formed, subjects encode the behaviors evaluatively and think about them with reference to this concept as well. This activity leads the behaviors to become associated with this concept as well as the concepts defining a trait-behavior cluster. When subjects encounter a behavior that is evaluatively inconsistent with their concept of the person, they think about it in relation to other behaviors in an attempt to understand why the person might have performed it. This cognitive activity leads the inconsistent behavior to become associated with the other behaviors that are organized around the person concept. Thus, in our example, three separate representations are formed. These representations can be conveyed metaphorically in network terms as shown in Figure 3. The representations are theoretically stored independently of one another in memory.

When subjects are later asked to report a judgment of the target, they theoretically search memory for a representation whose central concept has direct implications for the judgment. If they find such a representation, they base their judgment on the implications of its central concept without reviewing the features of the representation itself. Thus, in our example, subjects who are asked how well they would like the target should retrieve the evaluation-based person representation and use the implications of its central concept, judging the person as likeable. This is despite the fact that they would also rate him as stupid, based on the central concept of the trait-behavior cluster pertaining to this attribute.

Although the Person Memory model is only one of several possible conceptualizations of the way in which person information is organized in memory (for alternatives, see Carlston & Skowronski, 1986; Klein & Loftus, 1990; Seta & Seta, 1990), it has interesting implications in the context of the present discussion. In particular, it suggests that trait concepts of a target are not the basis for judging one's liking for the target. This is the case even though the behaviors of the person are encoded in terms of traits that have evaluative implications. If, of course, the initial information about the person being described consisted of trait adjectives rather than behaviors, an evaluative concept of the person might be formed on the basis of these adjectives. In this case, the adjectives would indirectly affect liking judgments. Nevertheless, there is theoretically no inherent relation between trait judgments and evaluative judgments. Indeed, trait concepts may not even be

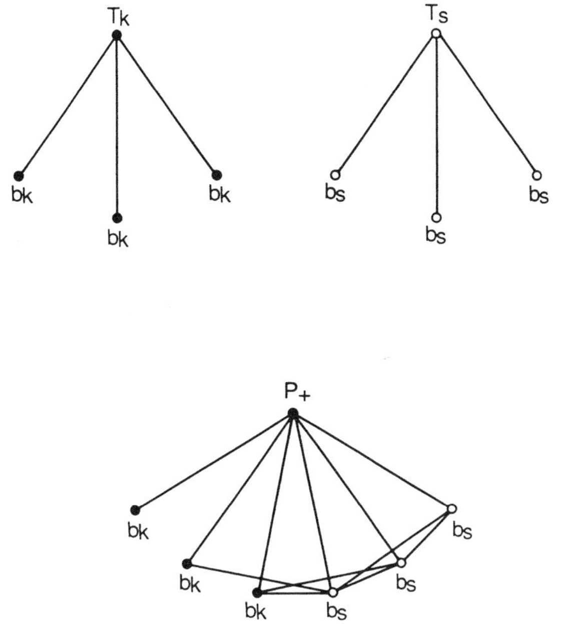

FIGURE 3.

Trait-behavior clusters and evaluation-based person representation formed form a sequence of 3 kind behaviors (b_k) followed by a sequence of 3 stupid behaviors (b_s). T_k and T_s denote trait concepts "kind" and "stupid," and P_+ denotes a favorable concept of the person that is formed on the basis of the initial (kind) behaviors presented.

contained in the same representation that is used as a basis for inferring the target's likeableness.

There is another, less direct implication of the assumption that several independent representations are formed of a person. That is, these representations are often formed at different points in time, each based on a different subset of information, and these representations may be stored in memory independently of one another. Therefore, more than one representation can often have implications for a given judgment. The likelihood of retrieving and using any particular representation depends on the frequency and recency with which it was formed and/or used in the past. Consequently, different representations may be retrieved and used as bases for judgments at different times, some of which are more likely to be formed from trait information about the person than are others.

Categorical versus Piecemeal Evaluation Processes

A rather different formulation of person impression formation focuses on the processes that underlie evaluative judgments and the type of information that is brought to bear on them. This conceptualization, proposed by Fiske and Neuberg (1990; see also Fiske & Pavelchak, 1986), recognizes that people often belong to a social group or category whose members are believed to have certain traits, and that subjects often base their judgments of an individual member on their liking for the group as a whole, without regard to the evaluative implications of the member's specific traits and behaviors. Two general conditions are considered.

In some cases, subjects receive specific trait and/or behavior information about a person whose membership in a social group or category is known. In such cases, subjects first use the *descriptive* implications of the trait and behavior information to determine whether the person is typical or atypical of the group to which he or she belongs.

a. If the person is typical, subjects base their liking for the person primarily on their attitude toward the group as a whole without regard to the evaluative implications of the specific information about the person.
b. If the person is atypical, subjects first attempt to identify a subcategory of the more general one whose associated features are more consistent with the person's traits and behaviors. If this attempt is unsuccessful, however, subjects default to a piecemeal assessment of the *evaluative* implications of the specific information about the person, computing an evaluation according to procedures akin to those postulated by Anderson (1981).

In other cases, a person's membership in a social group or category is not explicitly stated. If the individuating information about the person describes characteristics that are typical of such a group, however, a concept of the group member is spontaneously activated. If this occurs, subjects may base their evaluation of the target on their attitude toward this group without considering the favorableness of the target's individual attributes. (If such a category is not activated by the individuating information, a piecemeal assessment of the target's individual attributes is performed along the lines indicated in 1(B).)

In Fiske and Neuberg's formulation, like Wyer and Srull's, the role of trait information about a person on evaluations of the person is not as pervasive as earlier formulations assumed; that is, trait descriptions of a person (along with other information) are often used to infer the individual's membership in a social category, or to assess how typical the person is of category members. However, these descriptions are often not themselves the criterion for evaluating the individual. The use of trait information as a direct basis for the evaluation occurs under rather circumscribed conditions.

Summary

The general implications of these examples are clear. That is, current research and theory on the cognitive processes whereby information is used to form coherent impressions of a person have led to richer theoretical formulations of person impression formation and evaluative judgments than were previously available. In these formulations, traits often do not play the central role in arriving at global evaluations of persons. In some circumstances, inference and integration processes similar to those identified by research conducted within the Anderson paradigm may occur. However, these processes are only a small part of what we need to know about impression formation, and the occurrence of these processes is by no means universal. In many instances, the process may be more similar to that postulated by Asch (1946), many years before the Anderson paradigm was developed.

INFERENCES OF TRAITS FROM EVALUATIVE CONCEPTS

Then

The inference of specific traits of a person from more global evaluate concepts of the person has typically been attributed to a general "halo effect." That is, liked people are inferred to have favorable attributes, whereas disliked people are inferred to have unfavorable ones. These evaluation-based inferences are implied by cognitive balance theory (Heider, 1958), and their existence appears to be an implicit if not explicit assumption underlying the promotion of both commercial products and political candidates. Thus, for example, a candidate who creates a favorable image, and, therefore, is likeable, is attributed qualities of leadership and competence that are not directly implied by the information on which his likeableness is based (Riggle, Ottati, Wyer, Kuklinski, & Schwarz, 1989).

A traditional area of research in which halo effects appear to play a major role concerns the nature of individuals' "implicit personality theories" of what traits are interrelated (Rosenberg & Sedlak, 1972; Schneider, 1973). These theories presumably guide inferences of one trait of a person from information about another (Cohen & Ebbesen, 1979). As Rosenberg and Sedlak (1972) reported, however, these theories were based largely on evaluative considerations; that is, people believed that traits of similar favorableness were more likely to occur than traits of dissimilar favorableness. Although other descriptive criteria played a role (e.g., dominance–submissiveness, whether the traits reflected social behavior or intellectual behavior, etc.), the role of evaluation was clearly predominant. This suggested that subjects' trait inferences were governed largely by their common association with a more general evaluative ("good" or "bad") concept and might not have been directly related to one another.

The effects of global evaluations on trait inferences also came into play in research on prejudice and stereotyping (Allport, 1954). People often assign traits to members of a social group that are evaluatively consistent with their more general attitude toward the group. These attributions are presumably mediated by a group stereotype, or collection of traits that people apply to the group as a whole. The formation of a stereotype can often be guided by a desire to disparage a group that one dislikes (Allport, 1954). For this reason, the traits that typically compose a stereotype are often assumed to be unfavorable.

In a related vein, people generally have more unfavorable attitudes toward members of groups to which they do not belong than toward members of groups with which they are affiliated (Katz & Braly, 1933; Tajfel, 1970). In addition, they often attribute out-group members unfavorable characteristics. Such group-based trait attributions were often assumed to be irrational, and to be stimulated by negative affect toward the group itself. (See Ashmore & DelBoca, 1981, for a review of this research.)

Now

General attitudes toward a person, or toward a group to which the person belongs, can undoubtedly have an effect on inferences of the person's traits. However, the attribution of these inferences to a "halo effect" is more of a description than an explanation. Several areas of research and theory in social cognition provide insight into some of the processes that underlie these inferences and the conditions in which they occur. Two examples are provided below.

Person Memory and Judgment

Because judgments of a person are theoretically based on mental representations that are formed on the basis of the information that has been acquired about the person, conceptualizations of judgment processes are inextricably tied to assumptions about the nature of these representations. Therefore, for purposes of illustration, we will pursue the implications of the Person Memory model outlined in the previous section. Several contingencies on the effect of global evaluations on trait inferences are implied by this model.

To repeat, trait-behavior clusters are theoretically formed from the behavioral information about a person and are stored in memory separately from the evaluation-based person representation that is formed (see Figure 3). When subjects are later asked to make a trait judgment, they search for a trait-behavior cluster whose central concept has implications for the trait and, if they find one, base their judgment on this concept. Such trait judgments are consequently independent of the evaluative person concept on which liking for the person is based.

Subjects' evaluative concept of the person theoretically comes into play only when they do not find a trait behavior cluster whose central concept bears directly on the trait judgment to be made. In this case, subjects base their judgments on *both* (1) the implications of the evaluative person concept (producing a "halo effect") and (2) the descriptive implications of the behaviors that are associated with it and are identified in the course of a partial review of these behaviors. (For evidence supporting these assumptions, see Wyer & Budesheim, 1987; Wyer, Srull, & Gordon, 1984; Wyer & Unverzagt, 1985.) Therefore, in our earlier example, a person who is represented as shown in Figure 3 should be judged as kind and stupid. Subjects' estimates of their liking for this person should have no effect on either of these trait judgments. Suppose, however, that subjects are asked if the person is dependable (a trait for which the trait-behavior clusters have no implications). Then, they should use the evaluative implications of the person concept as a partial basis for judgments and, therefore, should respond affirmatively unless a large number of the specific behaviors associated with the concept imply otherwise.

It is again important to bear in mind that the Person Memory model used to generate these predictions is only one of several that might have implications for the issues discussed above. It nevertheless serves to exemplify our main point; that is, the general halo effect that was assumed to underlie judgments in earlier research has become more carefully circumscribed as a result of recent theorizing. Halo effects are now postulated to occur under somewhat limited conditions that can potentially be specified a priori.

Effects of Group Stereotypes on Judgments of Individuals

As noted earlier, the role of evaluative factors in trait judgments might also come into play when people infer traits of a person on the basis of the person's group membership; that is, people's liking for a group might determine the favorableness of traits that they attribute to the group as a whole and, therefore, might affect their inferences of the traits possessed by individual members. Although these processes undoubtedly occur, they have not been the primary focus of much current research on the cognitive and affective consequences of stereotyping. Because stereotyping is discussed in detail elsewhere in this volume, we will not consider it in detail here. A few observations of relevance to the particular concerns of this chapter are nonetheless worth noting.

Current stereotyping research has moved away from a consideration of the motivational factors that underlie stereotype-based inferences (i.e., the desire to disparage groups and individuals that one holds in low regard). Rather, it has considered the functional utility of using stereotypes to comprehend one's social world (Hamilton, 1981; Hamilton & Trolier, 1986). In this work, the descriptive rather than evaluative implications of stereotypes have been given the greatest attention.

Group stereotypes are generally considered to be abstract concepts whose trait and behavioral features have become associated with the group as a whole through learning. These features reflect the subjective "average" or modal values of group members along the attribute dimensions in question (but see Smith & Zárate, 1992). Although most of the attributes that are associated with a group are evaluatively similar to one's overall attitude toward the group, these attributes are nonetheless circumscribed. Thus, Nobel Prize winners are stereotyped as intelligent, but are not necessarily regarded as any more sociable than individuals in the general population. Correspondingly, sorority members are stereotyped as sociable but not as any more intelligent than nonmembers.

One focus of current stereotyping research has been on the conditions in which people base their judgments of a person on a group stereotype rather than using other available judgment-relevant criteria. In this research, stereotype-based inferences are seen as mediated by beliefs that the attributes that characterize group members "on the average" are reliable predictors of the attributes of a particular member.

A consequence of this conceptualization is the recognition that many attributes that compose a group stereotype have some basis in reality. More men than women are assertive; sorority members are actually more sociable on the average than are nonmembers; Republicans are less often concerned with social welfare than are Democrats. Because the attributes that compose a group stereotype obviously do not apply to *every* member of the group, it would be inappropriate to rely entirely on the stereotype to judge an individual member when other judgment-relevant information about the individual is available. On the other hand, other types of information about a person (e.g., the person's behavior) are *also* imperfect indicators of the person's attributes. Consequently, it would be equally irrational to rely entirely on behavioral information and ignore the implications of the person's membership.

It is obviously difficult, if not impossible, to determine the objective validity of beliefs about the attributes that are typically possessed by members of a group. (It is hard to know, for example, the actual proportion of women who are "assertive.") It is equally difficult to know the objective reliability of other information about a person. Consequently, an investigation of the weights that should "rationally" be given to these types of information is meaningless. Current research in stereotyping has therefore been devoted to an understanding of the conditions in which one or another type of information is more or less likely to be used, regardless of the rationality of doing so.

Several factors appear to have an impact. Bodenhausen and Lichtenstein (1987), for example, found that subjects are less likely to use a person's group membership when they are asked to infer a specific trait of the person (e.g., aggressiveness) than when they expect to make more complex judgments for which the trait has implications (whether the person is guilty of assault in a bar). Furthermore, Lambert and Wyer (1990) found that subjects used stereotypes in different ways, depending on their perceptions of the group's heterogeneity. Specifically, subjects used a person's group membership as a direct basis for judging a trait when they considered the group to be heterogeneous. When they perceived the group to be homogeneous, however, they used attributes they associated with the group as a whole as standards of comparison in judging a member with respect to traits for which the member's behavior had implications.

Other results obtained by Lambert and Wyer also argue against the assumption that evaluative factors were heavily involved in stereotype-based inferences. For example, subjects who liked Catholic priests in general sometimes judged a dishonest priest to be less likeable than a dishonest nonmember of this group, but also to be more likely to have a favorable stereotype-related trait (kindness) than the nonmember. Analogous to the previous situation, subjects who disliked sororities sometimes judged a socially independent sorority member to be more likeable than an independent nonmember, but also to be more likely to have an unfavorable stereotype-related trait (snobbishness).

The above research is only representative of the current shift away from the assumption that stereotype-based trait inferences are mediated by evaluative considerations. It would be a mistake to conclude from this shift, however, that attitudinal and evaluative factors do not play a role in these inferences. Evidence for the cognitive bases of stereotype-based judgments does not preclude the possibility that affective and motivational factors *also* have an impact on these judgments. A complete conceptualization of stereotype-based trait inferences will undoubtedly need to take into account these factors as well as the cognitive factors on which current research has been focused. Theory and research developed before the advent of social cognition is likely to be an important contributor to such a conceptualization.

THE PREDICTION OF BEHAVIORS FROM TRAIT INFORMATION

Then

The prediction of behaviors from traits has historically been more frequently considered in personality theory and research than in social psychology. Some research in social psychology is nevertheless worth noting. Certainly, people's social behavior is guided in part by their expectations of how others will respond, and these expectations, in turn, are often determined by perceptions of the others' general traits and dispositions. It is therefore surprising that so little research has directly considered the effects of trait attributions on predictions of behavior.

Perhaps the most provocative studies on this issue were conducted by Snyder and his colleagues (Snyder & Swann, 1978; Snyder, Tanke, & Berscheid, 1977). In these studies, subjects received information suggesting that another person possessed a trait, and then were asked to interact with the person. This information apparently led subjects to expect the person to behave toward them in a way that was consistent with this trait, and this expectancy in turn affected their own behavior. Specifically, subjects interacted with the other in a way that actually elicited the type of behavior they expected, thereby confirming their predictions. Although the influence of trait attributions on behavior predictions was not investigated directly in this research, these attributions seem likely to have mediated the effects that were observed.

Now

The past decade has unfortunately seen little increase in the amount of research performed to investigate the influence of trait information on behavior predictions. This could be due in part to a reconceptualization of trait constructs and their general role in cognitive functioning. It might also be due to a recognition that much of our knowledge of people is episodic. That is, it consists of cognitive representations of temporally or causally related sequences of actions. Each sequence, which constitutes a single unit of knowledge, is conceptually similar to a script (Abelson, 1976, 1981) or event schema (Wyer & Carlston, 1979; Wyer & Srull, 1989).

An event representation, which may pertain to a single individual or to a more general, prototypic one, theoretically comprises a series of "frames," each of which denotes a different action or event in a temporally related sequence. If elements of an event that one observes or learns about match a frame that is contained in such a representation, earlier frames in the sequence can be used to infer antecedents of the stimulus event and later frames can be used to infer events that will occur subsequently. This can be done without any mediating trait attributions whatsoever.

Abelson (1976, 1981) speculates that the use of event representations to make inferences and behavior predictions is more likely to be the rule than the exception in everyday life. The information we acquire about people is often interpretable in terms of concrete action and noun concepts of the sort that compose these representations, and trait encodings of the information have never been necessary. Although we sometimes hear people described in terms of traits, we are less likely to remember these abstract characterizations than to remember more vivid and detailed descriptions of their behavior (Nisbett & Ross, 1980). Thus, for example, I might hear a colleague described as "eccentric, multitalented, and brilliant." However, I am less likely to remember this description than to remember that he has decorated his living room ceiling with the stars of the northern hemisphere, that he walks around the hall performing magic tricks, and that he publishes three papers a year in mathematical psychology journals. These behavioral characterizations might therefore be retrieved and used to predict the individual's future behavior without making any trait attributions.

The event representation that has been formed of one person can often provide the basis for predicting the behaviors of a second person. Thus, a woman who has coffee with a man with the objective of deciding whether she wants to go out with him might identify features of the man's behavior that activate a previously formed event representation of an old boyfriend. The use of this representation may lead her to conclude that "this is the sort of guy who, if you give him any encouragement at all, winds up calling you up every half hour and gets into a blue funk whenever you want to spend 5 minutes by yourself." Although trait concepts could be used to describe the man's behaviors, these concepts are not themselves involved in predicting their occurrence.

In many instances, either an event representation or a trait concept could be used to predict another's behavior, and it is difficult to determine empirically which is actually employed. As we noted in earlier sections of this chapter, however, there are many indications that trait concepts are not the principal ingredients of person impressions. Moreover, there is evidence in other domains that event representations do play an important role in comprehension and inference (cf. Bower, Black, & Turner, 1979; Graesser, 1981; for a summary, see Wyer & Carlston, 1979; Wyer & Srull, 1989). Subjects are obviously able to generate predictions of behavior on the basis of trait descriptions when they are explicitly asked to do so (cf. Wyer et al., 1984). Nevertheless, these descriptions might not provide the basis for predicting the behavior of people that subjects encounter in daily life. (For a discussion of this possibility in close relationships, see Scott, Fuhrman, & Wyer, 1991.)

THE ROLE OF TRAITS IN PERCEPTIONS AND JUDGMENTS OF ONESELF

We have thus far ignored an extremely important object of people's perceptions and evaluations, namely, themselves. The role of traits in these judgments may be analogous to their role in perceptions and evaluations of others. That is, people conceivably infer their traits from their behavior, and use perceptions of themselves with respect to different traits as bases for their general self-evaluations. By the same token, they might sometimes use their overall self-evaluations as bases for judging themselves with respect to specific attributes. Moreover, people could use perceptions of their traits to predict how they would react to anticipated future situations. Thus, the four relations noted in Figure 2 could apply to judgments of oneself as well as others. Consequently, as one might expect, the change that has taken place in the role of trait constructs in research and theory on the perceptions of others is also evident in work on self-perception. Although space limitations preclude a detailed consideration of this shift, several observations are worth noting.

Then

It has long been assumed that one's self-concept, and the favorableness of this concept, is a major determinant of one's social adjustment (James, 1890; Mead, 1934). The self-concept is typically viewed as having two related components. One component is evaluative. People have either high or low self-esteem or conceptions of their self-worth. The other, descriptive component pertains to one's perceptions of one's specific traits and abilities. The descriptive and evaluative components of self are presumably related. That is, people who perceive themselves to have undesirable attributes are likely to evaluate themselves unfavorably in general.

Substantial research in both personality and social psychology has examined the factors that produce changes in the attributes that people use to describe themselves. Studies by Harvey, Kelley, and Shapiro (1957) and Steiner (1968), for example, examined the ways that subjects' self-perceptions of the traits they possess are influenced by others' judgments of them (see also Secord, Backman, & Eachus, 1964). Other research was concerned with the effect of feedback about one's performance on an achievement task on self-evaluations (cf. Wyer, Henninger, & Wolfson, 1975). An implicit assumption underlying this research was that traits per se, and their evaluative implications, are the fundamental ingredients of self-concepts that mediate one's responses to other persons and to events that occur in one's daily life. Moreover, people's perceptions that they do not possess traits they regard as desirable were postulated to elicit negative emotional reactions, and to decrease feelings of self-worth and general life satisfaction. (For a current theoretical formulation that also employs this assumption, see Higgins, 1987.)

Now

The emergence of interest in the cognitive representations of social information, and the influence of these representations on judgments, have broadened considerably our conception of self-knowledge and its impact on behavior. In this conception, trait constructs play a less important role than they had in previous research and theorizing. Moreover, the conception raises quite different questions concerning the influence of trait characterizations of oneself on inferences about oneself and others. A number of lines of research and theory exemplify the changes that have taken place.

We have come to recognize that the traits used by people to describe themselves may not be a major part of self-knowledge. Moreover, they may not even be important. This possibility was actually called to the attention of social psychologists some years ago by Bem (1965, 1972). He found evidence that people often do not have ready-made trait descriptions of themselves stored in memory. Even if they have these descriptions, they do not always use them when they are asked to judge themselves. Rather, they compute new self-judgments on the basis of whatever selective subset of self-knowledge happens to be easily accessible in memory at the time. Although this self-knowledge could in principle contain trait judgments one has made of oneself, it is more likely to include episodic representations of specific behaviors one has recently performed or thought about that have implications for the traits being judged. Support for this contention was obtained in a series of studies by Salancik (1974; Salancik & Calder, 1974). They found that subjects' judgments of their religiousness (an attribute that might be expected to be fairly stable) were influenced by the implications of whatever religiousness-relevant behaviors were called to mind as a result of reporting them in an earlier questionnaire. This does not mean, of course, that trait judgments of oneself are inherently unstable. However, a major determinant of their stability may be whether similar subsets of self-knowledge are likely to be activated and used to *compute* self-judgments at different points in time and not whether previously formed trait concepts of oneself have been stored in memory.

The results of research conducted by William and Claire McGuire (1987) are quite compatible with this view. The McGuires find that when people are asked to convey information about themselves without being given any indication of the type of information they should report, the likelihood that they spontaneously generate personality trait descriptions of themselves is quite low. Rather, subjects typically mention activities, significant others, and attitudes (McGuire & Padawer-Singer, 1976). Moreover, the things they report are ones that distinguish themselves from others in either their immediate social environment or their environment outside the laboratory. Quite aside from the specific implications of the McGuires' work for understanding the content and structure of self-knowledge, this research supports the conclusion that trait concepts per se play a relatively minor role in people's spontaneous thoughts about themselves.

Even though trait characterizations of oneself exist in memory, they could be stored and retrieved independently of specific behavior representations. Recent work by Klein and Loftus (1992) suggests that this is the case. Suppose subjects who are asked to make a trait judgment spontaneously retrieve an instance of behavior that exemplifies the trait to use as a basis for judgment. Then, they should be able to report such an instance more quickly after making the trait inference than they would otherwise. Klein and Loftus, however, found that making a trait inference had no effect at all on the accessibility of a trait-related behavior in memory. Furthermore, asking subjects to generate a trait-related behavior had no effect on the speed with which they judged themselves with respect to the trait that the behavior exemplified. In combination, these studies suggest that the trait and behavior knowledge one has about oneself is not interrelated in memory. Rather, each type of information is retrieved from memory independently to attain goals to which it is specifically relevant.

Finally, there is increasing evidence that people often base their evaluations of themselves and others in the affect or emotions they experience when they think about these persons (for a summary, see Schwarz & Clore, 1987). More specifically, pleasant or unpleasant experiences with a stimulus often lead affective reactions to become conditioned to this stimulus. If these reactions are reelicited by the stimulus when it is later encountered or thought about, the quality and intensity of these reactions may provide information about how one "feels" about the stimulus and, therefore, one's evaluation of it. Moreover, the affect that is elicited by the stimulus may often not be subjectively distinguishable from the affect one happens to be experiencing for reasons that have nothing to do with this stimulus. Therefore, this latter, extraneous affect may influence the judgment that is made.

It would obviously be a mistake to conclude that people do not have any previously formed concepts of the traits they possess, or that they never use these concepts as bases for their judgments and behavioral decisions. Klein and Loftus's (1992) research suggests that such trait concepts do exist. However, the role of these concepts has seldom been firmly established. Higgins (1987), for example, has used trait ratings to distinguish between subjects' "actual," "ideal," and "ought" selves, and has successfully predicted differences in subjects' emotional state from discrepancies between these various self-descriptions. Although the results he has obtained are impressive, they do not necessarily indicate that subjects' emotional reactions are directly produced by preexisting trait descriptions of themselves that they have stored in memory; that is, actual and ideal self-ratings they report could easily be computed at the time of judgment, based on episodic traces of their behavior in various situations and their perceptions of its desirability.[2]

Another conceptualization in which trait concepts of oneself are assumed to play a role was proposed by Markus (1977; Markus & Sentis, 1982). According to their theory, people are "schematic with respect to a trait if they both (1) describe themselves as having an extreme degree of a trait and (2) consider the trait to be important. These persons appear to process trait-relevant information about themselves and others more quickly than do people who consider the trait to be both less self-descriptive and less important (i.e., "aschematics"). Because of the confound of self-descriptiveness

[2]For example, a person might be depressed because he would like to go out on dates but becomes paralyzed whenever he reaches for the phone to call up a woman. If he is asked during the experiment, he might retrieve this self-knowledge and use it to report that he is more "shy" than he would like to be. However, these trait inferences might be computed at the time of judgment, and might not themselves be a direct source of the emotional reactions he experiences.

and importance in Markus's operationalization of "schematicity," her results do not necessarily reflect the role of traits in subjects' conceptions of themselves per se. Rather, the results could simply indicate that subjects who consider attributes to be *important* (regardless of whether they believe they personally possess the trait) have these attributes chronically accessible in memory and, therefore, are apt to process information they receive in terms of these concepts. (For evidence suggesting this possibility, see Bargh et al., 1986.)

Be that as it may, both Markus's and Higgins's research raise the question of when and under what conditions subjects retrieve previously formed trait concepts about themselves to use as a basis for judgments and decisions, and when they use more episodic knowledge about themselves instead. Although theoretical analyses of the contingency have been proposed (cf. Wyer & Srull, 1989), the question has not yet been answered empirically.

To the extent that people have fairly stable concepts of the traits they possess, these concepts could in principle be used in much the same way as trait concepts that exist in semantic memory to encode and organize new information. Evidence of the role of self-knowledge in memory for information was first investigated by Rogers, Kuiper, and Kirker (1977). They found that information was better remembered if it was thought about with reference to oneself than if it was processed in other ways (see also Bower & Gilligan, 1979; Keenan & Baillet, 1980). Although the cognitive processes underlying these effects were not clear from this early research, they have since been explicated in a series of studies by Klein and his colleagues (Klein & Kihlstrom, 1986; Klein & Loftus, 1988; Klein, Loftus, & Burton, 1989). They find that thinking about information with reference to oneself facilitates recall for two reasons. First, self-knowledge provides retrieval cues for individual pieces of information that have been thought about with reference to it. Second, self-knowledge can influence the way in which different pieces of stimulus information are organized in memory in relation to one another. Although the influence of trait concepts of oneself per se on this self-referential processing has not been directly established, these concepts may be part of the knowledge that is involved in this processing. To this extent, the effects of trait concepts that one applies to oneself on information processing are somewhat analogous to the effect of trait concepts that are retrieved from semantic memory, as discussed earlier in this chapter.

CONCLUDING REMARKS

Our discussion in this chapter is not intended to provide an exhaustive review of theory and research in which trait constructs have been applied. However, the examples we have provided suffice to exemplify the changes that have taken place in the role that these constructs are assumed to play in person perception and impression formation. In evaluating the implications of these changes, however, it is important to bear in mind that new conceptualizations of the role of trait constructs in person perception and judgment do not negate the empirical conclusions that were drawn on the basis of research performed within earlier conceptual frameworks. There is often a danger that contemporary theorizing loses contact with empirical phenomena identified in the past that may be equally if not more important. When this occurs, there is often motion without progress.

Our ultimate objective is obviously to develop a conceptualization of person perception and social judgment that can incorporate empirical phenomena that have been identified in the past, while at the same time providing insights into new phenomena that earlier conceptualizations did not address. An information-processing approach to understanding person perception, and the role of traits in person memory and judgment, is quite fruitful, as the work cited in this chapter testifies. However, in our desire to identify the contributions of social cognition to classical issues in social psychology (the general objective of this volume), we must not blind ourselves to the equally important contributions of classical social psychology to an understanding of contemporary issues in social cognition. Only in this way can we ultimately develop a conceptualization of person perception and impression formation that incorporates all of the empirical knowledge we have accumulated in our many years of work in this area.

ACKNOWLEDGMENTS

The writing of this chapter and much of the research described herein were supported by Grant MH3-8585 from the National Institute of Mental Health. Appreciation is extended to the University of Illinois Social Cognition Group for the stimulation of many of the ideas conveyed, and to Stephan Ahadi for insightful comments on an earlier draft of the manuscript.

REFERENCES

Abelson, R. P. (1976). Script processing in attitude formation and decision making. In J. S. Carroll & J. W. Payne (Eds.), *Cognitive and social behavior.* Hillsdale, NJ: Erlbaum.

Abelson, R. P. (1981). The psychological status of the script concept. *American Psychologist, 36,* 715–729.

Allport, G. W. (1937). *Personality.* New York: Holt, Rinehart & Winston.

Allport, G. W. (1954). *The nature of prejudice.* Reading, MA: Addison-Wesley.

Anderson, N. H. (1962). Application of an additive model to impression formation. *Science, 138,* 817–818.

Anderson, N. H. (1971). Integration theory and attitude change. *Psychological Review, 78,* 171–206.

Anderson, N. H. (1974). Information integration theory: A brief survey. In D. H. Krantz, R. C. Atkinson, R. D. Luce, & P. Suppes (Eds.), *Contemporary developments in mathematical psychology* (Vol. 2). New York: Academic Press.

Anderson, N. H. (1981). *Foundations of information integration theory.* New York: Academic Press.

Anderson, N. H., & Hubert, S. (1963). Effects of concomitant verbal recall on order effects in personality impression formation. *Journal of Verbal Learning and Verbal Behavior, 17,* 1–12.

Anderson, R. C., Reynolds, R. E., Schallert, D. L., & Goetz, E. T. (1976). *Framework for comprehending discourse* (Tech. Pre. No. 12). Urbana, IL: Laboratory for Cognitive Studies in Education, University of Illinois at Urbana-Champaign.

Asch, S. E. (1946). Forming impressions of personality. *Journal of Abnormal and Social Psychology, 41,* 258–290.

Ashmore, R. D., & DelBoca, F. K. (1981). Conceptual approaches to stereotypes and stereotyping. In D. L. Hamilton (Ed.), *Cognitive processes in stereotyping and intergroup behavior.* Hillsdale, NJ: Erlbaum.

Bargh, J. A. (1984). Automatic and conscious processing of social information. In R. S. Wyer & T. K. Srull (Eds.), *Handbook of social cognition* (Vol. 3). Hillsdale, NJ: Erlbaum.

Bargh, J. A., & Pietromonaco, P. (1982). Automatic information processing and social perception: The influence of trait information presented outside of conscious awareness on impression formation. *Journal of Personality and Social Psychology, 43,* 437–449.

Bargh, J. A., Bond, R. N., Lombardi, W., & Tota, M. E. (1986). The additive nature of chronic and temporary sources of construct accessibility. *Journal of Personality and Social Psychology, 50,* 869–878.

Bassili, J. N., & Smith, M. C. (1986). On the spontaneity of trait attributions: Converging evidence for the role of cognitive strategy. *Journal of Personality and Social Psychology, 50,* 239–245.

Bem, D. J. (1965). An experimental analysis of self-persuasion. *Journal of Experimental Psychology, 1,* 199–218.

Bem, D. J. (1972). Self-perception theory. In L. Berkowitz (Ed.) *Advances in experimental social psychology* (Vol. 6). New York: Academic Press.

Birnbaum, M. H. (1974). The nonadditivity of personality impressions. *Journal of Experimental Psychology, 102,* 543–561.

Block, J. (1971). *Lives through time.* Berkeley, CA: Bancroft Books.

Bodenhausen, G. V., & Lichtenstein, M. (1987). Social stereotypes and information processing strategies: The impact of task complexity. *Journal of Personality and Social Psychology, 52,* 871–880.

Bodenhausen, G. V., & Wyer, R. S. (1985). Effects of stereotypes on decision making and information processing strategies. *Journal of Personality and Social Psychology, 48,* 267–282.

Bower, G. H., & Gilligan, S. G. (1979). Remembering information related to one's self. *Journal of Research in Personality, 13,* 420–432.

Bower, G. H., Black, J. B., & Turner, T. J. (1979). Scripts in memory for text. *Cognitive Psychology, 11,* 177–220.

Bruner, J. S. (1951). Personality dynamics and the process of perceiving. In R. Blake & G. Ramsey (Eds.), *Perception: An approach to personality.* New York: Ronald.

Cantor, N., & Mischel, W. (1979). Prototypes in person perception. In L. Berkowitz (Ed.), *Advances in experimental social psychology* (Vol. 12). New York: Academic Press.

Carlston, D. E. (1980). Events, inferences and impression formation. In R. Hastie, T. Ostrom, E. Ebbesen, R. Wyer, D. Hamilton, & D. Carlston (Eds.), *Person memory: The cognitive basis of social perception.* Hillsdale, NJ: Erlbaum.

Carlston, D. E., & Skowronski, J. J. (1986). Trait memory and behavior memory: The effects of alternative pathways on impression judgment response times. *Journal of Personality and Social Psychology, 50,* 5–13.

Cattell, R. B. (1965). *The scientific analysis of personality.* Chicago: Aldine-Atherton.

Cohen, C. E., & Ebbesen, E. B. (1979). Observational goals and schema activation: A theoretical framework for behavior perception. *Journal of Experimental Social Psychology, 15,* 305–339.

Define, P. G. (1989). Stereotypes and prejudice: Their automatic and controlled components. *Journal of Personality and Social Psychology, 56,* 5–18.

Dreben, E. K., Fiske, S. T., & Hastie, R. (1979). The independence of item and evaluative information: Impression and recall order effects in behavior-based impression formation. *Journal of Personality and Social Psychology, 37,* 1758–1768.

Eysenck, H. (1952). *The structure of human personality.* London: Methuen.

Eysenck, H. J., & Eysenck, M. W. (1985). *Personality and individual differences.* New York: Plenum.

Fenigstein, A., Scheier, M. F., & Buss, A. H. (1975). Public and private self-consciousness: Assessment and theory. *Journal of Consulting and Clinical Psychology, 43,* 522–527.

Fiske, S. T., & Neuberg, S. L. (1990). A continuum model of impression formation from category-based to individuating responses: Influence of information on attention and interpretation. In M. P. Zanna (Ed.), *Advances in experimental social psychology* (Vol. 23). New York: Academic Press.

Fiske, S. T., & Pavelchak, M. A. (1986). Category-based vs. piecemeal-based affective responses: Developments in schema-triggered affect. In R. M. Sorentino & E. T. Higgins (Eds.), *Handbook of motivation and cognition.* New York: Guilford.

Fiske, S. T., & Taylor, S. E. (1984). *Social cognition.* Reading, MA: Addison-Wesley.

Fiske, S. T., Taylor, S. E., Etcoff, N. L., & Laufer, J. K. (1979). Imaging, empathy, and causal attribution. *Journal of Experimental Social Psychology, 15,* 356–377.

Funder, D. C. (1983). The "consistency" controversy and the accuracy of personality judgments. *Journal of Personality, 51,* 346–359.

Gordon, S. E., & Wyer, R. S. (1987). Person memory: Category-set-size effects on the recall of a person's behaviors. *Journal of Personality and Social Psychology, 53,* 648–662.

Graesser, A. C. (1981). *Prose comprehension beyond the word.* New York: Springer-Verlag.

Hamilton, D. L. (Ed.). (1981). *Cognitive processes in stereotyping and intergroup behavior.* Hillsdale, NJ: Erlbaum.

Hamilton, D. L., & Trolier, T. K., (1986). Stereotypes and stereotyping: An overview of the cognitive approach. In J. F. Dovidio & S. L. Gaertner (Eds.), *Prejudice, discrimination & racism.* Orlando, FL: Academic Press.

Hamilton, D. L., & Zanna, M. P. (1974). Context effects in impression formation: Changes in connotative meaning. *Journal of Personality and Social Psychology, 29,* 649–654.

Hamilton, D. L., Katz, L. B., & Leirer, V. O. (1980). Organizational processes in impression formation. In R. Hastie, T. Ostrom, E. Ebbesen, R. Wyer, D. Hamilton, & D. Carlston (Eds.), *Person memory: The cognitive basis of social perception.* Hillsdale, NJ: Erlbaum.

Harvey, O. J., Kelley, H. H., & Shapiro, M. M. (1957). Reactions to unfavorable evaluations of self made by other persons. *Journal of Personality, 25,* 393–411.

Hastie, R. (1980). Memory for behavioral information that confirms or contradicts a personality impression. In R. Hastie, T. Ostrom, E. Ebbesen, R. Wyer, D. Hamilton, & D. Carlston (Eds.), *Person memory: The cognitive basis of social perception.* Hillsdale, NJ: Erlbaum.

Heider, F. (1958). *The psychology of interpersonal relations.* New York: Wiley.

Higgins, E. T. (1987). Self-discrepancy: A theory relating self and affect. *Psychological Review, 94,* 319–340.

Higgins, E. T., & King, G. (1981). Accessibility of social constructs: Information processing consequences of individual and contextual variability. In N. Cantro & J. F. Kihlstrom (Eds.), *Personality, cognition and social interaction.* Hillsdale, NJ: Erlbaum.

Higgins, E. T., & Rholes, W. S. (1978). "Saying is believing": Effects of message modification on memory and liking for the person described. *Journal of Experimental Social Psychology, 14,* 363–378.

Higgins, E. T., Rholes, W. S., & Jones, C. R. (1977). Category accessibility and impression formation. *Journal of Experimental Social Psychology, 13,* 141–154.

Higgins, E. T., Bargh, J. A., & Lombardi, W. (1985). The nature of priming effects on categorization. *Journal of Experimental Psychology: Learning, Memory, and Cognition, 11,* 59–89.

Hogan, R., DeSoto, C. B., & Solano, C. (1977). Traits, tests, and personality research. *American Psychologist, 32,* 255–264.

James, W. (1890). *Principles of psychology.* New York: Holt.

Jones, E. E., & Davis, K. E. (1965). From acts to dispositions: The attributional process in person perception. In L. Berkowitz (Ed.), *Advances in experimental social psychology* (Vol. 2). New York: Academic Press.

Jones, E. E., Davis, K., & Gergen, K. (1961). Role playing variations and their informational value for person perception. *Journal of Abnormal and Social Psychology, 63,* 302–310.

Katz, D., & Braly, K. (1933). Racial stereotypes in one hundred college students. *Journal of Abnormal and Social Psychology, 28,* 280–290.

Keenan, J. M., & Baillet, S. D. (1980). Memory for personally and socially significant events. In R. S. Nickerson (Ed.), *Attention and performance* (Vol. 7). Hillsdale, NJ: Erlbaum.

Kelley, H. H. (1967). Attribution theory in social psychology. In D. Levine (Ed.), *Nebraska symposium on motivation* (Vol. 15, pp. 192–238).

Kelley, H. H. (1971). Causal schemata and the attribution process. In E. Jones, D. Kanouse, H. Kelley, R. Nisbett, S. Valins, & B. Weiner (Eds.), *Attribution: Perceiving the causes of behavior.* Morristown, NJ: General Learning Press.

Klein, S. B., & Kihlstrom, J. F. (1986). Elaboration, organization and the self-reference effect in memory. *Journal of Experimental Psychology: General, 115,* 26–38.

Klein, S. B., & Loftus, J. B. (1988). The nature of self-referent encoding: The contributions of elaborative and organizational processes. *Journal of Personality and Social Psychology, 55,* 5–11.

Klein, S. R., & Loftus, J. (1990). Rethinking the role of organization in person memory: An independent trace storage model. *Journal of Personality and Social Psychology, 59,* 400–410.

Klein, S. B., & Loftus, J. (1993). The mental representation of trait and behavioral knowledge about the self. In T. K. Srull & R. S. Wyer (Eds.), *Advances in social cognition, Vol. 5: The mental representation of trait and behavioral knowledge about the self.* Hillsdale, NJ: Erlbaum.

Klein, S. B., Loftus, J. B., & Burton, H. A. (1989). Two self-reference effects: The importance of distinguishing between self-descriptiveness judgments and autobiographical retrieval in self-referent encoding. *Journal of Personality and Social Psychology, 56,* 853–865.

Klinger, E. (1975). Consequences of commitment to and disengagement from incentives. *Psychological Review, 82,* 1–25.

Lambert, A. J., & Wyer, R. S. (1990). *Stereotypes and social judgment: The effect of typicality and perceived heterogeneity.* Unpublished manuscript, University of Illinois at Urbana-Champaign.

Levin, S. R., Wyer, R. S., & Schwarz, N. (1987). *Are you what you feel? The affective and cognitive determinants of self esteem.* Unpublished manuscript, University of Illinois at Urbana-Champaign.

Locksley, A., Hepburn, C., & Ortiz, V. (1982). Social stereotypes and judgments of individuals: An instance of the base-rate fallacy. *Journal of Experimental Social Psychology, 18,* 23–42.

Lombardi, W. J., Higgins, E. T., & Bargh, J. A. (1987). The role of consciousness in priming effects on categorization. *Personality and Social Psychology Bulletin, 13,* 411–429.

McGuire, W. J., & McGuire, C. V. (1987). Content and process in the experience of self. In L. Berkowitz (Ed.), *Advances in experimental social psychology* (Vol. 20). New York: Academic Press.

McGuire, W. J., & Padawer-Singer, A. (1976). Trait salience in the spontaneous self-concept. *Journal of Personality and Social Psychology, 33,* 743–754.

Manis, M., Nelson, T. E., & Shedler, J. (1988). Stereotypes and social judgment: Extremity, assimilation, and contrast. *Journal of Personality and Social Psychology, 55,* 28–36.

Markus, H. (1977). Self schemas and processing information about the self. *Journal of Personality and Social Psychology, 35,* 63–78.
Markus, H., & Sentis, K. (1982). The self in social information processing. In J. Suls (Ed.), *Psychological perspectives on the self* (Vol. 1). Hillsdale, NJ: Erlbaum.
Martin, L. L. (1986). Set/Reset: The use and disuse of concepts in impression formation. *Journal of Personality and Social Psychology, 51,* 493–504.
Mead, G. H. (1934). *Mind, self, and society.* Chicago: University of Chicago Press.
Mischel, W. (1968). *Personality and assessment.* New York: Wiley.
Nisbett, R. E., & Ross, L. (1980). *Human inference: Strategies and shortcoming of social judgment.* Englewood Cliffs, NJ: Prentice-Hall.
Petty, R. E., & Cacioppo, J. T. (1986). *Communication and persuasion: Central and peripheral routes to attitude change.* New York: Springer-Verlag.
Reeder, G. D., & Brewer, M. B. (1979). A schematic model of dispositional attribution in interpersonal perception. *Psychological Review, 86,* 61–79.
Regan, D., & Totten, J. (1975). Empathy and attribution: Turning observers into actors. *Journal of Personality and Social Psychology, 32,* 850–856.
Riggle, E. D., Ottati, V. C., Wyer, R. S., Kuklinski, J., & Schwarz, N. (1989). *Bases of political judgments: The role of a candidate's physical attractiveness, party membership, and voting record.* Unpublished manuscript, University of Illinois at Urbana-Champaign.
Rogers, T. B., Kuiper, N. A., & Kirker, W. S. (1977). Self-reference and the encoding of personal information. *Journal of Personality and Social Psychology, 35,* 677–688.
Rosenberg, S., & Sedlak, A. (1972). Structural representations of implicit personality theory. In L. Berkowitz (Ed.), *Advances in experimental social psychology* (Vol. 10). New York: Academic Press.
Ross, L. (1977). The intuitive psychologist and his shortcomings: Distortions in the attribution process. In L. Berkowitz (Ed.), *Advances in experimental social psychology* (Vol. 10). New York: Academic Press.
Salancik, G. R. (1974). Inference of one's attitude from behavior recalled under linguistically manipulated cognitive sets. *Journal of Experimental Social Psychology, 10,* 415–427.
Salancik, G. R., & Calder, B. J. (1974). *A non-predispositional information analysis of attitude expressions.* Unpublished manuscript, University of Illinois at Urbana-Champaign.
Schneider, D. J. (1973). Implicit personality theory: A review. *Psychological Bulletin, 79,* 294–319.
Schneider, D. J., Hastorf, A. H., & Ellsworth, P. C. (1979). *Person perception.* Reading, MA: Addison-Wesley.
Schwarz, N., & Clore, G. L. (1983). Mood, misattribution, and judgments of well-being: Informative and directive functions of affective states. *Journal of Personality and Social Psychology, 45,* 513–523.
Schwarz, N., & Clore, G. L. (1987). How do I feel about it? The informative function of affective states. In K. Fiedler & J. Forgas (Eds.), *Affect, cognition and social behavior.* Toronto: Hogrefe International.
Scott, C. K., Fuhrman, R. W., & Wyer, R. S. (1991). Information processing in close relationships. In G. O. Fletcher & F. D. Fincham (Eds.), *Cognition in close relationships.* Hillsdale, NJ: Erlbaum.
Secord, P. F., Backman, C. W., & Eachus, H. T. (1964). Effects of imbalance in the self-concept on the perception of persons. *Journal of Abnormal and Social Psychology, 68,* 442–446.
Seta, C. E., & Seta, J. J. (1990). Identifying the sources of social actions: The role of source cues in person memory. *Journal of Personality and Social Psychology, 58,* 779–790.
Sherman, S. J., Judd, C. M., & Park, B. (1989). Social cognition. *Annual Review of Psychology, 40,* 281–326.
Smith, E. R. (1990). Content and process specificity in the effects of prior experiences. In T. K. Srull & R. S. Wyer (Eds.), *Advances in social cognition, Vol. 3: Content and process specificity in the effects of prior experiences.* Hillsdale, NJ: Erlbaum.

Smith, E. R., & Zárate, M. A. (1992). Exemplar-based model of social judgment. *Psychological Review, 99,* 3–21.

Snyder, M. (1974). Self-monitoring of expressive behavior. *Journal of Personality and Social Psychology, 30,* 526–537.

Snyder, M., & Swann, W. B. (1978). Behavioral confirmation in social interaction: From social perception to social reality. *Journal of Experimental Social Psychology, 14,* 148–162.

Snyder, M., Tanke, E. D., & Berscheid, E. (1977). Social perception and interpersonal behavior: On the self-fulfilling nature of social stereotypes. *Journal of Personality and Social Psychology, 35,* 656–666.

Sorrentino, R. M., & Higgins, E. T. (Eds.). (1986). *Handbook of motivation and cognition.* New York: Guilford Press.

Srull, T. K., & Wyer, R. S. (1979). The role of category accessibility in the interpretation of information about persons: Some determinants and implications. *Journal of Personality and Social Psychology, 37,* 1660–1672.

Srull, T. K., & Wyer, R. S. (1980). Category accessibility and social perception: Some implications for the study of person memory and interpersonal judgment. *Journal of Personality and Social Psychology, 38,* 841–856.

Srull, T. K., & Wyer, R. S. (1989). Person memory and judgment. *Psychological Review, 96,* 58–83.

Steiner, I. D. (1968). Reactions to adverse and favorable evaluations of one's self. *Journal of Personality, 36,* 553–563.

Storms, M. (1973). Videotape and the attribution process: Reversing actors' and observers' point of view. *Journal of Personality and Social Psychology, 27,* 165–175.

Strack, F., Schwarz, N., & Gschneidinger, E. (1985). Happiness and reminiscing: The role of time perspective, affect, and mode of thinking. *Journal of Personality and Social Psychology, 49,* 1460–1469.

Tajfel, H. (1970). Experiments in intergroup discrimination. *Scientific American, 223,* 96–102.

Trope, Y. (1986). Identification and inferential processes in dispositional attribution. *Psychological Review, 93,* 239–257.

Winter, L., Uleman, J. S., & Cunniff, C. (1985). How automatic are social judgments? *Journal of Personality and Social Psychology, 49,* 904–917.

Wishner, J. (1960). Reanalysis of "Impressions of personality." *Psychological Review, 67,* 96–112.

Wyer, R. S. (1968). The effects of information redundancy on evaluations of social stimuli. *Psychonomic Science, 13,* 245–246.

Wyer, R. S. (1970). Information redundancy, inconsistency and novelty and their role in impression formation. *Journal of Experimental Social Psychology, 6,* 111–127.

Wyer, R. S. (1973). The effects of information inconsistency and grammatical context on evaluations of persons. *Journal of Personality and Social Psychology, 25,* 45–49.

Wyer, R. S. (1974). Changes in meaning and halo effects in personality impression formation. *Journal of Personality and Social Psychology, 29,* 829–835.

Wyer, R. S., & Budesheim, T. L. (1987). Person memory and judgments: The impact of information that one is told to disregard. *Journal of Personality and Social Psychology, 53,* 14–29.

Wyer, R. S., & Carlston, D. E. (1979). *Social cognition, inference and attribution.* Hillsdale, NJ: Erlbaum.

Wyer, R. S., & Gordon, S. E. (1982). The recall of information about persons and groups. *Journal of Experimental Social Psychology, 18,* 128–164.

Wyer, R. S., Henninger, M., & Wolfson, M. R. (1975). Informational determinants of females' self-perceptions and observers' perceptions of them in an achievement situation. *Journal of Personality and Social Psychology, 32,* 556–570.

Wyer, R. S., & Srull, T. K. (1984). *Handbook of social cognition* (Vols. 1–3). Hillsdale, NJ: Erlbaum.

Wyer, R. S., Srull, T. K., & Gordon, S. E. (1984). The effects of predicting a person's behavior on subsequent trait judgments. *Journal of Experimental Social Psychology, 20,* 29–46.

Wyer, R. S., & Srull, T. K. (1986). Human cognition in its social context. *Psychological Review, 93,* 322–359.

Wyer, R. S., & Srull, T. K. (1989). *memory and cognition in its social context.* Hillsdale, NJ: Erlbaum.

Wyer, R. S., & Unverzagt, W. H. (1985). The effects of instructions to disregard information on its subsequent recall and use in making judgments. *Journal of Personality and Social Psychology, 48,* 533–549.

Wyer, R. S., & Watson, S. F. (1969). Context effects in impression formation. *Journal of Personality and Social Psychology, 12,* 22–33.

6

Social Cognition of the Self

Patricia W. Linville
Donal E. Carlston

The "social cognition of the self" represents the intersection of the most pervasive approach in the field today (Wyer & Srull, 1984) with one of the most persistent domains of study in the field (cf. Sherman, Judd, & Park, 1989). Even the casual crossing of two such endeavors would necessarily command attention, and in the present instance, the juncture has been characterized as something special. Markus and Zajonc (1985), for example, suggest that self-concept theory is one of several important areas where the cognitive approach to social psychology has led directly to significant theoretical advances. Moreover, they argue that the cognitive approach has returned the self-concept to "the realm of legitimate empirical study." From this point of view, then, the joining of social cognition and self creates an avenue of study that reaches further than either field could have by itself.

Alternatively, a cynic might note that self research has encountered a number of new approaches in its long history, and that it has passed by each without much change in direction. In some ways, this history could be characterized as "one concept's search for self-definition." Along the way, self-concept has been understood as an attitude, a personality dimension, and a multidimensional structure. Currently, in keeping with the times, it is viewed as a schema, a prototype, a categorical structure, or an associative network. Will these current reconceptualizations represent important advances, or are they merely additional milestones along the road to self-understanding?

We will ultimately conclude that the merging of social cognition and self has led the field in fruitful new directions. But it is important to examine this conclusion carefully and critically, because, as we will suggest in our closing remarks, the contributions of social cognition may not be those that first come to mind. The general aim of our chapter is to consider how the theoretical and methodological developments known as "social cognition" have influenced how we conceive of and do research on the self.[1] One general theme that emerges is that issues of structure and content are inseparable from considerations of process. Assumptions about mental representations (structures) cannot be tested in isolation from assumptions about the cognitive processes that operate on those structures (Anderson, 1983; Barsalou, 1990). The social cognition approach provides both theoretical constructs and experimental tools for investigating the link between cognitive processes and the structure or content of knowledge about the self. It has also led to a much greater emphasis on process aspects of self cognition.

We begin this chapter by considering work on the self prior to the social cognition era. Then we consider the impact of social cognition on enduring issues of self, as well as its influence on the advent of new issues. We close by considering the conventional wisdom regarding the contributions of the social cognition approach.

HISTORICAL VIEW OF THE SELF

This history is a selective account of some major events in the psychological study of the self. Its primary objective is to provide a context for recent social cognition work on the self by reviewing the origin of some recurrent issues regarding the self, showing a transition from concerns with content to concerns with the interaction of content and process, noting some important methodological developments in self research, and highlighting the regularity with which the self gets reconceptualized in terms of the dominant concepts in social psychology.

Presocial Cognition Conceptualizations of Self

Most reviewers begin the modern history of self research with the century-old writings of William James (1890, 1910). James advanced the distinction between the self as knower and the self as that which is known, and tried to reconcile the two by conceiving of self as the stream of consciousness. Later, Allport (1955, 1961) would struggle with the idea of self as knower, first (1955) admitting it as the eighth facet of his self-structure, the proprium, but later (1961) banishing it as a theoretical homunculus. Recently there has been a renewed interest in process issues relating to the self as knower, which may partially reflect the availability of more concrete cognitive concepts (e.g., procedural knowledge) for understanding process.

[1]We benefited greatly from recent insightful reviews of the self literature (Greenwald & Pratkanis, 1984; Higgins & Bargh, 1987; Kihlstrom & Cantor, 1984; Kihlstrom et al., 1988; Markus & Wurf, 1987; Sherman, Judd, & Park, 1989; Fiske & Taylor, 1991; Wyer & Srull, 1989) as well as classic reviews (e.g., Gergen, 1971; Gordon & Gergen, 1967).

However, content issues relating to the "self as known" have engaged most attention during the past century. James identified three main components of this "empirical" self: the material, the social, and the spiritual. The latter two components have been prominently reflected in subsequent studies of the contents of the self-concept from a variety of different perspectives (e.g., Higgins, 1987; Jourard, 1964; McGuire, 1984; Wylie, 1974). More important, in advancing the notion of multiple selves, James anticipated questions regarding the complexity and the accessibility of self-conceptions that have since occupied much attention.

The impetus that the early writings of James (1890) and Cooley (1902) gave to self-studies was largely squelched by the ascendance of behaviorism (cf. Allport, 1943; Gordon & Gergen, 1968). During this dry spell, the concept of self was kept alive primarily in psychoanalytic approaches to personality (Freud, 1920), in the writings of sociologists (Mead, 1934), and in the writings of advocates such as Hilgard (1949), Rogers (1942), and Sherif and Cantril (1947).

From 1943 into the next decade, Allport encouraged the "[re]admittance of the ego to good standing in psychology" (p. 476), arguing for an approach to the self that would advance scientific progress through careful definition and discrimination of the concepts of self (1955, p. 37). Such pleas may have failed to stimulate sustained programs of research primarily because appropriate research methods had not yet been developed (Greenwald & Pratkanis, 1984).

The first half of the 1950s saw the emergence of several major approaches to the self that were centered on self-concept measurement. Research on self-esteem used a variety of structured self-report measures and found it to be somewhat related to a range of behaviors (see Wylie, 1974, for reviews). Other measures of self-concept developed during this era included the Q-sort (Rogers, 1951) and open-ended measures such as the "Who Are You?" test (Bugental & Zelen, 1950) and the "Twenty Statement" or "Who Am I?" questionnaire (Kuhn & McPartland, 1954). Although these latter measures provided a potentially rich reservoir of data on self-conceptions (e.g., Gordon, 1968), studies rarely exploited this potential until McGuire and Padawer-Singer's (1976) work on attribute distinctiveness in the spontaneous self-concept.

The prevalent conceptualizations during this era were of self as personality trait (e.g., Brownfain, 1952) and self as attitude (e.g., Kuhn & McPartland, 1954), although the latter metaphor was rarely pursued rigorously. Another conceptualization was Kelly's (1955) personal construct theory, which anticipated theoretical aspects of the social cognition approach, but preceded the methodological developments adequate to investigate them.

The next fifteen years saw continued emphasis on self-concept measurement and on self-esteem, the publication of several important books (e.g., Gordon & Gergen, 1968), and initiation of research on the public self including self-presentation (Goffman, 1959; Gergen, 1965; Jones, 1964) and self-disclosure (Jourard, 1958; Taylor & Oberlander, 1969). If any consensual conception of self existed in this era when impression formation research was taking root, it was self as impression, either formed about oneself or presented to others.

The 1970s saw an explosion of work directly or indirectly dealing with the self, including research on Bem's self-perception theory (1972), self-consciousness (Fenigstein, Scheier, & Buss, 1975), self-monitoring (Snyder, 1979), self-awareness (Duval & Wicklund, 1972), and attributional ego-defensiveness (Bradley [Weary], 1978). During the first half of the decade, the primary conceptualization of self was arguably the self as an attributional system.

The Social Cognition Approach to Self

The social cognition approach evolved in the latter half of the 1970s and achieved tangible credentials near the turn of the decade. These include the publication of several books on the topic (Wyer & Carlston, 1979; Hastie et al., 1980; Higgins, Herman, & Zanna, 1981), the designation of a subsection of the *Journal of Personality and Social Psychology* as "Attitudes and Social Cognition" in 1980, and establishment of the journal *Social Cognition* in 1982.

The social cognition perspective emerged simultaneously and independently in many places (see Wyer & Srull, 1984; Ostrom, 1984, for discussions). A number of different social psychologists began applying the concepts, theories, and methods of experimental cognitive psychology to issues arising in areas such as person perception, impression formation, stereotyping, attribution theory, and attitude change. Cognitive psychologists also moved toward realms of social psychology as their own work began to emphasize meaningful real-world materials and phenomena (cf. Holyoak & Gordon, 1984; Neisser, 1982; Wyer & Srull, 1984, preface). In the years that followed, social cognition researchers from these disciplines have increasingly collaborated and published in each others' journals, creating a truly hybrid discipline.

It is this hybrid discipline, and the orientation that it reflects, that we refer to as "social cognition." Schneider (1991) characterizes this approach in terms of three basic assumptions. First, the approach tends to emphasize cognitive process, which is assumed to be general and fundamental, regardless of particular content. This implies an equivalence between social and other forms of cognition (but see also Ostrom, 1984). Second, social cognition models adopt the general information processing model, in which memory plays a prominent role. Third, the encoding, storage, and retrieval of information is viewed as substantially affected by preexisting knowledge structures such as schemata, prototypes, scripts, and the like. These assumptions, in one form or another, underlie most of the work we review here.

The social cognition approach placed an early emphasis on the information processing effects of self. For example, research demonstrated that self-descriptive stimuli are attended to automatically (Bargh, 1982), processed quickly and confidently (e.g., Markus, 1977; Kuiper & Rogers, 1979; Mueller, 1982), and remembered readily (e.g., Bower & Gilligan, 1979; Kuiper & Rogers, 1979). Moreover, people make more confident behavioral predictions, attributions, and inferences in self-relevant domains (e.g., Markus, Crane, Bernstein, & Siladi, 1982; Andersen & Ross, 1984); and they make self-relevant judgments relatively quickly (Markus, 1977; Markus et al. 1982) or slowly (Kuiper, 1981; Markus, Hamill, & Sentis, 1987), depending on the novelty or complexity of the judgment to be make (Fiske & Taylor, 1991). The self may also affect the processing of information about other people (Fong & Markus, 1982) and the inferences made about them (Holmes, 1968; Ross, Greene, & House, 1977), although evidence for the latter is largely indirect. More generally, some argued that aspects of the self are inherently involved in the formation of episodic memories (Tulving, 1985; Greenwald, 1980). During this era, the self began to be conceptualized in terms of cognitive concepts such as schemata (Markus, 1977), prototypes (e.g., Kuiper, 1981; Rogers, 1981), associative networks (e.g., Bower & Gilligan, 1979) and hierarchical structures (Rogers, Kuiper, & Kirker, 1977). The social cognition work from this time into the 1980s is the focus of the remainder of this chapter.

Summarizing the History of Self

During each historical period, the self has been reconceptualized in terms of the concepts that were in vogue in social psychology as a whole. In this respect, social cognition conceptions are arguably only the latest in a long series of viewpoints that have taken hold first in other areas of social psychology, then emerged as reconceptualizations of the self. In a sense, then, the field has long been preoccupied with finding an appropriate way to conceptualize self. The most central and enduring issue in this area is reflected in the question: "What is the self?" We find it more useful to address this issue through a number of more specific questions that it subsumes, for example: Is there one self or many? Is the self stable or malleable? Is the self an ordinary construct or a unique one?

IMPACT OF SOCIAL COGNITION ON ENDURING ISSUES OF SELF

One way of measuring the impact of social cognition is to consider its influence on enduring issues of self. Another is to consider its influence on the advent of new issues. We begin with the enduring issues. These include whether the self is best characterized as unitary or multiple, as "knower or the known," and as stable or malleable (see Gordon & Gergen, 1968;

Gergen, 1971; Greenwald & Pratkanis, 1984). As we will see, current progress on these enduring issues derives in part from the influence of three key assumptions. (1) *Multiple selves:* The self is best viewed as consisting of multiple components, rather than as single and monolithic. (2) *Declarative plus procedural self-knowledge:* Self-perceptions and behavior are based not only on declarative (factual) knowledge of the self, but also on cognitive procedures (rules) for self-relevant inferences, evaluation, problem solving, and decision making. From this perspective, self-oriented processes involve the interaction of self as knower and known. (3) *Shifting activation:* We can understand the changing as well as stable nature of self by understanding the shifting activation of different aspects of self-knowledge. These three assumptions focus attention on a connection between cognitive structure and process, providing new perspectives on three classic issues regarding the self.

1. Is the Self Unitary or Multiple? The Role of Contextual Selves

The Debate

The debate over whether people have a single self or multiple selves has recurred regularly during the history of the self-concept. One early view pictured a single, unitary self (e.g., Allport, 1955; Rogers, 1951; Snygg & Combs, 1949). This view was reflected in self-esteem research (e.g., Wylie, 1961), which assumed that people have a single, global self-concept about which they feel good or bad. The unitary conception is also evident in a few more recent social cognitive models such as Rogers' (1977) concept of a single, prototypic self.

William James (1890) was an early proponent of the notion that people have multiple selves, identifying three aspects of the "self as known." The *material self* represents what we physically are and possess, the *social self* comprises our awareness of self as others see us, and the *spiritual self* reflects awareness of our thinking and feeling. Later, Gordon Allport (1943, 1955) proposed eight self-components, including *self-identity, self-enhancement, bodily sensations, self-extensions* identifying with people, groups, and possessions, *self-image* of current attributes and future ideals, *rational agent* balancing inner needs and outer reality through mental activities such as problem solving and coping, *future-directed strivings* or motivations, and the *knower* which monitors or experiences the other selves. More recently, Greenwald and Breckler (1985) identified four facets of the self tied to different ego-tasks, each providing a distinct basis for self-evaluation—a *diffuse self* seeking positive affect, a *public self* seeking others' approval, a *private self* with internalized evaluative standards, and a *collective self* with internalized goals of reference groups. The concept of multiplicity in these writings more accurately reflects *multiple functions* or components of a unitary self-conception rather than multiple contextual self-concepts.

Other early perspectives characterized multiplicity in terms of social selves connected to significant others or social roles (e.g., Gergen, 1971; Goffman, 1959). James (1890, p. 294) proposed that "a man has as many social selves as there are distinct groups of persons about whose opinion he cares." Similarly, sociologists suggested that people come to think about themselves in terms of others' views of themselves (Cooley, 1902; Mead, 1934). These proposals anticipated issues regarding the complexity and malleability of self-concepts as well as issues of self-presentation.

Most contemporary cognitive models have similarly adopted some assumption of multiple selves (e.g., Deaux, 1993; Higgins, 1987; Kihlstrom & Cantor, 1984; Kihlstrom et al., 1988; Linville, 1985, 1987; Markus, 1977; Markus & Nurius, 1986; Wyer & Srull, 1989). There has been a shift over time, however, in the nature of multiple selves. The social cognition perspective characterizes these multiple selves somewhat differently than did earlier approaches. First, it assumes that self-knowledge is cognitively organized in the same manner as knowledge of other cognitive domains. Second, these models take at least a beginning step toward specifying the memory and judgment processes that act on the representation of these multiple selves. Third, although earlier notions of multiplicity reflected different functions of self, recent notions tend to reflect *multiple contexts* of self. In other words, self-knowledge may be organized around specific contexts of one's life.

For example, Markus (1977) describes a system of personally relevant attribute schemas, each representing an important characteristic and its associated behaviors (e.g., extravert). Linville (1985, 1987) conceives of multiple self-aspects representing different contexts of experience (e.g., student, friend, at home, in small social gatherings). Kihlstrom and Cantor (1984) suggest a hierarchy of context-specific self-prototypes (e.g., self with mother vs. father vs. spouse). These approaches commonly assume that only a subset of selves will be active in cognition at any given time. A parallel movement in sociology focused on multiple identities or roles (e.g., parent, spouse, worker) (e.g., Burke, 1980; Stryker, 1980; Thoits, 1983). Thus, theoretical as well as empirical support for the concept of multiple selves has grown in the social cognitive era.

Theorists have identified several basic dimensions along which multiple self-concepts may vary. A *temporal* dimension reflecting past, present, and future selves (e.g., Gordon, 1968; Higgins, 1987; Rosenberg, 1979) can play motivational as well as emotional roles. For example, a future self representing what one hopes or fears one will become may provide both the motive and guide for specific behaviors (Higgins, 1987; James, 1910; Markus & Nurius, 1986; Showers & Cantor, 1985), and a past self may act as a reference point, influencing how satisfied one is with a current self (Strack, Schwarz, & Gschneidinger, 1985). A *centrality* dimension reflects the relative importance of different selves, with some being core selves and others being more peripheral (Gergen, 1968; Markus & Wurf, 1987; Stryker, 1980, 1986). An *evaluative* dimension reflects the fact that some self-concepts are relatively positive, some are more negative, and still others are evaluatively mixed (Linville, 1985, 1987; Showers, 1992a).

Implications of Multiple Selves for Issues of Self

The assumption that people have multiple selves has implications for classical as well as contemporary issues of self. Several of these are elaborated in later sections. First, the concept of multiple selves has different implications within different models of representation, for example, multiple self-schemas, self-bins, self-domains in associative network models, and prototype versus exemplar models of categorization. Second, the concept of multiple selves implies that the content and organization of self-knowledge is in part contextual. This explains how people represent the variability of their behavior along a given feature (e.g., one may be anxious at work yet relaxed around the kids). It also implies that inconsistent self-attributes can coexist—if they are parts of different selves (e.g., one may be competitive at sports but cooperative at work). The issue remains whether there is a general self that coexists apart from contextually specific selves. Third, the concept of multiple selves implies that interconnections among different selves are important. This raises structural issues (e.g., Are self-traits linked together? Are self-traits and their behavioral episodes linked?) as well as affective ones (e.g., What patterns of interconnectedness are characteristic of emotional vulnerability?). Fourth, the concept of multiple selves implies that momentary attention shifts from one self to another. Thus the self is dynamic rather than static, changeable as well as stable. This also implies that self-attention is focused on context-specific selves rather than on the self per se.

Representation of Multiple Selves in Different Cognitive Models

What has the social cognition approach contributed to this gelatinous yet heuristic concept of multiple selves? As we have seen, there has been a shift from relatively vague concepts (e.g., material, social, spiritual selves) to current conceptions of multiple structures that reflect specific self-contexts, domains, or central attributes. Here we elaborate how the concept "multiple selves" might be represented in several specific memory models. Each of these models gives specific meaning to the construct of multiple selves. Each offers at least a first step toward specifying memory (and in some cases judgment) processes that are applied to these self-representations.

Associative Network Models Associative memory network models typically represent self-knowledge as a set of propositions linking a "self node" to specific self-relevant episodes or attributes (e.g., Bower & Gilligan, 1979; Kihlstrom & Cantor, 1984). For example, in a simplified network model, a self node is associatively linked to trait concepts ("athletic," "adventuresome"), behavioral concepts ("play tennis often," "traveled to Nepal"), and other self-defining information ("like classic rock"). Much of this self-knowledge may be organized around domain concepts ("self as researcher,"

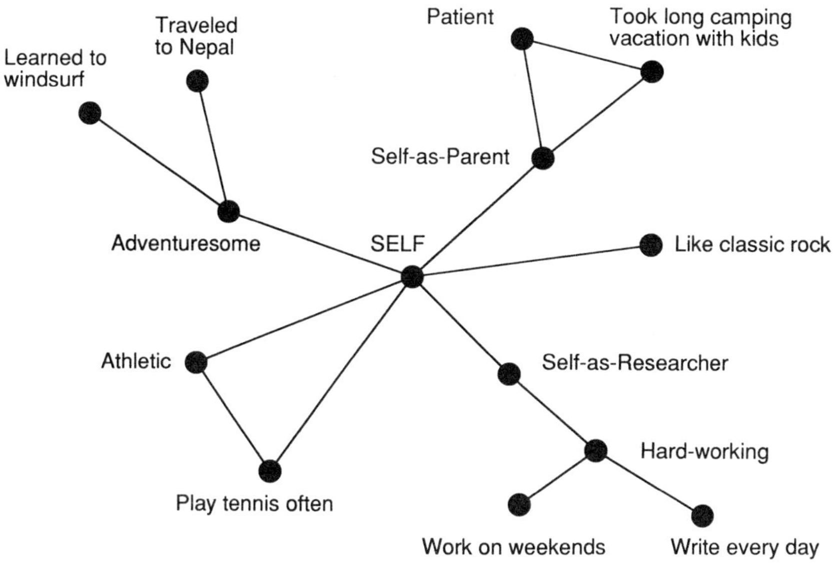

FIGURE 1.
An associative network representation of self-knowledge.

"self as parent"), consistent with the concept of multiple selves. A network representation allows associative links between various parts of self-knowledge (see Figure 1)—for example, traits linked with behaviors ("work on weekends" is associated with "hard working"); traits and behaviors linked with a domain ("hard working" is associated with "self as researcher"); traits linked with other traits and behaviors with other behaviors; the general semantic knowledge ("researchers do experiments and write papers") linked with self-knowledge. Schematic traits may be those directly linked to a central "self" node in a network model (e.g., "adventuresome"), accounting for subjects' quick access and response to questions regarding schematic traits (Kihlstrom et al., 1988). In a semantic network, retrieval of self-knowledge occurs via spreading activation (Anderson, 1983). For example, asking subjects to judge themselves in terms of specific attributes activates the corresponding nodes in memory. Activation then spreads from activated nodes along connecting paths to nodes representing associated knowledge.

Bin Model Wyer and Srull's (1989) bin model involves concept bins in which information is sequentially stored and retrieved. Multiple selves may be represented as multiple self-bins, each with a header describing a specific domain of experience such as "self as father" or "self at parties." Each bin may include abstract trait information as well as individual behaviors. In addition to context-specific self-bins, a general self-bin may exist containing features associated with the self in general. Units of information in any bin are stored and retrieved independently from one another. Thus the subset of self-knowledge retrieved at the moment depends on the specific probe as well as on which information is near the top of that self-bin. Factors such as priming or recent use of a concept lead self-information to be near the top of its storage bin and thus more accessible.

Self-Schemas Schemas and related abstract knowledge structures (e.g., scripts, frames, prototypes) have played a major explanatory role in most of the social cognitive areas represented in this book (e.g., person perception, stereotyping, attitudes, affect, attribution). The schema concept has also proven heuristic in understanding the structure and processing of self-knowledge, and it may be credited in part for revitalizing current interest in the self (Markus, 1977; Rogers et al., 1977).

A schema is an abstract knowledge structure that represents the typical features of a domain. Schemas guide the selection of incoming information and the abstraction of its meaning. They also guide interpretation by filling in missing features and by distorting other features to make them schema consistent. Finally, schemas integrate incoming with prior information to generate a single, unified representation (see Alba & Hasher, 1983, for a critical review).

Investigators differ in how they characterize and measure the self-schema construct. Rogers et al. (1977) conceptualize a single, stable self-schema or list of traits and behaviors that helps organize and interpret incoming information. Beck proposes a similar concept of a unitary depressive schema consisting of negative beliefs about the self and the world that negatively distorts the meaning of self-relevant information, resulting in negative emotional experience (Beck, Rush, Shaw, & Emery, 1979).

Markus' (1977) emphasis on a system of self-schemas elaborates the concept of multiple selves. A self-schema, or cognitive generalization about the self, contains trait and behavioral information about a personally descriptive and important attribute. For example, "independent" schematics perceive themselves to be extremely independent and consider being independent to be important, whereas aschematics do not perceive themselves as either independent or dependent, or they consider the attribute to be unimportant. Self-schemas result in the efficient processing of relevant information. For example, "independent" schematics have well-organized and highly accessible knowledge about their independence, resulting in rapid access and efficient processing of information. Schematics make quick and confident judgments or predictions about their schematic trait, easily retrieve examples, and resist evidence contrary to their self-schema (e.g., Markus, 1977; Markus et al., 1982).

Self-schemas may be organized around attributes (e.g., sociable) or social relationships (e.g., self-as-spouse). Markus and Kitayama (1991) suggest that the tendency to view the self in terms of relationships is greater in Asian cultures, which emphasize the interdependence of self and others, whereas the tendency to view the self in terms of internal attributes is greater in Northern European and North American cultures, which emphasize the role of the self as independent agent.

Prototype Models Self-knowledge can be represented within categorization models. Two broad classes are prototype and exemplar models (Smith & Medin, 1981). According to simple prototype models, knowledge of a category is represented by a list of prototypic feature values summarizing the central tendency of the category (e.g., Posner & Keele, 1968; Reed, 1972). Categorization judgments are based on the similarity of new instances to the prototype. From the self-as-prototype perspective, the self may be represented by a summary list of most typical or modal self-characteristics including traits, attitudes, and typical behavior (e.g., Kihlstrom & Cantor, 1984; Kuiper, 1981; Rogers, 1981).

The self as a stable prototype acts as a fixed reference point enabling efficient self-relevant judgments. For example, when judging the self-descriptiveness of traits, the prototype becomes active, and those that fit the prototype are easily integrated into the prototype and thus better recalled. Consequently, self-descriptive traits are better recalled than those not self-descriptive, and traits rated in a self-referent task ("Describes you?") are better recalled than those rated in other tasks such as semantic tasks ("Means the same as XXX?") (Rogers et al., 1977).

Additional findings supporting the self-as-prototype model include faster judgment times for highly self-descriptive and highly non-self-descriptive traits than for moderately self-descriptive traits (e.g., Klein, Loftus, Trafton, & Fuhrman, 1992; Kuiper, 1981), and an increase in false alarm rates (identifying an unpresented adjective as one previously presented) as traits became more self-descriptive (Rogers, Kuiper, & Rogers, 1979). However, a self-as-prototype model cannot easily account for self-reference results found in episodic, autobiographical retrieval tasks (see Greenwald & Pratkanis, 1984; Higgins & Bargh, 1987; Klein, Loftus, & Burton, 1989).

One difficulty with a simple prototype model of self-knowledge is that there is no natural way of representing contextual information (e.g., myself as a researcher, teacher, father). A related difficulty is that there is no natural characterization of feature variability such as being sociable with close friends, shy in unfamiliar groups, and distant with colleagues.[2] One way of representing multiple selves is within a more complex prototype model such

[2]One strategy for capturing variability information within a prototype framework is to assume that self-prototypes encode variability information as well as information about most typical characteristics. This approach has been used to model beliefs about variability within social groups (Park & Hastie, 1987; Judd & Park, 1988). However, this approach does not really capture the notion of the clustering of self-knowledge into distinct contexts of the self such as "self at work" or "self with family."

as Kihlstrom and Cantor's (1984) hierarchical prototype model containing a general self-prototype at a superordinate level, with contextual self-prototypes abstracted from specific situations at a subordinate level (e.g., self with acquaintances vs. friends).

Multiple Exemplar Models According to multiple exemplar models, knowledge of a category is represented by a collection of memory traces representing exemplars of the category (e.g., Hintzman, 1986; Medin & Schaffer, 1978; Nosofsky, 1986). Categorization judgments are based on the similarity of new instances to specific stored exemplars. Knowledge of a domain consists largely of a set of specific memory traces corresponding to prior experiences in that domain. If those experiences have been variable, then memory naturally represents variability. If the experiences fall into a variety of contexts, then memory naturally incorporates context. Exemplar models explain a variety of categorization phenomena (e.g., sensitivity to context and to correlations among attributes) that are not predicted by classical prototype models (Smith & Medin, 1981).

Although exemplar models have been applied in the stereotyping and intergroup perception literature (e.g., Linville, Fischer, & Salovey, 1989; Linville & Fischer, 1993; Smith & Zarate, 1992), there has been little application to issues of self-representation. In a multiple exemplar model, knowledge of the self is represented by a large set of self-exemplars or instances. Each self-exemplar might consist of a list or string of attributes or propositions describing the self and the context. Some exemplars might describe specific episodic memories. Others might describe context-specific generalizations about the self. Structure is imposed on this huge store of self-memories in the process of retrieving information from long-term memory. For example, to retrieve knowledge relevant to a specific role or context, one might form the memory probe <self, school> which would activate memory traces that include both concepts; for example, <self, school, A in geometry> and <self, school, rebellious, disagreed with teacher's politics>. To retrieve information about oneself as a family member, a different probe is needed, such as <self, family>, which would activate a different set of exemplars in memory. In this manner, an exemplar representation allows one to retrieve and structure information about the self along many dimensions (e.g., situations, traits, time periods) depending on task demands, and to represent variability about the self within each context. Thus, multiple exemplar representations hold considerable promise for representing knowledge of a multifaceted and variable self.

These examples illustrate an important property of exemplar models. An exemplar may encode details regarding specific behavioral episodes ("I disagreed with my teacher about politics"), abstracted trait information about the self ("I am rebellious at school"), or both. These abstractions may be generated on-line by the actor or suggested by others at the time. Some researchers have interpreted exemplar models more narrowly as applying only to specific behavioral episodes (e.g., Klein & Loftus, 1993), but exemplar models have routinely been interpreted as encoding abstracted properties of instances or subtypes of a category (e.g., Medin, 1989; Nosofksy, 1986; Smith & Medin, 1981, pp. 144–146).

It seems likely that people extract the typical features of sets of experiences as well as show context sensitivity to the details of specific experiences. The complexity of self-knowledge probably requires a model of self that accounts for both. (For related arguments in various contexts, see Klein & Loftus, 1993; Medin, Altom, & Murphy, 1984; Smith & Zarate, 1992).

Parallel Distributed Processing Models The neurally inspired parallel distributed processing (PDP) models of memory may prove useful in representing both abstracted as well as instance knowledge about self, although no one has yet modeled self-processes in this manner. PDP models represent memory as patterns of activation over a set of units in a highly interconnected network (McClelland & Rumelhart, 1986; Rumelhart & McClelland, 1986). The basic elements of this network are units and connection strengths among units. In associative network models, a meaningful concept corresponds to a node reserved for that knowledge, and retrieval of that concept is the activation of that node. In PDP models, a unit does not individually correspond to a concept but rather to a microfeature of the concept. Each concept thus corresponds to a pattern of activation among a collection of units. Each unit typically is involved in representing many different concepts, and different patterns of activation over the same collection of units represent different concepts. The network typically comprises at least three layers, an input layer in which units are activated by inputs from perceptual channels, an output level in which units receive activation from lower levels and then activate response mechanisms, and one or more intermediate layers of "hidden units" in which units receive input from lower levels and transmit it upward.

Each unit has an activation level that it passes on to other units through connections. Each connection between a pair of units has a strength (or weight) that determines the effect that activating the first unit has on the second. Connection strengths may be positive or negative, reflecting either an excitatory or inhibitory effect that an activated unit has on another unit. Thus, the signal transmitted from unit x to unit y depends on both the activation level of unit x and the connection strength from x to y. The current activation pattern over a set of units captures what the system is representing at the present moment. In this way, knowledge is represented in a distributed fashion in the connection strengths among large sets of units. Learning occurs by modifying the connection strengths among units.

In a distributed self-representation, each item of self-knowledge may correspond to a different pattern of activation among a set of units. Figure 2 illustrates how a very simple self-knowledge structure of this type could represent three specific instances of self-knowledge in memory. (To simplify,

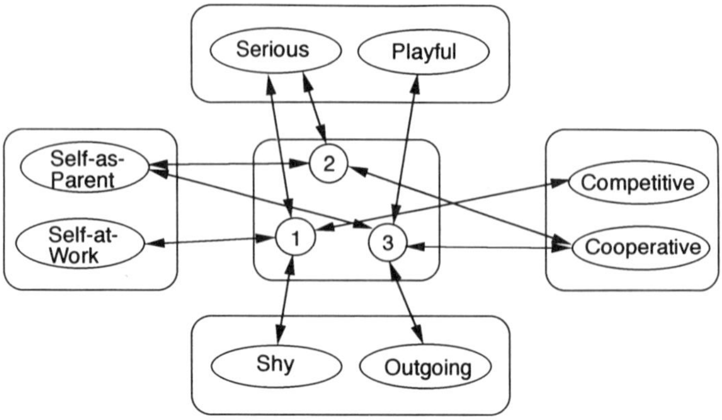

FIGURE 2.

Units and connections in a simple PDP representation of multiple self-instances and multiple selves. Units connected by arrows are mutually excitatory. (Not all connections are shown.) Units within the same grouping are mutually inhibitory (e.g., shy and outgoing). Circled numbers represent specific memory episodes. To simplify this figure, individual units are depicted as representing entire concepts (e.g., competitive) rather than elementary microfeatures.

this figure adopts a convention common in many expositions of PDP models in that individual units are depicted as representing entire concepts [e.g., "competitive"] rather than elementary microfeatures). Circled numbers represent specific memory episodes. Units connected by arrows are mutually excitatory. (Not all connections are shown.) Units within the same grouping are mutually inhibitory (e.g., shy and outgoing). Thus, instance 1 involves an episode of the "self-at-work" in which one was competitive, shy, and serious. Instance 2 represents an episode of the "self-as-parent" in which one was cooperative and serious. Instance 3 represents another episode of the "self-as-parent" in which one was cooperative, outgoing, and playful.

The network represents connections among these units and predicts which aspects of self are instantiated. For instance, positive activation of the "self-as-parent" unit evokes memory instances 2 and 3. It also strongly evokes the trait cooperative and weakly evokes the trait outgoing. In this manner, a PDP model can represent both specific instances as well as generalizations about sets of instances having a common property (e.g., "self-as-parent" is cooperative). It also predicts which self-aspect is more likely to be activated; for example, activating "cooperative" is more likely to activate "self-as-parent" than "self-at-work." By including units that encode different contexts or roles of the self (e.g., "self-as-parent" and "self-at work"), it is possible to represent multiple self-concepts as different patterns of activation over the same set of units. If two self-concepts are similar, for example sharing many traits, then the representation of the two will have similar activation patterns. To reflect that all self-concepts have something in common—they each represent the self—part of each pattern might be identical for each of the various selves.

Testing Models of Multiple Selves As we have seen, researchers have proposed a variety of representations of self including schemas, prototypes, bins, and semantic networks. However, despite the sophistication of these models, empirical tests are difficult and "multiple selves" remains a somewhat gelatinous concept.

First, the field lacks strong empirical tests of specific models. Because representation is defined in terms of the processes that operate on it, one cannot test representational assumptions in isolation (Anderson, 1983). Rather, to test a model of self, one must specify both a representation of self in memory and a set of memory and judgment processes that act on that representation. Further, it is probably not possible to empirically test and reject broad classes of models (e.g., prototype models, exemplar models, schema models). However, one can test well-specified instances of a class of models, such as Hintzman's MINERVA model of exemplar memory. To further complicate matters, there is no obvious signature empirical finding that compels us to accept or reject the concept of multiple selves within specific models. Nonetheless, the possibility of such tests seems more promising given recent empirical tests of specific assumptions of self-knowledge (e.g., Are self-traits linked to one another? Are behaviors retrieved with their associated traits?) (e.g., Higgins, Van Hook, & Dorfman, 1988; Klein et al., 1989).

Second, the nature of self-knowledge makes testing cognitive models of the self difficult. The field of social cognition offers a variety of sophisticated experimental paradigms for testing models of person perception, social judgment, or stereotyping processes. Many of these paradigms rely on the existence of consensual social knowledge (e.g., social concepts, categories, or stereotypes) as a basis for experimental manipulations. But the fact that self-knowledge is relatively idiosyncratic compared to consensual knowledge about librarians, social groups, and restaurant scripts makes it difficult to apply paradigms that experimentally manipulate various aspects of self-knowledge (e.g., trait vs. behavioral or exemplar vs. prototypic self-knowledge) (cf. Klein & Loftus, 1990b).

Interconnections among Components of Self-Knowledge

These general models of self-representation (e.g., network models, self-schemas, self-prototypes) suggest specific assumptions regarding the interconnections among different components of self-knowledge; for instance, among self-descriptive traits, among traits and their related behaviors, among domains of self-knowledge, and among positive and negative aspects of self. Does the activation of one part of self-knowledge imply increased accessibility to another part of self-knowledge? Do linkages among certain selves have affective consequences?

Interconnections among Traits and Behaviors A common assumption is that semantic self-knowledge (e.g., I am shy) is abstracted from behavioral episodes (e.g., I did not talk in class, I was quiet on a date), resulting in interconnections between traits and their exemplary behaviors. Consistent with this, most network models of self depict trait knowledge (e.g., kind) as directly linked with their trait-relevant behaviors (e.g., I gave up my seat on the train to an elderly person) (e.g., Kihlstrom et al., 1988; Kihlstrom & Cantor, 1984; Markus, 1977, 1980; Rogers et al., 1977). There are at least two complications with this view. First, research suggests that the link between self-traits and related behavioral instances may be weak. For example, although both general traits and autobiographical episodes are available in memory, activating a trait (e.g., judging the self-descriptiveness of the trait "honest") does not facilitate the retrieval of autobiographical instances exemplifying that trait (e.g., Klein & Loftus, 1993; Klein et al., 1989). Second, different behavioral instances of a trait may be encoded in different context-specific self-structures (e.g., cheating on one's taxes encoded with self as business person; honest responses to a child's questions encoded with self as parent). This diminishes any connection between the two and between the instances and a general abstracted trait inference node (e.g., honest).

Interconnections among Self-Attributes Another common suggestion is that self-descriptive traits are structurally linked with one another. This suggests that the activation of one self-attribute should increase the activation of other self-attributes. In research discussed later in this chapter, Higgins et al. (1988) found evidence of such interconnections only for self-attributes that represented problem areas for the respondents. This suggests that strong linkages are most likely to exist among self-attributes about which people ruminate. On the other hand, it is also possible that the trait terms activated general semantic concepts, rather than specifically self-referent ones, except when they referred to areas that were problematic for subjects.

Interconnections among Self-Domains: Self-Complexity and Affective Consequences The organization and interconnections among self-structures, not simply their content, is important. Assuming that self-knowledge is organized in terms of multiple, context-specific selves, some may be interlinked, whereas others may not. Two self-domains that share many common features or are often simultaneously activated may share rich connections. The interconnections among self-domains may have affective consequences, suggesting types of self-structures that predict affective vulnerability.

The self-complexity model (Linville, 1985, 1987) assumes that there are individual differences in the number of domain-specific self-structures and in the degree to which these structures are interconnected. Those high in self-complexity organize self-knowledge in terms of a greater number of self-aspects and maintain greater distinctions (less feature redundancy) between self-aspects than those low in self-complexity. Interconnections among the various self-structures have evaluative and emotional consequences. According to the model, thoughts and feelings about one self-aspect tend to spread and color thoughts and feelings about related self-aspects. But with greater self-complexity, a smaller proportion of self-aspects is likely to be affected by a self-relevant event in any particular domain of life, leaving unaffected self-aspects as buffers. Thus, those high in self-complexity are less affected by the ups and downs of life. In contrast, those low in self-complexity are likely to experience this spread, thus having a smaller proportion of self-aspects unaffected by a self-relevant event. As a result, a positive or negative experience in one domain of life is likely to have greater impact on their self-perception, evaluation, mood, or self-esteem.

Several types of evidence support the model. First, self-complexity acts as a moderator of affect and self-appraisal. Those lower in self-complexity experienced greater swings in affect and self-appraisal following success or failure; and they experienced greater variability in mood over a two-week period (Linville, 1985). In addition, complexity of "present selves" mediated affective reactions to feedback about current goals, whereas complexity of "possible selves" mediated reactions to feedback about future goals (Niedenthal, Setterlund, & Wherry, 1992). Second, self-complexity acts as a moderator or protective buffer against the adverse physical and mental health consequences of stress (Linville, 1987; Kalthoff & Neimeyer, 1993; Smith & Cohen, 1993). For example, following high levels of stressful events, those lower in self-complexity were more prone to depression, perceived stress, physical symptoms, and occurrence of the flu and other illnesses (Linville, 1987). Similarly, "relationship complexity" buffered reactions to a romantic breakup (Smith & Cohen, 1993). Third, high self-complexity makes it easier to "face oneself after failure" (Dixon & Baumeister, 1991). Because a failure threatens a greater proportion of self-aspects for those low in self-complexity, Dixon and Baumeister reasoned that low self-complexity people are more motivated to escape from self-awareness following failure. In support of this, those low in self-complexity were the quickest to finish an essay on self-goals in front of a mirror following failure.

Self-complexity also has implications for self-esteem. The notion of multiple cognitive selves suggests that people also possess multiple affective selves—or multiple self-esteems. Further, because high self-complexity involves greater cognitive differentiation among self-aspects, these self-aspects may also be affectively and evaluatively distinct as well. In support of this, those higher in self-complexity do not simply experience higher or lower self-esteem, but rather show greater differentiation (less correlation) among their domain-specific self-esteems (Linville, 1994). For example, one might feel excellent about one's family-self, good about one's career-self, but bad about one's physical-self. Also, higher self-complexity moderated the impact of low as well as high self-esteem in one domain on one's global self-esteem. In sum, high self-complexity buffers you against bad times but also keeps your feet on the ground in good times.

Interconnections among Discrepant Self-Beliefs: Self-Discrepancy and Affective Vulnerability In Higgins' (1987, 1989) self-discrepancy model, interconnections among certain types of selves also predict affective vulnerability. Higgins proposes five types of self-beliefs—an actual self (beliefs about one's actual attributes), an ideal self (attributes one hopes or wishes to attain), an ought self (attributes one has a duty or responsibility to possess), a can self (beliefs about one's capabilities or potential), and a future self (expectations of one's future attributes). It is the type of interconnections or discrepancies between different types of self-beliefs that are more important than their content per se, because it is the discrepancies that produce different kinds of emotional distress. For example, an actual/ideal discrepancy is related to depression, whereas an actual/ought discrepancy is related to anxiety (Higgins, Bond, Klein, & Strauman, 1986; Strauman & Higgins, 1987). As the magnitude of the specific discrepancy increases, so do the specific symptoms. Symptoms can also be induced by simply priming the self-discrepancy, or even one part of the discrepancy, suggesting that self-discrepancies are cognitive structures that can be automatically activated to produce emotional problems.

Interconnections between Positive and Negative Self-Knowledge Interconnections between positive and negative self-knowledge also have affective consequences. *Within* a particular self-domain such as one's social life, people who intermix positive and negative self-items have higher self-esteem than do those who cluster items of the same valence together (Showers, 1992b). Linking positive and negative items within a domain increases the ease of focusing on a positive feature if a negative one is activated within the same structure, thus limiting the impact of negative items and protecting self-esteem. Showers (1992a) also looked at the distribution of items *across* different self-domains. Compartmentalizing one's negative and positive traits into separate self-domains is related to higher self-esteem for those whom their positive self-domains are most important. However, compartmentalizing is related to lower self-esteem for those depressed persons for whom their negative self-aspects are most important. Thus, for those who frequently activate important positive self-domains, isolating negative features into a few self-domains allows them to avoid or devalue them. But for those who frequently activate important negative self-domains, it's better to have some positive features in those domains to buffer the negative.

In summary, historically there has been a debate over whether the self is a unified, single structure or whether it is best characterized in term of multiple self-structures. Most contemporary cognitive approaches assume some form of multiple selves. The debate is now over the nature of these selves and the processes acting on them. The concept of multiplicity has raised a number of new issues for researchers, such as how self-knowledge is interconnected, and these are now the focus of much research.

2. Knower versus Known: Declarative versus Procedural Self-Knowledge

Knower versus Known Distinction

The classic distinction between the self as knower and the self as known dates back at least to the turn of the century. William James (1890) set the stage for dual functions of the self, making a distinction between the self as a body of knowledge known about the self (termed the *known* or *me*) versus the self as subject who actively experiences (termed the *knower* or *I*). From a more current perspective, the self as known can be viewed as the content of self-representation; and the self as knower can be viewed as the mental processes monitoring and operating from moment to moment on this self-representation, controlling thoughts, emotions, and actions. However, a continuing problem has been: What is the knower? The very notion suggests a homunculus or a "self within a self" that guides behavior. James tried to bring this philosophical problem into the domain of psychology, but after struggling with it, neither he nor Allport (1961) found a satisfying solution. Most theorists abandoned the knowing self and focused on the known self. Recent resurrections related the self as knower to the experience of conscious awareness (Kihlstrom, 1984), to processes of self-regulation (Markus & Wurf, 1987), and to schematic processes (Greenwald & Pratkanis, 1984).

Cognitive science provides one approach for understanding this classic distinction. A production system framework, such as Anderson's (1983, 1987) ACT* model, makes a distinction between declarative and procedural knowledge that parallels in many respects this classic content/process dichotomy. The basic cognitive architecture in ACT* includes a *declarative* long-term memory to represent factual knowledge, and a *procedural* long-term memory to represent mental rules regarding how to do things (see Figure 3 for a representation of self-knowledge). Viewing the self from a production system framework, what James termed the *self as known* corresponds to *declarative knowledge* structures, which includes factual knowledge about the self; and the *self as knower* corresponds to *procedural knowledge*, which controls the processing of information including self-oriented processes (see Greenwald & Pratkanis, 1984, for an early analogy between the process–content and procedural–declarative distinctions). For example, a declarative fact might be "social support helps people under stress," a procedural rule might be "IF UNDER STRESS, THEN TALK TO A FRIEND." As this example illustrates, elements of knowledge can be represented both declaratively and procedurally. Moreover, these are not simply two different types of self-knowledge. Rather, Linville and Clark (1989) suggest how the interaction of declarative and procedural self-knowledge

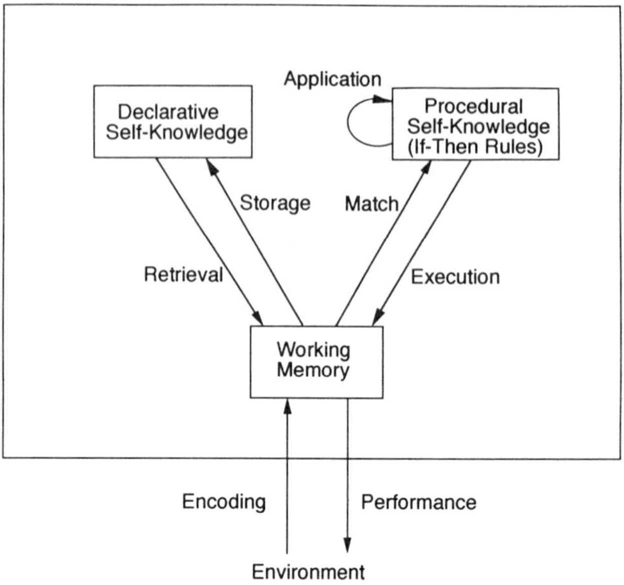

FIGURE 3.
Declarative and procedural self-knowledge represented in the ACT* framework. (Adapted from Anderson, 1983.)

guides the flow of cognition involved in self-perception, self-evaluation, self-presentation, causal attributions, perceptions of control, social comparison, social interactions, affective reactions, social problem solving, and coping behavior.

Declarative versus Procedural Self-Knowledge

Declarative Knowledge In ACT*, declarative knowledge is organized as a network of nodes representing concepts or facts that are linked together by associations (as in associative network models described earlier). Declarative self-knowledge may include traits, physical and social identities, behavioral episodes, typical responses to situations, attitudes, or self-relevant events. The interconnections among these units or nodes form a network structure. Collectively, these stored memory traces regarding the self define what James would term the "self as known."

Memory retrieval occurs via *spreading activation*—that is, activation spreads automatically along links from currently active knowledge to associated knowledge. Retrieving declarative information can be thought of as activating that information. *Working memory* is that part of declarative memory that is currently highly activated. Because the capacity to maintain information in working memory is limited, only limited parts of declarative self-knowledge are accessible at any given moment.

Procedural Knowledge Procedural knowledge is a set of mental rules for how to do things. Procedural knowledge is represented by sets of condition–action (If–Then) rules referred to as productions. The *condition* component of the rule is an "IF statement" that specifies under what conditions the rule applies. The *action* component of the rule is a "THEN statement" that specifies what mental or physical action should be taken when the rule applies. For example, an attribution rule might be represented in a fairly simple production: "IF I FAIL, AND OTHERS SUCCEED, THEN INFER I'M NOT SMART."[3] Production systems guide cognitive activity through a *matching* process that matches declarative knowledge in working memory to relevant rules and an *execution* process that deposits the action of a matched rule into working memory. For example, consider when the attribution production above might apply. If the current pattern of knowledge in working memory matches information in the IF statement (the knowledge "I failed a math test" and "my friends did well" are in working memory), the production executes, carrying out the actions specified in the THEN statement by placing the action into working memory (infer that "I'm not smart"). (See Figure 3.) An "action" may add new knowledge to memory, activate existing knowledge, set subgoals, or cause motor behavior. The sequence of thoughts involved in most self-oriented processes, such as inferences or problem-solving tasks, can be modeled as a linked sequence of productions. That is, executing the action of one production (infer "I'm not smart") might satisfy the condition of another production ("IF I'M NOT SMART, THEN INFER I'M WORTHLESS"), and so on, resulting in the firing of a sequence of productions that directs complex mental processes.

Productions gain strength as they are successfully used, resulting in their frequent and quick execution. A production may compete with other productions for execution, but preference is given to the production that has the greatest strength and that best matches the knowledge and goal currently active in working memory. In this way, priority is given to goal-directed processing.

Production systems specify the learning mechanisms by which people develop productions that automatically guide mental activity. Knowledge starts out as declarative knowledge, but it can be built through use and practice into specialized, automatic productions. For example, people initially solve new problems by applying general problem-solving productions (such as analogy or means–ends analysis) to active declarative knowledge

[3]Productions in this chapter appear in nontechnical notation and in a compact form that omits many procedural details. More specifically, first, productions here are written using ordinary English, whereas computer simulations of production systems are written in standard computer languages such as LISP. Second, most tasks, even simple ones like adding several numbers or dialing a telephone number, involve a series of productions that specify processing details (see Anderson, 1983). Thus, productions can be broken down into finer and finer processing steps. Most of the productions in this chapter omit most of these details.

about a problem. This is slow, conscious, and makes heavy demands on working memory. But with practice, they incorporate the specific problem solution into productions that are specialized for doing that task. When the same circumstances arise again, these task-specific productions apply directly, automatically, and with great speed and efficiency. Productions that repeatedly prove useful continue to acquire strength, which increases the likelihood of their automatic and continued use.

Linville and Clark (1989) suggest that people develop a variety of mental rules or productions for interpreting and responding to self-relevant information. For example, failing at a task may activate rules for making causal attributions, for perceiving personal control over the situation, and for inferring self-worth. In addition, rules may play a role in inferring and generating emotional reactions, for example, "IF I EXPERIENCE A NEGATIVE, SELF-RELEVANT OUTCOME, AND THE EVENT WAS CAUSED BY ME, AND THE EVENT WAS CONTROLLABLE BY ME, THEN FEEL ANGER TOWARD MYSELF." Others develop to regulate emotions: "IF THE GOAL IS TO BE OPTIMISTIC ABOUT A FUTURE OUTCOME, THEN MENTALLY SIMULATE POTENTIAL PATHS TOWARD POSITIVE OUTCOMES." Rules aid in coping: "IF THE GOAL IS TO BOOST MY SELF-IMAGE, THEN SEARCH FOR A COMPARISON OTHER WHO IS WORSE THAN I AM ON A RELEVANT DIMENSION." Others guide escape behavior: "IF MY ANXIETY IS TOO HIGH, THEN TAKE A DRINK." Interpersonal behavior can also be represented in a production framework. For example, rules guide self-presentations: "IF THE GOAL IS TO CREATE A POSITIVE IMPRESSION FOR PERSON X, THEN MIMIC THE ATTITUDES OF PERSON X."

In short, a variety of self-oriented cognitive processes and resulting behaviors can be viewed as resulting from the execution of production rules. This approach does not assume that people consciously apply such rules or that they have access to the rules that guide their behavior, only that such rules implicitly underlie their thoughts, feelings, and actions.

Implications of Procedural Aspects of the Self

A production system framework adds specificity to several issues in the self literature by drawing on features of procedural knowledge such as its tendency to be relatively automatic, inaccessible, domain specific, and learned only through practice. First, although most recent reviews suggest that "the self-structure guides behavior," it is not clear exactly how this happens. Activation of declarative knowledge, including facts about the self, does not directly initiate cognitive or behavioral actions. Rather, processes must convert activated knowledge into behavior. In ACT* and other production system frameworks, these interfacing processes have been specified—namely, activation of declarative self-knowledge results in behavior by matching and executing relevant productions that guide mental and physical activity. For example, knowledge in working memory that you tripped another person may execute a production such as: "IF A NEGATIVE EVENT OCCURS TO ANOTHER, AND I AM TO BLAME, THEN SAY 'I AM SORRY'." In this manner, procedural knowledge acts as the controller of behavior, providing an understanding of motivation and goal-directed behavior without the need for a homunculus. Thus the interaction of declarative and procedural knowledge gives specificity to the notion of an interaction between self-structure and the processes that act on it.

Although James set the stage for linkages between knowledge structure and process aspects of self, subsequent researchers tended not to pursue these links. For example, Markus and Wurf (1987) observed that work on self-representation and work on self-regulatory processes tend to be treated in two separate literatures. However, the interaction of declarative and procedural self-knowledge provides a link between these areas, viewing processes of self-regulation discussed by Markus and Wurf such as goal setting, planning, strategy selection, adjusting behavior toward a goal, and affect regulation as social problem-solving productions that are cued by specific patterns of knowledge and goals in working memory.

Second, a production framework suggests that rules for guiding self-oriented processes will tend to be task or context specific rather than general in nature (Linville & Clark, 1989). The learning mechanisms in ACT* and other common production systems lead to context-specific productions. Productions develop through problem solving on specific tasks and are fine-tuned for successful use in that task. This suggests that general productions may be used for relatively unfamiliar tasks or contexts, but that our productions for dealing with familiar tasks will tend to be specialized. For example, rather than having only one general rule for dealing with anger, people are likely to develop several, context-specific rules, for example, "IF I FEEL ANGRY, AND I AM AT WORK, THEN COUNT TO 10 AND SUPPRESS MY FEELINGS"; and "IF I FEEL ANGRY, AND I AM WITH FAMILY, THEN EXPRESS MY FEELINGS." This is consistent with our earlier discussion of multiple context-specific selves. Each self-concept, when currently active, may automatically activate a set of context-specific rules or productions. Thus the "self as knower" is likely to contain context-specific knowledge just as the "self as known" does.

Third, procedural knowledge provides a framework for understanding the seemingly "unconscious" or automatic nature of many self-oriented processes. Productions develop gradually, only with the repeated practice of a procedure. Once established, however, productions control behavior rather directly by automatically executing a sequence of actions when certain data are in working memory. Increased practice of a procedure (or *proceduralization*) has several consequences related to increased automaticity—a speedup in performance of the procedure, a decrease in awareness and verbalization of the process, and a decrease in interference with the performance of concurrent tasks (see Anderson, 1983, 1987). These consequences can be seen in interpersonal perception and behavior (e.g., Langer, 1978; Lewicki, 1986; Nisbett & Wilson, 1977; Smith & Lerner, 1986). These consequences also have implications for self-oriented processes (see Linville & Clark, 1989). One implication is that processes such as self-evaluation, self-attribution, and social problem-solving solutions are so frequently practiced that they are likely to occur automatically. Quick, automatic responses are especially likely in contexts where a person has sufficient experience to have developed well-practiced procedures. Another implication is that, because many self-oriented inferences are well practiced and automatic, people will show little ability to verbalize the processes underlying their inferences or to identify the conditions triggering them. Finally, the automatic nature of many self-oriented processes makes them less demanding on the cognitive system, allowing people to simultaneously address other goals or tasks.

Fourth, the declarative–procedural distinction helps us understand how self-knowledge may appear inconsistent at times. For example, a person may store declaratively the belief that "I am an optimistic person," despite having automatic production rules that produce pessimistic assessments, for example, "IF AN UNCERTAIN SELF-RELEVANT EVENT WILL OCCUR IN THE NEAR FUTURE, THEN MENTALLY SIMULATE PATHS TOWARD A NEGATIVE OUTCOME."

Fifth, a production system framework helps explain the persistence of ineffective ways of coping and thinking about ourselves such as distorted self-evaluations and maladaptive coping and problem-solving strategies (Linville & Clark, 1989). Well-practiced responses become proceduralized and thus performed automatically without conscious awareness of the conditions that evoke them, making them hard to change. Similarly, procedural knowledge provides a model for depression, accounting for the automatic inference rules that lead to distortions such as overgeneralization and personalization (Beck et al., 1979). For example, "IF I AM CRITICIZED, THEN INFER THAT I AM WORTHLESS."

Finally, a production system approach suggests how to teach people better coping or social problem-solving strategies. People learn procedural skills only by performing them. Thus coping productions develop only in the process of active coping, that is, only by repeatedly performing a specific procedure. Therefore, advising someone to think or to behave differently (e.g., "Have a more positive attitude") is likely to be ineffective in competing with well-used productions (e.g., procedures for forming negative expectations). In contrast, specific "how to do it" instruction integrated with repeated practice of the new procedure should be more beneficial than "formal instruction" or "why explanations" in modifying maladaptive self-inferences, coping responses, or social problem-solving strategies (Linville & Clark, 1989). This is consistent with the approach taken in cognitive therapy.

3. Is the Self Stable or Malleable? Shifting Activation of Contextual Selves

Psychologists have shown a continuing interest in the paradox of how the self can be both stable and malleable. Historically, the concept of a stable self guided theorizing and measurement of specific aspects of self. For example, a predominant focus of research in prior decades was on self-esteem, viewed as one of the most stable components of the self. William James (1890) suggested that the self, especially the social self, is inherently malleable yet retains a sense of stability or unity by the knower's knowledge that the same person underlies any changes. Backman and Secord (1968) suggested that stability comes from our selection of roles that are compatible with the attributes of our self-concept, whereas malleability comes from incorporating the attributes of our roles into the self.

The degree of stability of self-concepts remains an issue actively debated in social psychology. On one hand, self-concepts maintain a degree of stability over time and context. People seek information that verifies their self-view and actively resist information that challenges it (e.g., Greenwald, 1980; Markus, 1977; Swann, 1983; Tesser & Campbell, 1983). Many cognitive models of self assume that the self is a stable, well-organized structure (e.g., Kihlstrom & Cantor, 1984; Kihlstrom et al, 1988; Markus & Sentis, 1982; Rogers, 1977). On the other hand, self-concepts also reflect a degree of malleability. One's active self-concepts are influenced by the subset of information made salient by the immediate situation (e.g., Bern, 1972; Fazio, Effrein, & Falender, 1981; Jones et al., 1981; McGuire, 1984; Salancik & Conway, 1975). The changeable nature of the self stems in part from its social quality and origins, being influenced by our social roles and how others see us (James, 1890; Mead, 1934), and by our self-presentations and use of impression management (Baumeister, 1982; Jones & Pittman, 1982; Schlenker & Trudeau, 1990). These two different perspectives are combined in recent work emphasizing a dynamic self that is both stable and malleable (e.g., Markus & Wurf, 1987; Markus & Kunda, 1986; Rhodewalt, 1986).

The social cognition perspective contributes in several ways to our understanding of how self-knowledge changes over time and across situations yet also maintains some stability. First, apparent changes in stable self-concepts may reflect the momentary activation of different subsets of self-knowledge. Second, several sources of activation influence which parts of self are likely to be active at any given time. Third, self-attention may not reflect attention on the self per se, but rather on particular self-aspects. Each of these three suggestions builds on our earlier discussion of multiple selves. Fourth, actual changes in self-concept are presumed to reflect processes that are common to other kinds of knowledge. Fifth, the sense of stability that people have about themselves is partly driven by the way people search and interpret self-information. All five suggestions concern the interaction between self-representations and the processes that operate on them.

Shifting Activation

Not all ways of defining ourselves are relevant in any particular context. In fact, people could not consciously access their entire repertoire of self-conceptions at once. Rather, specific self-aspects are activated when they are currently relevant (e.g., Linville, 1987; Markus & Wurf, 1987; McGuire, 1984; Rhodewalt, 1986). Contextual and motivational factors make certain self-aspects more accessible. Apparent changes in relatively stable self-concepts can thus be understood in terms of shifts in the momentary accessibility of different aspects of self-knowledge (see Markus & Wurf, 1987). Prior to the advent of these activation models, claims of momentarily inaccessible selves required allusion to Freudian models of the repressed subconscious. In current models, individual self-aspects may be stable, but their content may differ from one another, and their relative accessibility may change. This allows relative stability of self-knowledge, yet malleability in which self-knowledge is currently activated. This implies that self-descriptions may be fairly consistent given a context that activates the same self-structure, yet they may vary across contexts that activate different self-structures (McGuire, 1984; Wyer & Srull, 1989).

What Self-Knowledge is Activated?

Currently activated self-aspects are most likely to play a role in current inferences, judgment, and evaluations. The subset of self-structures active at a given moment has been described as our phenomenal self (Jones et al., 1981) or our working self (Cantor, Markus, Niedenthal, & Nurius, 1986; Markus & Kunda, 1986). The phenomenal self may consist of latitudes of acceptable and unacceptable self-characteristics (Rhodewalt & Agustsdottir, 1986). A primary contribution of social cognition has been to identify mechanisms that explain which parts of self are active at any given time. These sources of activation include chronic accessibility, contextual accessibility, distinctiveness, and representativeness of various parts of self-knowledge.

Chronic and Contextual Construct Accessibility Accessibility of knowledge reflects the ease with which that knowledge is brought into consciousness or working memory. The accessibility of self-knowledge may derive from contextual cues or momentary priming in the immediate environment. For example, one's current activity may automatically activate a certain self-concept (e.g., writing a paper may activate one's "researcher" or "hard-working" self-representation; talking to one's mother may activate one's "daughter" or "dependent" self-representation). Similarly, internal factors such as one's current goals or needs also influence the accessibility of specific self-constructs (Bruner, 1957; Higgins & King, 1981; Wyer & Srull, 1981; Srull & Wyer, 1986). For example, for a student who is a top athlete, a current goal to make oneself feel competent may activate "self-as-athlete" representation. Additionally, accessibility of self-knowledge may derive from the frequent long-term use of certain self-structures such as chronically accessible constructs (Higgins, King, & Mavin, 1982), self-discrepancies (Higgins, 1987), or self-schemas (Markus, 1977).

There is ample evidence that more accessible chronic and primed trait constructs influence the processing of social information, and they appear to do so automatically (e.g., Higgins et al, 1982; Higgins, Bargh, & Lombardi, 1985; Bargh, Bond, Lombardi, & Tota, 1986; Srull & Wyer, 1979, 1980). Similarly, the accessibility of chronic self-schemas results in quick and confident self-relevant judgments, easily retrievable examples, confident self-predictions, and resistance to contrary evidence (e.g., Markus, 1977; Markus et al., 1982).

Distinctiveness Distinctive self-features are more accessible, because of either their frequent long-term use or their immediate saliency (see McGuire, 1984; McGuire & Padawer-Singer, 1976). In spontaneous self-descriptions, students tend to describe features that distinguish themselves from others in their immediate social context. For example, students are more likely to mention their gender, race, or physical characteristics (e.g., hair color) when these features are in the minority in their class. They also tend to describe features that distinguish themselves from others in their more permanent environment. For example, they are more likely to mention their gender if they are in the gender minority at home (e.g, a male with more female siblings than male siblings).

Representativeness People appear to adopt behavior that is representative of particular aspects of their self-concepts, either to maintain their current self-concept or to achieve a desired one (see Sherman et al., 1989). For example, students' intention to smoke is predictable from the degree of match between their self-image and their prototype of a smoker (Barton, Chassin, Presson, & Sherman, 1982; Chassin, Presson, Sherman, Cotty, & Olshavsky, 1981). Likewise, housing preferences reflected the degree of match between their own traits and their perception of a person who would be happy in various kinds of living settings (Niedenthal et al., 1985). People especially engage in behavior representative of their self-image when that image is threatened or contradicted (Sherman & Gorkin, 1980; Mori et al., 1987; Swann, 1983).

Behavioral Implications of Activated Self-Concepts The self-aspect accessible at the moment may influence current behavior, self-perception, mood, and self-evaluation. For example, accessing "myself-as-lawyer" representation may evoke competitive behavior, whereas accessing "myself-as-friend" may evoke cooperative behavior. Likewise, activating a self-aspect that implicates low rather than high esteem, or success rather than failure, should effect one's current mood and self-evaluation. Finally, activating particular past memories influences current self-judgments (Salancik & Conway, 1975). For example, accessing past proreligious or antireligious thoughts and feelings influenced people's current self-perceptions of religiosity (Salancik & Conway, 1975).

Shifting Self-Attention

The social cognition approach contributes to our understanding of self-attention. The classic issue has been the degree to which the self is the focus of attention. The accessibility of the self varies, depending on contextual cues such as mirrors that make the self salient and individual differences in the tendency to focus on oneself. Greater self-focused attention has behavioral consequences, such as making one's ideal standards accessible to guide behavior. For example, greater self-attention due to the presence of a mirror leads people to "self-regulate" or adjust their behavior to be more in line with their ideal-standards (Carver & Scheier, 1981). The concept of multiple selves that shift from moment to moment in relative accessibility has implications for the concept of self-attention. Attention may not focus on the self per se, but rather on particular self-aspects. And each self-aspect may have its own ideal standard. This implies that self-attention leads to behavior more consistent with the ideals of that particular self-aspect (cf. Sherman et al., 1989). Different self-aspects may have differing, even conflicting, ideals. Thus the relative accessibility of "self as independent business manager" compared to "self as dependent spouse" influences the standards available to guide behavior.

How Do Self-Conceptions Change?

The social cognition approach suggests how actual changes or enduring revisions in the self may occur. First, actual changes in self-knowledge are presumed to reflect basic processes that are common to other kinds of knowledge. Second, new self-knowledge is acquired socially from others (your boss mentions that you are clever) (Lord, Desforges, Chacon, Pere, & Clubb, 1992) as well as inferred from behavior (Bem, 1967), thoughts and feelings (Andersen, 1984; Andersen & Ross, 1984), internalized self-presentations (Jones et al., 1981), and physiological reactions (Bandura, 1977). Third, changes in self may be local rather than global, reflecting changes in specific self-concepts rather than changes in the self in general. Fourth, self-structures can be added or reduced in salience through major life changes such as parenthood, retirement, or death of a spouse. Fifth, changes in the way children define themselves in different domains (e.g., their social or school lives) reflects normal cognitive development. For example, self-definitions show increasing differentiation, integration, and abstraction with age (Dweck & Elliott, 1983; Harter, 1983, 1986; Rosenberg, 1986).

Drives toward Stability in Self-Representations

Finally, a sense of stability is also driven by the way people seek, recall, and interpret self-information. Three different, and sometimes competing, motives underlie the search and interpretation of self-knowledge and thus the degree of its stability—self-consistency, self-enhancement, and accuracy. First, people seek information that is *consistent* with their existing view of themselves and resist information that challenges that view. Swann's (1983, 1987) self-verification model proposes a drive toward maintaining a current self-concept, even at the expense of verifying a negative self-image. People maintain consistency in their self-concepts not by passively denying feedback that challenges their self-view, but rather by selecting, interpreting, and recalling self-confirming information and by selecting situations and companions that affirm their self-view.

Another way that people maintain consistency and hence stability in their self-conceptions is through reconstructed memories of their past. People tend to reconstruct past memories of their behavior to be in line with their present behavior or self-image, resulting in a perception of consistency over time (Ross & Conway, 1986). Thus the sense of consistency or stability that people have about themselves may be partly illusory, reflecting biased memory. Reconstructive processes can also lead to illusory change, as when people reconstruct what they were like before they began a self-improvement program.

Second, people seek information that is *self-enhancing;* that is, they try to maintain the most positive self-evaluation possible. Tesser's (1986, 1988; Tesser & Campbell, 1983) self-evaluation maintenance model proposes that people interpret the performances of others in a manner that makes them feel good about themselves. People can feel good by doing relatively well compared to similar others on a personally relevant dimension (e.g., surpassing professional rivals). They can also enhance their own self-esteem by "basking in the reflected glory" of the accomplishments of a close other on a personally irrelevant dimension (e.g., mentioning the marathon time of a sibling if one is not a runner). People vary their closeness to the other or the perceived relevance of the dimension to their self-definition in order to maintain positive self-evaluations.

Most people tend to hold positive, self-enhancing views of themselves, but they tend to have an exaggerated and illusory quality (see Greenwald, 1980; Taylor & Brown, 1988, for reviews). These distorted positive perceptions of one's social and intellectual skills, personal control, and future predictions appear, in some respects, to be adaptive in promoting one's mental health.

Third, people also seek self-information that is *accurate.* Trope's self-assessment theory proposes that people seek information about themselves that is likely to be diagnostic regarding their uncertain features (Trope,

1983, 1986). This concern with assessing abilities accurately leads people to choose tasks on which their performance is most likely to be informative about abilities of greatest uncertainty.

Motives of self-consistency and self-enhancement should contribute to a sense of self-stability, whereas the consequences of motives of accuracy, while not as clear, may not necessarily produce unstable self-definitions. As Fiske and Taylor (1991) note in reconciling these three motives, most behavior is positive and self-enhancing most of the time, so our positive self-conceptions also fulfill consistency and accuracy needs. Also, drives toward accurate self-information appear to be strongest on attributes about which one is most uncertain (Sorrentino & Roney, 1986; Trope, 1986). Thus changes in self-definition may occur most often on attributes that are already ambiguous and unstable. Drives toward consistent information appear to be strongest on attributes about which one is most certain, adding further to the stability of self-conceptions. People seek consistent feedback regarding negative attributes they already hold with certainty, but self-enhancing feedback on negative attributes about which they are less sure (Pelham, 1991).

Summary of Enduring Issues

In summary, social cognition provides a perspective for resolving many classic paradoxes of the self. The definition of these issues, as well as their methodological investigation, has taken on a decidedly different flavor in recent times. For example, theorizing about multiple selves has shifted from content to the interaction of representation and process. This interaction fits naturally with models of the interaction between declarative and procedural self-knowledge. Finally, theorizing about stability and malleability of self has shifted to process issues of priming and shifting accessibility.

IMPACT OF SOCIAL COGNITION ON EMERGING ISSUES OF SELF

Another way of measuring the impact of social cognition is to consider its influence on the advent of new issues. Here we discuss four emerging issues.

1. Is the Self a (Special) Cognitive Structure?

In recent years, one of the most central questions raised about the self is whether it is an ordinary cognitive structure or whether it is somehow special, unique, or distinct from other such structures (Greenwald & Pratkanis, 1984; Higgins & Bargh, 1987). In some respects, self-knowledge obviously is special. Relative to most perceptual objects, we possess more information about ourselves, we derive the information more from our own unique perspective, we tend to care more about this information and the object it describes (our selves), and we reference aspects of this information more frequently in the course of everyday thinking and behavior. At the same time, however, we often know and care a lot about other people and objects, we often have a unique perspective on these objects, and we may commonly reference them during ruminations and activities. Whatever the properties of the self, these same properties can undoubtedly be found in other perceptual objects. Thus their effects may vary in degree but probably not in their essential nature. Consequently, the self is almost certainly ordinary in the sense that it must obey the same general laws of cognition that govern other cognitive structures.

So, if the self is in some ways special and in other ways ordinary, then the critical question is not "whether the self is a special, unique, or distinct cognitive structure" but rather "precisely what are the (special or ordinary) structural properties of the self?" Three possible answers are that self-knowledge is especially elaborate, that self-attributes are interconnected, and that self-attributes are separate from non-self-attributes. Recent research on these possibilities represents some of the most thoughtful and innovative work on the self done from the social cognition perspective. We review it here not only to address the special/ordinary question, but also to illustrate the manner in which social cognition researchers have imported cognitive methods to test the current, cognitive conceptualization of self.

Klein and Kihlstrom (1986)

The notion that the self is uniquely elaborate was an early explanation for the seemingly superior recall of words encoded self-referently (Keenan & Baillet, 1980; Kendzierski, 1980; Rogers et al., 1977). The experimental paradigm for studying the self-reference effect compares recall under different types of learning conditions. In the self-reference condition, subjects are asked questions such as "Does this word describe you?" In the semantic condition, subjects are asked questions such as "Does this word fit the following sentence?" Later subjects in both conditions are asked to recall the words they saw earlier. The self-reference condition typically leads to superior recall. The original explanation was that the self provides a highly elaborated memory structure that can facilitate recall for information encoded self-referently by providing multiple, readily accessible cognitive links.

Klein and Kihlstrom (1986) argued that the usual superiority of self-referent encoding reflects the involvement of a preexisting categorical discrimination ("me" vs. "not me") in the self-reference task that is lacking in the usual semantic tasks. They demonstrated that the organizational benefit of requiring a categorical discrimination, and not the self-referent nature of the task, accounts for the superiority of recall. In one experiment, for example, they orthogonally manipulated the organizational and the self-referent properties of their encoding tasks. In addition to the usual (organized) self-reference and (disorganized) semantic conditions, some subjects were asked disorganized self-referent questions ("Does this word fit in the following [self-referent] sentence?") and some were asked organized semantic questions ("Does this word describe a body part?").

The results indicated that organization significantly facilitated recall for target words, whether or not they were encoded self-referently, whereas self-reference had no effect. This implies that superior memory for self-referently processed words reflects organizational properties of the self-referent questions, not deeper processing of self-related material. Klein and Kihlstrom concluded that "although it may well be that the self is a highly elaborate memory structure, the SRE [self-reference effect] does not give evidence to support this conclusion. . . " (p. 36). Similarly, research on the "self-generation effect" indicates that the advantage in recall of self-generated names versus names generated by others is due to ordinary memory processes rather than some special property of the self (Greenwald & Banaji, 1989).

McDaniel, Lapsley, and Milstead (1987)

McDaniel et al. (1987) address the question of whether people automatically encode self-attributes in a manner that is categorically different from the way they encode non-self-referent material. The suggestion that self-attributes are special in this regard derives both from conceptions of the self as a memory schema (Keenan & Baillet, 1980; Markus, 1977; Rogers et al., 1977) and from suggestions that stimuli are automatically screened for self-relevance (Hull & Levy, 1979; Kuiper & Derry, 1981; see also Bargh, 1984).

McDaniel et al. used a release from proactive interference paradigm (Zechmeister & Nyberg, 1982). The central feature of this paradigm is that when subjects are given small categorically related sets of stimuli to memorize, performance declines across each set due to proactive interference from preceding sets. But if a set is then encountered that represents a new category, subjects are released from the proactive interference, and performance on that trial rebounds to normal levels.

McDaniel et al. presented three sets of self-referent traits to subjects and then switched on the fourth trial to non-self-referent traits, or they began with the non-self-referent traits and switched to self-referent ones. In both cases, recall performance failed to rebound. Memory remained poor on the fourth trial, as though subjects did not "recognize" that a switch in category had occurred. This implies that self-relevant and self-irrelevant traits are categorically indistinguishable, providing no evidence for the special or distinct categorization of self-referent attributes.

Higgins, Van Hook, and Dorfman (1988)

Higgins et al. (1988) investigated the claim that the self is a special cognitive structure in the sense that different self-attributes are highly interconnected (cf. Greenwald & Pratkanis, 1984; Kuiper & Derry, 1981;

Markus & Sentis, 1982; Rogers, 1981). To do so, they conducted several studies using a modified Stroop task, in which subjects' ability to name the color of a printed target word is inhibited when an immediately preceding prime is a close associate of the target (Warren, 1972). Higgins et al. reasoned that if self-attributes were closely associated with each other, then priming subjects with one self-attribute would inhibit immediately subsequent color-naming performance for another self-attribute. No such effect emerged, even when the self was made salient through use of a mirror and video camera. Instead, they found inhibited response times only for semantically related control words and for "problematic" self-attributes. In other words, although the paradigm was sufficiently sensitive to detect semantic associates, it provided little support for the argument that self-attributes are similarly associated. Higgins et al. concluded that their results failed to support the self as cognitive structure proposal. However, it is possible that the trait terms were encoded semantically and not self-referently, and that greater connectivity would be found if subjects interpreted the traits as their own attributes.

Summary

These studies currently tell us more about what the self is not than they do about what it is. However, these studies do illustrate the importation of cognition theory and methods into the study of self. Moreover, the mere fact that such sophisticated methods are being employed to explore the nature of self represents a significant advance over earlier eras, when the validity of self-conceptualizations depended more on conceptual than empirical considerations.

2. Are People Selectively Self-Attentive?

A wide variety of studies provide support for the proposition that people tend to selectively attend to and encode self-related information (for reviews, see Greenwald, 1980; Markus & Wurf, 1987). For example, people invariably detect their own name when it is presented in their unattended ear during a dichotic listening task. Moreover, self-related trait adjectives interfere with performance when similarly presented in the unattended ear (Bargh, 1982). People tend to prefer the alphabetic letters in their own name (Nuttin, 1985). In the "next-in-line effect," people in a group tend to focus on their own performance at the expense of immediately preceding or following performances (Brenner, 1973). Moreover, self-descriptive information is processed more efficiently and confidently (e.g., Markus, 1977) and is ultimately better recalled (e.g., Bower & Gilligan, 1979; Kuiper & Rogers, 1979) than non-self-descriptive information or information about others. This body of evidence suggests preferential processing of self-related information.

However, much of this evidence is either indirect or confounded with the importance or frequency of past exposure to the information (cf. Wyer & Srull, 1989, for a similar argument). There is surprisingly little evidence that such information is processed preferentially when it is mixed with equivalently useful self-irrelevant information.

3. Why Does Self-Reference Enhance Recall for Material?

Rogers and his colleagues (Kuiper & Rogers, 1979; Rogers et al., 1977) first demonstrated that subjects who judged stimulus words for their self-descriptiveness (e.g., "Describes you?") had better incidental recall for those words than subjects who engaged in structural (e.g., "Printed in big letters?") or semantic (e.g., "Means the same as XXX?") processing tasks. This self-reference effect (SRE) was initially interpreted in terms of the greater depth of processing (cf. Craik & Tulving, 1975) accorded self-relevant material. The notion that self-reference results in a deeper, more elaborated memory trace remains a common interpretation today (Brown, Keenan, & Potts, 1986; Ganellen & Carver, 1985; Katz, 1987).

A number of alternative explanations have been proposed, including arguments that the SRE reflects such cognitive processes as evaluation (Ferguson, Rule, & Carlston, 1983), cognitive cuing (Bellezza, 1984), distinctiveness (Friedman & Pullyblank, 1982), and organization (Klein & Kihlstrom, 1986). This explanatory diversity is probably encouraged by certain discrepancies in attempts to replicate the SRE. For example, some studies have found that self-reference tasks produce better recall than tasks that refer to a well-known other (e.g., Lord, 1980), whereas others have not (e.g., Bower & Gilligan, 1979). Klein et al. (1989) recently argued that many of these apparent inconsistencies can be resolved by distinguishing between reference tasks that are descriptive (e.g., "Does this trait describe you [your mother]?") and those that are autobiographical (or episodic) (e.g., "Recall an episode in which you [your mother] exemplified this trait."). As a rule, they suggest, self-reference is superior to encoding with regard to well-known others when descriptive tasks are used, but not when autobiographical ones are used.

The distinction between descriptive and autobiographical tasks also clarifies a second set of findings. Early research on the SRE focused on adjectives as descriptors. Attempts to replicate the effect with nouns produced mixed results. Klein et al. (1989) note that when autobiographical tasks were used, the SRE effect generally held for nouns, whereas when descriptive tasks were used, the SRE effect often failed to replicate for nouns.

Klein et al. (1989) also present direct evidence that descriptive and autobiographical (episodic) tasks involve different cognitive processes. First, neither task is facilitated by immediately preceding it with the other; and second, combining the two tasks leads to an additional increment in recall.

They conclude that SREs on trait-descriptive tasks can be accounted for by the self-as-prototype model (Kuiper, 1981; Rogers, 1981), whereas SREs on episodic tasks are best explained by either an elaborative-organizational processing model (Klein & Loftus, 1988) or a cognitive cueing model (Bellezza, 1984).

Taken as a whole, the research on the self-reference effect reflects many of the strengths of the social cognition approach. Because this approach emphasizes the continuity of cognitive processes across domains, the SRE work draws nicely on cognitive theories of memory. This has been true from Rogers et al.'s (1977) initial theorizing in terms of depth of processing to Klein et al.'s (1989) recent work. This continuity benefits self research by allowing theorists to make use of concepts and ideas borrowed from the cognitive literature, but it also makes the self research more relevant to issues regarding memory for other kinds of social and nonsocial information. Additionally, the linkages with traditional cognitive research have suggested new research methodologies that allow researchers to go beyond simple demonstrations of memory facilitation to investigations of the processes and structures involved (cf. Klein & Loftus, 1988). The concern with process and structure, which is also characteristic of the social cognition approach (Hastie & Carlston, 1980; Schneider, 1991), has transformed the SRE from mere phenomenon to an important tool in defining the self.

4. What is the Nature of Autobiographical Memory?

Wyer and Srull (1989) suggest that the most common type of self-information that we communicate to others involves particular experiences that we have had. Despite this seeming centrality, autobiographical self has only recently been subjected to careful examination (for an early review, see Greenwald, 1980). Research on autobiographical memory has gone in many different directions, and thus it lacks the thematic consistency of the self-reference literature. However, a sampling of this work serves to highlight some of the contributions made by the social cognition perspective.

Is Autobiographical Memory Reconstructive?

Ross and his colleagues have explored autobiographical memories that are biased by the implicit belief that one has or has not changed (see Ross & Conway, 1986, for a review). For example, people's recall of their evaluations of their dating partners and their relationship two months earlier were reconstructed from their current evaluations, resulting in more consistency in liking and relationships than was actually warranted (McFarland & Ross, 1987). On the other hand, participants in a study skills improvement program misreported more change than actually occurred. They misremembered their initial study skills as having been worse than they really were, and they eventually exaggerated their postprogram academic performance (see Ross & Conway, 1986). Ross and Conway view such effects as examples of reconstructive biases such as those first postulated by Bartlett (1932). They posit "relatively minor editorial revisions" (p. 139) that bring one's past more in line with one's current self-image.

Is Autobiographical Memory Temporally Organized?

Tulving (1985) postulated that a central characteristic of episodic memory is that it includes information about the temporal order of experiences. This has been recently examined on both autobiographical (e.g., Wyer, Shoben, Fuhrman, & Bodenhausen, 1985; Thompson, Skowronski, & Lee, 1988) and nonautobiographical memory (e.g., Brown, Rips, & Shevell, 1985; Loftus & Marburger, 1983). Some of this work suggests that autobiographical memories are organized temporally, at least within broad epochs such as during high school (Chew, 1983, cited in Kihlstrom et al., 1988; Fuhrman & Wyer, 1988). However, research also suggests that information about the order and dates of events is not an inherent part of the episodic memory trace, but it is often inferred using various heuristics (Thompson et al., 1988; for a review, see Wyer & Srull, 1989). For example, people may compute the apparent date for an event by considering its relation to a particularly important "landmark" event for which a date was stored (cf. Loftus & Marburger, 1983). Neisser (1982) argued that some events of this character serve a special "benchmark" function by linking people's personal histories to socially important historic events.

Do People Rely on Autobiographical Memory?

When people make judgments of others, they may use retrieved event memories or rely on past judgments of that individual (Carlston, 1980; Carlston & Skowronski, 1986; Lingle & Ostrom, 1979). Klein and Loftus (1990a) suggest that although people can retrieve and use behavioral knowledge when making trait judgments about themselves, they generally rely on abstracted trait knowledge. Such "dual memory" formulations raise issues regarding the interrelationship between episodic and trait memories. Some cognitive models of the self assume a hierarchical structure in which summary traits are directly linked to the specific behaviors and events that they subsume (cf. Greenwald & Pratkanis, 1984; Kihlstrom & Cantor, 1984; Wyer & Srull, 1989).

Albright & Kihlstrom (1986, described in Kihlstrom et al., 1988) examined whether retrieving an autobiographical memory cued by one trait (e.g., ambitious) would facilitate the retrieval latency for a subsequent memory cued by a related trait (e.g., dominant). Their failure to find any priming effect for similar traits led them to suggest that autobiographical memory is not primarily organized hierarchically in terms of traits. Klein and Loftus (1990a) conducted a similar series of experiments in which the autobiographical judgment task (to retrieve a specific behavioral incident) was preceded by either a descriptive task (to judge the relevant trait for its self-descriptiveness) or a semantic task (to generate a definition of the trait). The descriptive task failed to facilitate the generation of a specific related behavior. That is, the time required to retrieve a specific behavior was not differentially affected by the previous descriptive or semantic task, regardless of whether the traits were self-descriptive. From these results, they also concluded that evidence is lacking for direct links between abstracted trait knowledge about oneself and relevant behavioral episodes.

Such studies suggest a marked independence between autobiographical memories and self-ascribed traits. However, this does not mean that autobiographical memories are unimportant. Even if unrelated to self-ascriptions of personality traits, such memories may represent an important aspect of the way that people think about themselves, generate self-perceptions, and disclose themselves to others. In fact, given that people seem as likely to tell self-relevant anecdotes as to engage in self-description, the role of autobiographical memories may have been *under*emphasized, at least with regard to the public self-concept.

Summary of Emerging Issues

Social cognition research on the self has a number of distinctive characteristics. First, although it has been concerned with issues regarding the structure of self-representation, it also has emphasized the cognitive processes operating on these structures. For instance, researchers have examined structural issues such as whether the self is a unique or distinct category, the linkages among self-attributes, and the organization of autobiographical memory in terms of processes such as encoding, elaboration, inhibition, and reconstruction. Similarly, researchers have gone beyond the demonstration that self-encoding facilitates memory to investigate the processes responsible for this effect. Second, it tends to take the prevailing "cognitive structure" metaphors for self seriously, testing their fundamental properties rather than tacitly accepting their suitability. This is evident in the research programs on the uniqueness of the self-structure, as well as in work on temporal and trait organization in autobiographical memory. Third, in examining the precise nature of the self-structure, it adapts methods and models from cognitive psychology. As Kihlstrom et al. (1988) noted, this allows researchers in both domains to benefit from the achievements and errors of the other, and it brings us closer to unified theories of self (and of cognition). Finally, research has generally failed to support many of the "special" properties commonly ascribed to the self-structure, instead suggesting a continuity with similar structures not involving the self (see Higgins & Bargh, 1987). There are certainly other ways in which the representation of self may be special, although some of these currently fall outside of the realm confidently addressed by social cognition approaches. For example, the self may be special in terms of how its representation incorporates affective or behavioral properties, or how frequently and in what ways it is retrieved and used during rumination, decision making, or behavior.

Recent research on the self demonstrates a number of interesting effects and raises some important questions about the self and about cognitive organization more generally. It does not, however, at this point, provide many definitive answers to these questions. Nonetheless, the social cognition approach has proven useful both in defining the issues in testable terms, and in suggesting many of the novel research methodologies that have been used to investigate them.

CONTRIBUTIONS OF SOCIAL COGNITION TO THE STUDY OF SELF

For purposes of summary, it may be useful to reconsider the general contributions of the social cognition approach to the study of self. As a rhetorical device, we consider these in relation to the conventional wisdom regarding these contributions.

1. Has Social Cognition Contributed New Answers to Enduring Questions or Enduring Answers to New Questions?

It is clear from this review that social cognition has shed new light on that most enduring issue, What is the self? as well as on subsidiary questions such as Are there multiple selves?, Is there a self as knower and known?, and Is the self-concept stable or malleable? Current progress on these traditional issues derives in part from newer frameworks involving, for example, the declarative versus procedural knowledge distinction and the notion of shifting patterns of knowledge activation. Of course, new answers are offered by each new theoretical approach to the self, and the critical question is whether these new answers will endure longer than those provided by prior conceptualizations. At present many seem tentative, but the fact that they are now being explored systematically and empirically is encouraging.

However, many of the most interesting and important questions being asked about the self today are new ones, questions that flow directly from the social cognition perspective. For example, some of the best of this research addresses the question "Is the self an ordinary or a unique cognitive structure?" The question of uniqueness arises from the social cognition premise that common structures and processes are implicated in both social and object cognition (cf. Hastie & Carlston, 1980; Ostrom 1984; Schneider, 1991). It is thus not a question that was likely to arise from the attitude, impression, or attribution approaches that preceded it. The answers provided to these new questions are also tentative, and it is too early to ask whether they will endure. But the fact that they have been asked at all, and the precision with which such questions can now be framed, are valuable contributions to the study of self.

2. Is the Contribution of Social Cognition to Self Research Primarily Methodological?

Methodological innovation has certainly played an important role in the history of self studies. The most productive eras for the self have been those in which new methodologies flourished (the 1950s and the 1980s), and correspondingly, the least productive have been those in which new methodologies were scarce (e.g., the 1940s and, perhaps, the 1960s). This has led some to characterize the contribution of social cognition as a methodological one.

Social-cognition-oriented researchers have brought many promising new research methodologies to bear on questions regarding the self, often by transplanting procedures developed within experimental cognitive psychology. A partial list would include Warren's modified Stroop effect (Higgins et al., 1988), release from proactive interference (McDaniel et al., 1987), cued recall (Barclay & Subramaniam, 1987), encoding specificity (Klein, Loftus, & Plog, 1992), reaction time methods (Kuiper, 1981), often coupled with priming methods (Klein et al., 1989), and memory load procedures (Bargh & Tota, 1988). These research efforts have made a substantial contribution, and they promise even more for the future.

However, it seems inappropriate to characterize the contribution of the social cognition approach as singularly, or even primarily, methodological. Some of these methodologies have been around for some time, including, for example, reaction time methods (e.g., Donders, 1868) and various forms of recognition and recall measures (Ebbinghaus, 1885). Such methods were not previously brought to bear on questions regarding the self primarily because they had little apparent utility, given the prevailing conceptualizations of self. The way that the self was construed, and the questions that were raised about it, mandated use of alternative techniques.

We suggest that the new methods for examining the self are natural outgrowths of the social cognition perspective. Within the tenets of this perspective lie the justifications for borrowing cognitive methodologies, for emphasizing encoding and memory measures, and for assessing or priming cognitive structures to clarify process and organizational issues about the self. These new methods were a logical consequence of the social cognition conceptualization of self, not a cause of it. Thus, although we value the innovative methodologies contributed by social cognition researchers to the study of self, we must emphasize that these methodologies were not developed in a vacuum. They should not be singled out as though they represented fortuitous discoveries that changed our conception of self.

3. Is the Contribution of Social Cognition Simply That It Provides a New Language or New Concepts for Describing the Self?

The self has been eagerly labeled a prototype, a schema, procedural knowledge, semantic memory, episodic memory, and more. Such characterizations can be beneficial when they stimulate empirical efforts at validation or the derivation of unique new hypotheses. But they can also be detrimental when they import unvalidated surplus meaning into thinking about an area or create unnecessary rifts between alternative approaches that differ less in content than in terminology. The positive and negative effects of such scientific rhetoric has been documented elsewhere (cf. Schachtel, 1947; Carlston, 1987).

A primary concern is that the rhetoric in vogue is often used in a fairly nonrigorous way. Although examples abound, the notion of self as a rich and highly organized cognitive structure (e.g., a schema or prototype) is representative. As several reviewers have noted (Greenwald & Banaji, 1989; Higgins & Bargh, 1987), direct evidence to support these conceptions over plausible alternatives has been lacking. Given that many predictions generated by this point of view derive equally well from alternative viewpoints (Higgins & Bargh, 1987), it sometimes appears that social cognition has contributed more verbiage than substance. Indeed, the schema concept itself has been criticized as often being theoretically ill defined and connoting an aura of specificity that it often does not live up to (Alba & Hasher, 1983; Fiske & Linville, 1980). Moreover, as noted previously, recent efforts to directly assess the structural nature of the self have failed to support several of the "self-as-cognitive structure" assumptions. Nonetheless, our point is not that such conceptualizations have failed to benefit the field of self-study. In fact, modern theories of the self (including schema and prototype approaches) have done exactly what theories are supposed to do—help organize research findings and suggest directions for future research.

This history serves to highlight yet another contribution of the social cognition perspective. Current researchers have not simply applied new labels to the study of the self. They have taken these labels seriously, and they have used them to explore the specific properties of self, as well as the relationships between the self and definitionally similar structures. Thus, their achievement lies not only in their new conceptualizations or labels, but also in the systematic empirical examination that these have stimulated.

4. Does Social Cognition Explain What the Self "Really" Is?

There is a temptation to believe that the social cognition approach is bringing us closer to truth about the nature of the self. Perhaps this is because social cognition models incorporate a broader domain, encompassing not only the self, but other social and nonsocial phenomena as well. These models of self thus seem more "real" because they are consistent with much of what is already known about cognitive process and structure. Or perhaps it is because social cognition methodologies rely less than earlier methods on subjects as informants about their self-conceptions.

In any case, it is important (if humbling) to remind ourselves from time to time that the models of social cognition, and of cognitive psychology more broadly, are just that—models. We hope that current ones are better models—more intuitively reasonable, more heuristic, and more consistent with the rapidly expanding research literature than their predecessors. However, given the state of the art, they are still just models, and they need to be reconstructed from time to time as a pillar here or there crumbles in the face of new empirical evidence. Even the cognitive bedrock on which they are built shifts occasionally as challenges arise to notions such as depth of processing (cf. Cermak & Craik, 1979), semantic memory, and associative structure. It is therefore wise to carefully couch our discussions in terms of how best to conceive of the self, rather than in terms of what the self really is. As Gordon and Gergen suggested some time ago (1968): "although one may be convinced privately that [some aspects of self] are real, it is not good science to assume their actuality or that what one is measuring is an adequate index of underlying reality" (p. 5).

5. Is the Social Cognition Approach to Self Another Evolutionary Change or a Revolutionary Advance in Theory and Research?

We have noted the tendency for the self to be reconceptualized every decade or so, framed in terms of the perspective that dominates social psychology at the time. These transitions tend to be somewhat predictable and orderly, much more like the periodic change in United States presidents than the sudden and violent upheavals of a revolution. Moreover, like new presidents, new viewpoints on the self often campaign with novel phrases and ideas, but they ultimately seem to see things, and to leave things, much as their predecessors did. Thus there is a temptation to view the social cognition approach as just another place holder to the orderly succession of self-conceptions.

Given past history, it is difficult to deny the possibility that the social cognition conceptualization of self will eventually be supplanted by the next orientation to take hold of social psychology. Nonetheless, there are aspects of this "administration" that are different, that have revolutionary importance with regard to the study of self, and that will seemingly have impact long after the phrase "social cognition" has fallen from vogue. First, the social cognition approach has taken its metaphors for the self more seriously than have most past approaches. Attempts to test rigorously the assumptions and implications of self-conceptions represent a revolutionary development that is likely to create new expectations for future theorists.

Second, social cognition theorists have utilized models of the self that apply more generally to a variety of other social and nonsocial knowledge structures. As a consequence, self research now both benefits from, and speaks to, research involving other cognitive constructs and processes. Third, social cognition models of the self implicate theories and methods from both social psychology and traditional experimental psychology. This has resulted in a virtual revolution in the kinds of research methods used to investigate the self.

Finally, the social cognition approach provides an opportunity to integrate the myriad facets and concerns of self theories within a single model. For example, a production system model or a PDP model might well be able to capture the essence of multiple selves, self-affect, procedural self-knowledge, goal-oriented behavior, and self-presentation. Alternative models have been proposed that may provide similar integrative potential (e.g., Wyer & Srull, 1989). The potential for such models to parsimoniously deal with a wide range of self phenomena is a tribute to their utility and versatility (though this potential is only partly realized at this time). Therefore, even if the social cognition approach should prove to be just one more stage in the reconceptualization of self, it seems likely to be an important stage, which has an enduring influence on the study of self.

REFERENCES

Alba, J. W., & Hasher, L. (1983). Is memory schematic? *Psychological Bulletin, 93,* 203–231.

Albright, J. S., & Kihlstrom, J. F. (1986). *Motivation, visual perspective, and the self–other difference in causal attribution: A study of autobiographical memory.* Unpublished manuscript, Northwestern University.

Allport, G. W. (1943). The ego in contemporary psychology. *Psychological Review, 50,* 451–478.

Allport, G. W. (1955). *Becoming.* New Haven: Yale University Press.

Allport, G. W. (1961). *Pattern and growth in personality.* New York: Holt, Rinehart and Winston.

Andersen, S. M. (1984). Self-knowledge and social inference: II. The diagnosticity of cognitive/affective and behavioral data. *Journal of Personality and Social Psychology, 46,* 294–307.

Andersen, S. M., & Ross, L. (1984). Self-knowledge and social influence: I. The impact of cognitive/affective and behavioral data. *Journal of Personality and Social Psychology, 46,* 280–293.

Anderson, C. A. (1983). Abstract and concrete data in the perseverance of social theories: When weak data lead to unshakable beliefs. *Journal of Experimental Social Psychology, 19,* 93–108.

Anderson, J. R. (1987). Skill acquisition: Compilation of weak-method problem solutions. *Psychological Review, 94,* 192–210.

Backman, C. W., & Secord, P. F. (1968). In C. Gordon & K. J. Gergen (Eds.), *The self in social interaction: Volume I: Classic and contemporary perspectives* (pp. 289–296). New York: Wiley.

Bandura, A. (1977). *Social learning theory.* Englewood Cliffs, NJ: Prentice-Hall.

Barclay, C. R., & Subramaniam, G. (1987). Autobiographical memories and self-schemata. *Applied Cognitive Psychology, 1,* 169–182.

Bargh, J. A. (1982). Attention and automaticity in the processing of self-relevant information. *Journal of Personality and Social Psychology, 43,* 425–436.

Bargh, J. A. (1984). Automatic and conscious processing of social information. In R. S. Wyer & T. K. Srull (Eds.), *Handbook of social cognition* (Vol. 3, pp. 1–43). Hillsdale, NJ: Erlbaum.

Bargh, J. A., & Tota, M. E. (1988). Context-dependent automatic processing in depression: Accessibility of negative constructs with regard to self but not others. *Journal of Personality and Social Psychology, 54,* 925–939.

Bargh, J. A., Bond, R. N., Lombardi, W. L., & Tota, M. E. (1986). The additive nature of chronic and temporary sources of construct accessibility. *Journal of Personality and Social Psychology, 50,* 869–879.

Barsalou, L. W. (1990). On the indistinguishability of exemplar memory and abstraction in category representation. In T. K. Srull and R. S. Wyer, Jr. (Eds.), *Advances in social cognition: Content and process specificity in the effects of prior experiences* (Vol. 3, pp. 61–88), Hillsdale, NJ: Erlbaum.

Bartlett, F. C. (1932). *Remembering.* Cambridge: Cambridge University Press.

Barton, J., Chassin, L., Presson, C. C., & Sherman, S. J. (1982). Social image factors as motivators of smoking initiation in early and middle adolescence. *Child Development, 53,* 499–511.

Baumeister, R. F. (1982). A self-presentational view of social phenomena. *Psychological Bulletin, 91,* 3–26.

Beck, A. T., Rush, A. J., Shaw, B. F., & Emory, G. (1979). *Cognitive therapy of depression.* New York: Guilford.

Bellezza, F. S. (1984). The self as a mnemonic device: The role of internal cues. *Journal of Personality and Social Psychology, 47,* 506–516.

Bem, D. J. (1967). Self-perception: An alternative interpretation of cognitive dissonance phenomena. *Psychological Review, 74,* 183–200.

Bem, D. J. (1972). Self-perception theory. In L. Berkowitz (Ed.), *Advances in experimental social psychology* (Vol. 6, pp. 1–62). New York: Academic Press.

Bower, G. H., & Gilligan, S. G. (1979). Remembering information related to one's self. *Journal of Research in Personality, 13,* 420–461.

Bradley, G. W. [Weary, G.] (1978). Self-serving biases in the attribution process: A reexamination of the fact and fiction question. *Journal of Personality and Social Psychology, 36,* 56–71

Brenner, M. (1973). The next-in-line effect. *Journal of Verbal Learning and Verbal Behavior, 12,* 320–323.

Brown, N. R., Rips, L. J., & Shevell, S. K. (1985). The subjective dates of natural events in very-long-term memory. *Cognitive Psychology, 17,* 139–177.

Brown, P., Keenan, J. M., & Potts, G. R. (1986). The self-reference effect with imagery encoding. *Journal of Personality and Social Psychology, 51,* 897–906.

Brownfain, J. J. (1952). Stability of the self-concept as a dimension of personality. *Journal of Abnormal and Social Psychology, 47,* 597–605.

Bruner, J. S. (1957). On perceptual readiness. *Psychological Review, 64,* 123–152.

Bugental, J. F. T., & Zelen, S. L. (1950). Investigations into the self-concept. *Journal of Personality, 18,* 483–498.

Burke, P. J. (1980). The self: Measurement requirements from an interactionist perspective. *Psychology Quarterly, 43,* 18–29.

Cantor, N., Markus, H., Niedenthal, P., & Nurius, P. (1986). On motivation and the self-concept. In R. M. Sorrentino & E. T. Higgins (Eds.), *Handbook of motivation and social cognition: Foundations of social behavior* (pp. 96–121). New York: Guilford Press.

Carlston, D. E. (1980). The recall and use of traits and events in social inference processes. *Journal of Experimental Social Psychology, 16,* 303–329.

Carlston, D. E. (1987). Turning psychology on itself: The rhetoric of psychology and the psychology of rhetoric. In J. S. Nelson, A. Megill, & D. N. McClosky (Eds.), *The rhetoric of the human sciences: Language and argument in scholarship and public affairs* (pp. 211–235). Madison: University of Wisconsin Press.

Carlston, D. E., & Skowronski, J. J. (1986). Trait memory and behavior memory: The effects of alternative pathways on impression judgment response times. *Journal of Personality and Social Psychology, 50*, 5–13.

Carver, C. S., & Scheier, M. F. (1981). *Attention and self-regulation: A control theory approach to human behavior.* New York: Springer-Verlag.

Cermak, L. S., & Craik, F. I. M. (Eds.). (1979). *Levels of processing in human memory.* Hillsdale, NJ: Erlbaum.

Chassin, L., Presson, C. C., Sherman, S. J., Cotty, E., & Olshavsky, R. W. (1981). Self-images and cigarette smoking in adolescence. *Personality and Social Psychology Bulletin, 7*, 670–676.

Chew, B. R. (1983). *Selective recall of self- and other-references information.* Unpublished doctoral dissertation, Harvard University.

Cooley, C. H. (1902). *Human nature and the social order.* New York: Scribner's.

Craik, F. I. M., & Tulving, E. (1975). Depth of processing and the retention of words in episodic memory. *Journal of Experimental Psychology: General, 104*, 268–294.

Deaux, K. (1993). Reconstructing social identity. *Personality and Social Psychology Bulletin, 19*, 4–12.

Dixon, T. M., & Baumeister, R. F. (1991). Escaping the self: Moderating effects of self-complexity. *Personality and Social Psychology Bulletin, 17*, 363–368.

Donders, F. E. (1868). Die schnelligkeit psychischer processe. *Archiv Anatomie und Psysiologie, 23*, 657–681.

Duval, S., & Wicklund, R. A. (1972). *A theory of objective self-awareness.* New York: Academic Press.

Dweck, C., & Elliott, E. S. (1983). Achievement motivation. In E. M. Hetherington (Ed.), *Handbook of child psychology: Socialization, personality, and social development* (Vol. 4). New York: Wiley.

Ebbinghaus, H. (1885). *Memory: A contribution to experimental psychology* (translated by H. A. Ruger & C. E. Bussenues, 1913). New York: Teachers College, Columbia University.

Fazio, R. H., Effrein, E. A., & Falender, V. J. (1981). Self-perceptions following social interaction. *Journal of Personality and Social Psychology, 41*, 232–242.

Fenigstein, A., Scheier, M. F., & Buss, A. H. (1975). Public and private self-consciousness: Assessment and theory. *Journal of Consulting and Clinical Psychology, 43*, 522–527.

Ferguson, T. J., Rule, G. R., & Carlston, D. E. (1983). Memory for personality relevant information. *Journal of Personality and Social Psychology, 44*, 251–261.

Fiske, S. T., & Linville, P. W. (1980). What does the schema concept buy us? *Personality and Social Psychology Bulletin, 6*, 543–557.

Fiske, S. T., & Taylor, S. E. (1991). *Social cognition* (2nd ed.). New York: McGraw-Hill.

Fong, G. T., & Markus, H. (1992). Self-schemas and judgments about others. *Social Cognition, 1*, 191–205.

Freud, S. (1920). *A general introduction to psychoanalysis.* New York: Boni and Liveright.

Friedman, A., & Pullyblank, J. (1982). *Remembering information about oneself and others: The role of distinctiveness.* Paper presented at the Psychonomic Society, Minneapolis, MN.

Fuhrman, R. W., & Wyer, Jr., R. S. (1988). Event memory: Temporal-order judgments of personal life experiences. *Journal of Personality and Social Psychology, 54*, 365–384.

Ganellen, R. J., & Carver, C. S. (1985). Why does self-reference promote incidental encoding? *Journal of Experimental Psychology, 21*, 284–300.

Gergen, K. J. (1965). Interaction goals and personalistic feedback as factors affecting the presentation of self. *Journal of Personality and Social Psychology, 1*, 413–424.

Gergen, K. J. (1968). Personal consistency and presentation of self. In C. Gordon & K. J. Gergen (Eds.), *The self in social interaction* (Vol. 1, pp. 299–308). New York: Wiley.

Gergen, K. J. (1971). *The concept of self.* New York: Holt, Rinehart, and Winston.

Goffman, E. (1959). *The presentation of self in everyday life.* Garden City, NY: Doubleday Anchor Books.

Gordon, C. (1968). Self-conceptions: Configurations of content. In C. Gordon & K. J. Gergen (Eds.), *The self in social interaction: Volume I: Classic and contemporary perspectives* (pp. 115–136). New York: Wiley.

Gordon, C., & Gergen, K. J. (Eds.). (1968). *The self in social interaction: Volume I: Classic and contemporary perspectives.* New York: Wiley.

Greenwald, A. G. (1980). The totalitarian ego: Fabrication and revision of personal history. *American Psychologist, 35,* 603–618.

Greenwald, A. G., & Banaji, M. R. (1989). The self as a memory system: Powerful, but ordinary. *Journal of Personality and Social Psychology, 57,* 41–54.

Greenwald, A. G, & Breckler, S. J. (1985). To whom is the self presented? In B. R. Schlenker (Ed.), *The self and social life* (pp. 126–145). New York: McGraw-Hill.

Greenwald, A. G., & Pratkanis, A. R. (1984). The self. In R. S. Wyer & T. K. Srull (Eds.), *Handbook of social cognition* (Vol. 3, pp. 129–178). Hillsdale, NJ: Erlbaum.

Harter, S. (1983). Developmental perspectives on the self-esteem. In P. H. Mussen (Ed.), *Carmichael's manual of child psychology* (Vol. 4). New York: Wiley.

Harter, S. (1986). Processes underlying the construction, maintenance, and enhancement of the self-concept in children. In J. Suls & A. G. Greenwald (Eds.), *Psychological perspectives on the self* (Vol. 3, pp. 136–182). Hillsdale, NJ: Erlbaum.

Hastie, R., & Carlston, D. E. (1980). Theoretical issues in person memory. In R. Hastie, T. M. Ostrom, E. B. Ebbeson, R. S. Wyer, D. L. Hamilton, & D. E Carlston (Eds.), *Person memory: The cognitive basis of social perception.* Hillsdale, NJ: Erlbaum.

Hastie, R., Ostrom, T., Ebbeson, E., Wyer, R., Hamilton, D., & Carlston, D. E. (1980). *Person memory: The cognitive bases of social perception.* Hillsdale, NJ: Erlbaum.

Higgins, E. T. (1987). Self-discrepancy: A theory relating self and affect. *Psychological Review, 94,* 3, 319–340.

Higgins, E. T. (1989). Self-discrepancy theory: What patterns of self-beliefs cause people to suffer? In L. Berkowitz (Ed.), *Advances in experimental social psychology* (Vol. 22, pp. 93–136). New York: Academic Press.

Higgins, E. T., & Bargh, J. A. (1987). Social cognition and social perception. In M. R. Rosenweig & L. W. Porter (Eds.), *Annual review of psychology* (Vol. 38, pp. 369–425). Palo Alto, CA: Annual Reviews.

Higgins, E. T., & King, G. A. (1981). Accessibility of social constructs: Information-processing consequences of individual and contextual variability. In N. Cantor & J. F. Kihlstrom (Eds.), *Personality, cognition and social interaction* (pp. 69–122). Hillsdale, NJ: Erlbaum.

Higgins, E. T., Herman, C. P., & Zanna, M. P. (Eds.). (1981). *Social cognition: The Ontario Symposium* (Vol. 1). Hillsdale, NJ: Erlbaum.

Higgins, E. T., King, G. A., & Mavin, G. H. (1982). Individual construct accessibility and subjective impressions and recall. *Journal of Personality and Social Psychology, 43,* 35–47.

Higgins, E. T., Bargh, J. A., & Lombardi, W. (1985). The nature of priming effects on categorization. *Journal of Experimental Psychology: Learning, Memory, and Cognition, 11,* 59–69.

Higgins, E. T., Bond, R. N., Klein, R., & Strauman, T. (1986). Self-discrepancies and emotional vulnerability: How magnitude, accessibility, and type of discrepancy influence affect. *Journal of Personality and Social Psychology, 51,* 5–15.

Higgins, E. T., Van Hook, E., & Dorfman, D. (1988). Do self-attributes form a cognitive structure? *Social Cognition, 6,* 177–207.

Hilgard, E. R. (1949). Human motives and the concept of the self. *American Psychologist, 4,* 374–382.

Hintzman, D. L. (1986). "Schema abstraction" in a multiple-trace memory model. *Psychological Review, 93,* 411–428.

Holmes, D. S. (1968). Dimensions of projection. *Psychological Bulletin, 69,* 248–268.
Holyoak, K. J., & Gordon, P. C. (1984). Information processing and social cognition. In R. S. Wyer, Jr. & T. K. Srull (Eds.), *Handbook of social cognition* (Vol. 1, pp. 39–70). Hillsdale, NJ: Erlbaum.
Hull, J. G., & Levy, A. S. (1979). The organizational functions of the self: An alternative to the Duval and Wicklund model of self-awareness. *Journal of Personality and Social Psychology, 37,* 756–768.
James, W. (1890). *The principles of psychology.* New York: Holt.
James, W. (1910). *Psychology: The briefer course.* New York: Holt.
Jones, E. E. (1964). *Ingratiation.* New York: Irvington.
Jones, E. E., & Pittman, T. S. (1982). Toward a general theory of strategic self-presentation. In J. Suls (Ed.), *Psychological perspectives on the self* (pp. 231–262). Hillsdale, NJ: Erlbaum.
Jones, E. E., Rhodewalt, F., Berglas, S., & Skelton, J. A. (1981). Effects of strategic self-presentation on subsequent self-esteem. *Journal of Personality and Social Psychology, 41,* 407–421.
Jourard, S. M. (1958). A study of self-disclosure. *Scientific American, 198,* 77–82.
Jourard, S. M. (1964). *The transparent self.* Princeton, NJ: Van Nostrand.
Judd, C. M., & Park, B. (1988). Out-group homogeneity: Judgments of variability at the individual and group levels. *Journal of Personality and Social Psychology, 54,* 778–788.
Kalthoff, R. A., & Neimeyer, R. A. (1993). Self-complexity and psychological distress: A test of the buffering model. *International Journal of Personal Construct Psychology, 6,* 327–349.
Katz, A. N. (1987). Self-reference in the encoding of creative-relevant traits. *Journal of Personality, 55,* 97–120.
Keenan, J. M., & Baillet, S. D. (1980). Memory for personally and socially significant events. In R. S. Nickerson (Ed.), *Attention and performance* (Vol. 8, 651–669). Hillsdale, NJ: Erlbaum.
Kelly, G. A. (1955). *The psychology of personal constructs.* New York: Norton.
Kendzierski, D. (1980). Self-schemata and scripts: The recall of self-referent and scriptal information. *Personality and Social Psychology Bulletin, 6,* 23–29.
Kihlstrom, J. F. (1984). Conscious, subconscious, unconscious: A cognitive perspective. In K. S. Bowers & D. Meichenbaum (Eds.), *The unconscious reconsidered.* New York: Wiley.
Kihlstrom, J. F., & Cantor, N. (1984). Mental representations of the self. In L. Berkowitz (Ed.), *Advances in experimental social psychology* (Vol. 17, pp. 1–47). New York: Academic Press.
Kihlstrom, J. F., Cantor, N., Albright, J. S., Chew, B. R., Klein, S. B., & Niedenthal, P. M. (1988). Information processing and the study of the self. In L. Berkowitz (Ed.), *Advances in experimental social psychology* (Vol. 21, pp. 145–180). New York: Academic Press.
Klein, S. B., & Kihlstrom, J. F. (1986). Elaboration, organization and the self-reference effect in memory. *Journal of Experimental Psychology: General, 115,* 26–38.
Klein, S. B., & Loftus, J. (1988). The nature of self-referent encoding: The contributions of elaborative and organizational processes. *Journal of Personality and Social Psychology, 55,* 5–11.
Klein, S. B., & Loftus, J. (1990a). Rethinking the role of organization in person memory: An independent trace storage model. *Journal of Personality and Social Psychology, 59,* 400–410.
Klein, S. B., & Loftus, J. (1990b). The role of abstract and exemplar-based knowledge in self-judgments: Implications for a cognitive model of the self. In T. K. Srull & R. S. Wyler (Eds.), *Advances in social cognition* (Vol. 3, pp. 131–139). Hillsdale, NJ: Erlbaum.
Klein, S. B., & Loftus, J. (1993). The mental representation of trait and autobiographical knowledge about the self. In T. R. Srull & R. S. Wyler (Eds.), *Advances in social cognition* (Vol. 5, pp. 1–49). Hillsdale, NJ: Erlbaum.
Klein, S. B., Loftus, J., & Burton, H. A. (1989). Two self-reference effects: The importance of distinguishing between self-descriptiveness judgments and autobiographical retrieval in self-referent encoding. *Journal of Personality and Social Psychology, 56,* 853–865.

Klein, S. B., Loftus, J., & Plog, A. E. (1992). Trait judgments about the self: Evidence from the encoding specificity paradigm. *Personality and Social Psychology Bulletin, 18,* 730–735.

Klein, S. B., Loftus, J., Trafton, J. G., & Fuhrman, R. W. (1992). The use of exemplars and abstractions in trait judgments: A model of trait knowledge about the self and others. *Journal of Personality and Social Psychology, 63,* 739–753.

Kuhn, M. H., & McPartland, T. S. (1954). An empirical investigation of self-attitudes. *American Sociological Review, 19,* 68–76.

Kuiper, N. A. (1981). Convergent evidence for the self as a prototype: The "Inverted-U RT effect" for self and other judgments. *Personality and Social Psychology Bulletin, 7,* 438–443.

Kuiper, N. A., & Derry, P. A. (1981). The self as a cognitive prototype: An application to person perception and depression. In N. Cantor & J. F. Kihlstrom (Eds.), *Personality, cognition, and social interaction* (pp. 215–232). Hillsdale, NJ: Erlbaum.

Kuiper, N. A., & Rogers, T. B. (1979). Encoding of personal information: Self–other differences. *Journal of Personality and Social Psychology, 37,* 499–514.

Langer, E. J. (1978). Rethinking the role of thought in social interaction. In J. H. Harvey, W. J. Ickes, & R. F. Kidd (Eds.), *New directions in attribution research* (Vol. 2, pp. 36–58). Hillsdale, NJ: Erlbaum.

Lewicki, P. (1986). *Nonconscious social information processing.* New York: Academic Press.

Lingle, J. H., & Ostrom, T. M. (1979). Retrieval selectivity in memory-based impression judgments. *Journal of Personality and Social Psychology, 37,* 180–194.

Linville, P. W. (1985). Self-complexity and affective extremity: Don't put all your eggs in one cognitive basket. *Social Cognition, 3,* 94–120.

Linville, P. W. (1987). Self-complexity as a cognitive buffer against stress-related illness and depression. *Journal of Personality and Social Psychology, 52,* 663–676.

Linville, P. W. (1994). Self-complexity and multiple self-esteems. Unpublished manuscript. Duke University, Durham, NC.

Linville, P. W., & Clark, L. F. (1989). Can production systems cope with coping? *Social Cognition, 7,* 195–236.

Linville, P. W., & Fischer, G. W. (1993). Exemplar and abstraction models of perceived group variability and stereotypicality. *Social Cognition, 11,* 92–125.

Linville, P. W., Fischer, G. W., & Salovey, P. (1989). Perceived distributions of the characteristics of in-group and out-group members: Empirical evidence and a computer simulation. *Journal of Personality and Social Psychology, 57,* 165–188.

Loftus, E. F., & Marburger, W. (1983). Since the eruption of Mt. St. Helens, has anyone beaten you up? Improving the accuracy of retrospective reports with landmark events. *Memory and Cognition, 11,* 114–120.

Lord, C. G. (1980). Schemas and images as memory aids: Two modes of processing social information. *Journal of Personality and Social Psychology, 38,* 257–269.

Lord, C. G., Desforges, D. M., Chacon, S., Pere, G., & Clubb, B. (1992). Reflections on reputation in the process of self-evaluation. *Social Cognition, 10,* 2–29.

McClelland, J. L., & Rumelhart, D. E. (Eds.). (1986). *Parallel distributed processing: Explorations in the microstructure of cognition* (Vol. 2). Cambridge, MA: MIT Press.

McDaniel, M. A., Lapsley, D. K., & Milstead, M. (1987). Testing the generality and automaticity of self-reference encoding with release from proactive interference. *Journal of Experimental Social Psychology, 23,* 269–284.

McFarland, C., & Ross, M. (1987). The relation between current impressions and memories of self and dating partners. *Personality and Social Psychology Bulletin, 13,* 228–238.

McGuire, W. J. (1984). Search for the self: Going beyond self-esteem and the reactive self. In R. A. Zucker, J. Aronoff, & A. I. Rabin (Eds.), *Personality and the prediction of behavior.* New York: Academic Press.

McGuire, W. J., & Padawer-Singer, A. (1976). Traits salience in the spontaneous self-concept. *Journal of Personality and Social Psychology, 33,* 743–754.

Markus, H. (1977). Self-schemata and processing information about the self. *Journal of Personality and Social Psychology, 35*, 63–78.
Markus, H. (1980). The self in thought and memory. In D. M. Wegner & R. R. Vallacher (Eds.), *The self in social psychology.* New York: Oxford University Press.
Markus, H. R., & Kitayama, S. (1991). Culture and the self: Implications for cognition, emotion, and motivation. *Psychological Review, 98*, 224–253.
Markus, H., & Kunda, Z. (1986). Stability and malleability of the self-concept. *Journal of Personality and Social Psychology, 51*, 858–866.
Markus, H., & Nurius, P. (1986). Possible selves. *American Psychologist, 41*, 954–969.
Markus, H., & Sentis, K. (1982). The self in social information processing. In J. Suls (Ed.), *Psychological perspectives on the self* (Vol. 1). Hillsdale, NJ: Erlbaum.
Markus, H., & Wurf, E. (1987). The dynamic self-concept: A social psychological perspective. In M. R. Rosenzweig & L. W. Porter (Eds.), *Annual review of psychology* (Vol. 38, pp. 299–337). Palo Alto, CA: Annual Reviews.
Markus, H., & Zajonc, R. B. (1985). The cognitive perspective in social psychology. In G. Lindzey & E. Aronson (Eds.), *The handbook of social psychology* (3rd ed.) (Vol. 1, pp. 137–230). New York: Random House.
Markus, H., Crane, M., Bernstein, S., & Siladi, M. (1982). Self-schemas and gender. *Journal of Personality and Social Psychology, 42*, 38–50.
Markus, H., Hamill, R., & Sentis, K. (1987). Thinking fat: Self-schema for body weight and the processing of weight relevant information. *Journal of Applied Social Psychology, 17*, 50–71.
Mead, G. H. (1934). *Mind, self, and society.* Chicago: University of Chicago Press.
Medin, D. L. (1989). Concepts and conceptual structure. *American Psychologist, 44*, 1469–1481.
Medin, D. L., & Schaffer, M. M. (1978). Context theory of classification learning. *Psychological Review, 85*, 207–238.
Medin, D. L., Altom, M. W., & Murphy, T. D. (1984). Given versus induced category representations: Use of prototype and exemplar information in classification. *Journal of Experimental Psychology: Learning, Memory and Cognition, 10*, 333–352.
Mori, D., Chaiken, S., & Pliner, P. (1987). "Eating lightly" and the self-presentation of femininity. *Journal of Personality and Social Psychology, 53*, 693–702.
Mueller, J. H. (1982). Self-awareness and access to material rated as self-descriptive or nondescriptive. *Bulletin of Psychonomic Soc., 19*, 323–326.
Neisser, U. (1982). *Memory observed.* San Francisco: Freeman.
Niedenthal, P. M., Cantor, N., & Kihlstrom, J. F. (1985). Prototype matching: A strategy for social decision making. *Journal of Personality and Social Psychology, 48*, 575–584.
Niedenthal, P. M., Setterlund, M. B., & Wherry, M. B. (1992). Possible self-complexity and affective reactions to goal-relevant evaluation. *Journal of Personality and Social Psychology, 63*, 5–16.
Nisbett, R. E., & Wilson, T. D. (1977). Telling more than we can know: Verbal reports on mental processes. *Psychological Review, 84*, 231–259.
Nosofsky, R. M. (1986). Attention, similarity, and the identification-categorization relationship. *Journal of Experimental Psychology: General, 115*, 39–57.
Nuttin, Jr., J. M. (1985). Narcissism beyond gestalt and awareness: The name-letter effect. *European Journal of Social Psychology, 15*, 353–361.
Ostrom, T. M. (1984). The sovereignty of social cognition. In R. S. Wyer & T. K. Srull (Eds.), *Handbook of social cognition* (Vol. 1, pp. 1–38). Hillsdale, NJ: Erlbaum.
Park, B., & Hastie, R. (1987). Perception of variability in category development: Instance- versus abstraction-based stereotypes. *Journal of Personality and Social Psychology, 53*, 621–635.
Pelham, B. W. (1991). On confidence and consequence: The certainty and importance of self-knowledge. *Journal of Personality and Social Psychology, 60*, 518–530.
Posner, M. I., & Keele, S. W. (1968). On the genesis of abstract ideas. *Journal of Experimental Psychology, 77*, 353–363.

Reed, S. K. (1972). Pattern recognition and categorization. *Cognitive Psychology, 3,* 382–407.

Rhodewalt, F. T. (1986). Self-presentation and the phenomenal self: On the stability and malleability of self-conceptions. In R. Baumeister (Ed.), *Public and private selves* (pp. 117–142). New York: Springer-Verlag.

Rhodewalt, F., & Agustsdottir, S. (1986). Effects of self-presentation on the phenomenal self. *Journal of Personality and Social Psychology, 50,* 47–53.

Rogers, C. R. (1942). *Counseling and psychotherapy.* Boston: Houghton-Mifflin.

Rogers, C. R. (1951). *Client-centered therapy.* New York: Houghton-Mifflin.

Rogers, T. B. (1977). Self-reference in memory: Recognition of personality items. *Journal of Research in Personality, 1,* 295–305.

Rogers, T. B. (1981). A model of the self as an aspect of the human information processing system. In N. Cantor & J. F. Kihlstrom (Eds.), *Personality, cognition, and social interaction* (pp. 193–214). Hillsdale, NJ: Erlbaum.

Rogers, T. B., Kuiper, N. A., & Kirker, W. S. (1977). Self-reference and the encoding of personal information. *Journal of Personality and Social Psychology, 35,* 677–688.

Rogers, T. B., Kuiper, N. A., & Rogers, J. P. (1979). Symbolic distance and congruity effects for paired-comparisons judgments of degree of self-reference. *Journal of Research in Personality, 13,* 433–449.

Rosenberg, M. (1979). *Conceiving the self.* New York: Basic Books.

Rosenberg, M. (1986). Self-concept from middle childhood through adolescence. In J. Suls & A. G. Greenwald (Eds.), *Psychological perspectives on the self* (Vol. 3, pp. 107–135). Hillsdale, NJ: Erlbaum.

Ross, M., & Conway, M. (1986). Remembering one's own past: The construction of personal histories. In R. M. Sorrentino & E. T. Higgins (Eds.), *Handbook of motivation and cognition: Foundations of social behavior* (pp. 122–144). New York: Guilford Press.

Ross, L., Greene, D., & House, P. (1977). The "false consensus effect": An egocentric bias in social perception and attribution processes. *Journal of Experimental Psychology, 13,* 279–301.

Ross, M., McFarland, C., Conway, M., & Zanna, M. P. (1983). Reciprocal relation between attitudes and behavior recall: Committing people to newly formed attitudes. *Journal of Personality and Social Psychology, 45,* 257–267.

Rumelhart, D. E., & McClelland, J. L. (Eds.). (1986). *Parallel distributed processing: Explorations in the microstructure of cognition* (Vol. 1). Cambridge, MA: MIT Press.

Salancik, G. R., & Conway, M. (1975). Attitude inference from salient and relevant cognitive content about behavior. *Journal of Personality and Social Psychology, 32,* 829–840.

Schachtel, E. G. (1947). On memory and childhood amnesia. *Psychiatry, 10,* 1–26.

Schlenker, B. R., & Trudeau, J. V. (1990). Impact of self-presentations on private self-beliefs and misattribution. *Journal of Personality and Social Psychology, 58,* 22–32.

Schneider, D. J. (1991). Social cognition. In M. R. Rosenzweig & L. W. Porter (Eds.), *Annual review of psychology* (Vol. 42, pp. 527–561). Palo Alto, CA: Annual Reviews.

Sherif, M., & Cantril, H. (1947). *The psychology of ego-involvements.* New York: Wiley.

Sherman, S. J., & Gorkin, I. (1980). Attitude bolstering when behavior is inconsistent with central attitudes. *Journal of Experimental Social Psychology, 16,* 388–403.

Sherman, S. J., Judd, C. M., & Park, B. (1989). Social cognition. In M. R. Rosenzweig & L. W. Porter (Eds.), *Annual review of psychology* (Vol. 40, pp. 281–326). Palo Alto, CA: Annual Reviews.

Showers, C. (1992a). Compartmentalization of positive and negative self-knowledge: Keeping bad apples out of the bunch. *Journal of Personality and Social Psychology, 62,* 1036–1049.

Showers, C. (1992b). Evaluatively integrative thinking about characteristics of the self. *Personality and Social Psychology Bulletin, 18,* 719–729.

Showers, C., & Cantor, N. (1985). Social cognition: A look at motivated strategies. In M. R. Rosenzweig & L. W. Porter (Eds.), *Annual review of psychology* (Vol. 36, pp. 275–305). Palo Alto, CA: Annual Reviews.

Smith, E. E., & Medin, D. L. (1981). *Categories and concepts*. Cambridge, MA: Harvard University Press.
Smith, E. R., & Lerner, M. (1986). Development of automatism of social judgments. *Journal of Personality and Social Psychology, 50*, 246–259.
Smith, E. R., & Zárate, M. A. (1992). Exemplar-based model of social judgment. *Psychological Review, 99*, 33–21.
Smith, H. S., & Cohen, L. H. (1993). Self-complexity and reactions to a relationship breakup. *Journal of Social and Clinical Psychology.*
Snyder, M. (1979). Self-monitoring processes. In L. Berkowitz (Ed.), *Advances in experimental social psychology* (Vol. 12, pp. 86–131). New York: Academic Press.
Snygg, D., & Combs, A. W. (1949). *Individual behavior*. New York: Harper and Row.
Sorrentino, R. M., & Roney, C. J. R. (1986). Uncertainty orientation, achievement-related motivation, and task diagnosticity as determinants of task performance. *Social Cognition, 4*, 420–436.
Srull, T. K., & Wyer, Jr., R. S. (1979). The role of category accessibility in the interpretation of information about persons: Some determinants and implications. *Journal of Personality and Social Psychology, 37*, 1660–1672.
Srull, T. K., & Wyer, Jr., R. S. (1980). Category accessibility and social perception: Some implications for the study of person memory and interpersonal judgments. *Journal of Personality and Social Psychology, 38*, 841–856.
Srull, T. K., & Wyer, Jr., R. S. (1986). The role of chronic and temporary goals in social information processing. In R. M. Sorrentino & E. T. Higgins (Eds.), *Handbook of motivation and cognition: Foundations of social behavior* (pp. 503–549). New York: Guilford.
Strack, F., Schwarz, N., & Gschneidinger, E. (1985). Happiness and reminiscing: The role of time perspective, affect and mode of thinking. *Journal of Personality and Social Psychology, 49*, 1460–1469.
Strauman, T. J., & Higgins, E. T. (1987). Automatic activation of self-discrepancies and emotional syndromes: When cognitive structures influence affect. *Journal of Personality and Social Psychology, 53*, 1004–1014.
Stryker, S. (1980). *Symbolic interactionism*. Menlo Park, CA: Benjamin/Cummings.
Stryker, S. (1986). Identity theory: Developments and extensions. In K. Yardley & T. Honess (Eds.), *Self and Identity*. New York: Wiley.
Swann, Jr., W. B. (1983). Self-verification. Bringing social reality into harmony with the self. In J. Suls & A. G. Greenwald (Eds.), *Psychological perspectives on the self* (Vol. 2, pp. 33–66). Hillsdale, NJ: Erlbaum.
Swann, Jr., W. B. (1987). Identity negotiation: Where two roads meet. *Journal of Personality and Social Psychology, 53*, 1038–1051.
Taylor, D. A., & Oberlander, L. (1969). Person-perception and self-disclosure: Motivational mechanisms in interpersonal processes. *Journal of Experimental Research in Personality, 4*, 14–28.
Taylor, S. E., & Brown, J. D. (1988). Illusion and well-being: A social psychological perspective on mental health. *Psychological Bulletin, 103*, 193–210.
Tesser, A. (1986). Some effects on self-evaluation maintenance on cognition and action. In R. M. Sorrentino & E. T. Higgins (Eds.), *Handbook of motivation and cognition: Foundations of social behavior* (pp. 435–464). New York: Guilford.
Tesser, A. (1988). Toward a self-evaluation maintenance model of social behavior. In L. Berkowitz (Ed.), *Advances in experimental social psychology* (Vol. 21, pp. 181–227). New York: Academic Press.
Tesser, A., & Campbell, J. (1983). Self-definition and self-evaluation maintenance. In J. Suls & A. G. Greenwald (Eds.), *Psychological perspectives on the self* (Vol. 2, pp. 1–32). Hillsdale, NJ: Erlbaum.
Thoits, P. A. (1983). Multiple identities and psychological well-being: A reformulation and test of the social isolation hypothesis. *American Sociology Review, 48*, 174–187.

Thompson, C. P., Skowronski, J. J., & Lee, D. J. (1988). Reconstructing the date of a personal event. In M. M. Gruneberg, P. E. Morris, & N. Sykes (Eds.), *Practical aspects of memory: Current research and issues* (pp. 241–246). New York: Academic Press.

Trope, Y. (1983). Self-assessment in achievement behavior. In J. Suls & A. G. Greenwald (Eds.), *Psychological perspectives on the self* (Vol. 2, pp. 93–122). Hillsdale, NJ: Erlbaum.

Trope, Y. (1986). Self-enhancement and self-assessment in achievement behavior. In R. M. Sorrentino & E. T. Higgins (Eds.), *Handbook of motivation and cognition: Foundations of social behavior* (pp. 350–378). New York: Guilford.

Tulving, E. (1985). *Elements of episodic memory.* London: Oxford University Press.

Warren, R. E. (1972). Stimulus encoding and memory. *Journal of Experimental Psychology, 94,* 90–100.

Wyer, Jr., & R. S., Carlston, D. E. (1979). *Social cognition, inference, and attribution.* Hillsdale, NJ: Erlbaum.

Wyer, Jr., R. S., & Srull, T. K. (1981). Category accessibility: Some theoretical and empirical issues concerning the processing of social stimulus information. In E. T. Higgins, C. P. Herman, & M. P. Zanna (Eds.), *Social cognition: The Ontario Symposium* (Vol. 1, pp. 161–198). Hillsdale, NJ: Erlbaum.

Wyer, Jr., R. S., & Srull, T. K. (Eds.). (1984). *Handbook of social cognition* (Vol. 1–3). Hillsdale, NJ: Erlbaum.

Wyer, Jr., R. S., & Srull, T. K. (1989). *Memory and cognition in its social context.* Hillsdale, NJ: Erlbaum.

Wyer, Jr., R. S., Shoben, E. J., Fuhrman, R. W., & Bodenhausen, G. V. (1985). Event memory: The temporal organization of social action sequences. *Journal of Personality and Social Psychology, 49,* 857–877.

Wylie, R. (1961). *The self-concept: A critical survey of pertinent research.* Lincoln, NE: University of Nebraska Press.

Wylie, R. (1974). *The self-concept* (Vol. 1). Lincoln, NE: University of Nebraska Press.

Zechmeister, E. B., & Nyberg, S. E. (1982). *Human memory.* Monterey, CA: Brooks/Cole.

7

The Cognitive Foundation of Attitudes: It's a Wonderful Construct

Thomas M. Ostrom
John J. Skowronski
Andrzej Nowak

In the classic 1946 Christmas movie, *It's a Wonderful Life,* a depressed George Bailey (played by Jimmy Stewart) tells his guardian angel he wishes he had never been born. George's wish is granted. As George later walks through his old home town, visiting long-familiar people and places, he finds himself in a different reality. He encounters a world in which George Bailey had never been. His town, its people and places, and its history were dramatically altered. The home George shared with his wife and family was an abandoned shell. A man he had once helped was a drunken derelict. Even his warm and loving mother was hostile and suspicious. George came to realize his life was important, not just for himself, but for the entire fabric of his social world. The movie provides a sentimental, but evocative, reminder that each of us makes a difference.

Consider, if you will, a social psychology, without the construct of *attitude.* Imagine that Thomas and Znaniecki (1918) had never delved into the diaries of Polish peasants who had immigrated to America, that Thurstone (1928) had never proclaimed "attitudes can be measured," and that Allport's (1935) chapter in the field's first *Handbook of Social Psychology* had been on instincts and urges instead of attitudes.

Without these contributions, our counterfactual world might have found the field during the 1950s and 1960s to be aggressively behaviorist, as was the bulk of work in experimental psychology. Our theorizing might be ignorant of cognitive consistency processes (such as congruity theory, Osgood & Tannenbaum, 1955; and dissonance theory, Festinger, 1957), of information processing principles of communication and persuasion (Hovland, Janis, & Kelley, 1953), of assimilation–contrast processes (Sherif & Hovland, 1961), and of models of belief and information integration (Anderson, 1974; Fishbein & Ajzen, 1975). These foundational theories of attitudes and beliefs, which constitute the bedrock of current work in the field, may have never existed.

Jumping to contemporary times, we would not have the elaboration likelihood analysis of cognitive responses to persuasion (see Petty, Priester, & Wegener, in press) that has encouraged the distinction between central and peripheral processing modes. Furthermore, applied fields, such as consumer psychology, health psychology, organizational psychology, and political psychology would be substantially altered. Given these considerations, it seems reasonable to conclude that social psychology, if visited without the past contributions of attitude to the field, would be as pallid and dreary as was Jimmy Stewart's town. Attitude is a concept that has made a difference.

OBJECTIVES OF THE CHAPTER

The impact of attitudes has been widely recognized. Allport described attitudes as "the most distinctive and indispensable concept in American social psychology" and one that has "virtually established itself as the keystone in the edifice of American social psychology." This claim is as true today as it was in 1935. Attitudes and beliefs provided the mentalistic dynamic that propelled social psychology through the behaviorist era into the present.

Because of their focus on the attitude construct, social psychologists rightfully take pride in having, from the very beginning, taken a "cognitive" approach to the study of psychology. This focus substantially predated the information processing approach, which led the area of "experimental psychology" to reconstrue itself as "cognitive psychology."

But social psychologists should not be too proud of their embracing cognitive concepts so early. There has been a little-recognized cost associated with the fact that attitudes have always been conceptualized in a cognitive manner. The nature of the conceptual primitives adopted by many contemporary attitude theorists frequently reflects the zeitgeist of the 1920's and 1930's. The concern we raise here is that many of those original metatheoretic assumptions have been uncritically retained. One objective of this chapter is to identify and, in light of recent advances in cognitive psychology, analyze the implicit assumptions that have remained unchanged over the years.

Such an analysis is essential. In contrast to the unchanging history of the attitude construct, researchers in the field of cognitive psychology almost completely abandoned the conceptual assumptions held by their intellectual ancestors in experimental psychology. The antimentalistic concepts of behaviorism are largely irrelevant to the information processing constructs employed by contemporary cognitive psychologists. This change has even been described as a Kuhnian "paradigm shift" (Lachman, Lachman, & Butterfield, 1979).

Some progressive attitude theorists have noted the emerging developments in cognitive psychology, and have used those contemporary ideas in their theory and research. Because of this, substantial advances have already been achieved in our understanding of attitudinal processes. A second objective of this chapter, then, is to review some of the literature illustrating how modern cognitive constructs have been integrated into the study of attitudes.

Despite the fact that some assimilation of information processing constructs has taken place, we believe these modern cognitive constructs remain seriously underutilized by attitude theorists. Consequently, the third purpose of this chapter is to review a number of core cognitive constructs and show their relevance to our understanding of attitudinal processes.

ATTITUDE AS A TRADITIONAL LATENT VARIABLE

Attitude has been historically viewed as a point on a continuum. The continuum is an evaluative one, ranging from very positive to very negative. Once an attitude object has been identified, each person's attitude can be located somewhere on that continuum, indicating the extent to which the person is "for" or "against" the attitude object. This notion of attitudes as falling on an evaluative dimension has traditionally been the focus of attitude theory and attitude measurement (Ostrom, 1989). This metatheoretical fixation by social psychologists on dimensions spreads far beyond the study of attitudes. It has been noted in research on attribution theory (Ostrom, 1981), impression formation (Devine & Ostrom, 1988), social judgment (Ostrom, 1988), and questionnaire design (Ostrom, 1987).

The "point-on-a-continuum" assumption is shared with many traditional constructs in psychology at large, and has been an article of faith since the work of Fechner and Weber. Most latent variables of a psychometric nature (such as intelligence, need for achievement, and locus of control) posit an implicit dimension on which individuals can be located and their differences specified. Classic test theory and the development of factor analytic techniques encouraged the use of continua (involving either interval or ratio properties; see Stevens, 1946) for the representation of all sorts of other individual differences. This approach to the study of individual differences was historically contemporaneous with the emergence of the construct of attitude, and clearly had an impact on that construct's development.

Using this approach to attitudes, not only can persons be located as points on a continuum, but so can attitude-relevant knowledge, feelings, beliefs, and actions. This can most clearly be seen in the attitude theories that emphasize belief and information integration (e.g., Anderson, 1974, 1981; Fishbein & Ajzen, 1975). In these models, attitude is a summary response to the mixture of beliefs, judgments, inferences, and knowledge that people have about the attitude object. Each constituent cognitive element has two defining parameters, both of which are conceptualized as points on continua.

The first of the two parameters is the "scale value." The scale value reflects the point on the evaluative continuum at which the cognitive element is located. Beliefs reflect characteristics of the attitude object that vary in valence from very positive to very negative. The second of the two parameters reflects the functional weight or belief strength that characterizes each cognitive element's contribution to the overall attitude. This weight parameter is also conceptualized as a point on a continuum. In this case, the continuum varies from zero weight to a large weight.

Thurstone (1928) first articulated this "point-on-a-continuum" metatheoretical assumption about the nature of attitudes. Although this basic assumption has remained unchanged (McGuire, 1989), subsequent theorists qualified the idea in several ways. For example, the idea of attitude as a single point was challenged by Sherif, Sherif, and Nebergall (1965), who argued that the notion of a point should be expanded to a "region of acceptance." This region reflects a range of points on the evaluative continuum that the respondent finds personally acceptable. This revision is reasonable, especially given instabilities and uncertainties in attitude, but it does not alter the presumption that the task of attitude researchers is to locate cognitions on the evaluative continuum.

Another modification of the strict "point-on-a-continuum" metatheory has been to argue that attitudes are multidimensional, and that attitude-relevant beliefs can be located in multidimensional space. For example, beliefs about a presidential candidate may jointly fall on the dimensions of competence, integrity, liberal versus conservative political philosophy, and concern about the environment. However, this multidimensional approach does not represent a substantial deviation from the "point-on-a-continuum" frame of reference. Locating cognitions on dimensions is still at the core of this approach.

Despite such minor revisions, then, the task of most attitude theorists, from the 1920s to the present, has been to develop a model of what leads a person to change his or her attitude from one point on the continuum to another. The approach was viewed as "cognitive" because first, the concept of attitude is itself mentalistic, and second, beliefs and other cognitions play a fundamental role in attitudinal dynamics. By comparison, the field of cognitive psychology has blossomed over the past 20 years, introducing many new conceptions of cognitive structures and cognitive processes. Only a few of the new concepts from cognitive psychology have been seriously studied by attitude researchers. Yet, whenever these concepts have been explored, important new insights about attitudes have emerged.

RECENT ADVANCES IN THE COGNITIVE ANALYSIS OF ATTITUDES

The view of this chapter is that attitudes are imbedded in an information processing system, and that to understand attitudes we must understand this cognitive host. The cognitive approach views the person as a flexible and imaginative information processor that both acts on and reacts to the surrounding social and physical environment. In broadest brush strokes, the information processing view starts with information being generated either peripherally through sensory experience, or centrally through either active memory search (e.g., inference and decisional activity) or activation of implicit processes (e.g., unconscious priming and implicit memory). This information is operated on through some limited capacity working memory function. And based on this activity, responses are generated at both the cognitive (e.g., goals, plans, and judgments) level and the motor (e.g., facial expressions, donating money to the church, and aggressive actions) level. The focus of this section is on the kinds of centrally located (i.e., in the brain) constructs that have been proposed by cognitive psychologists to mediate information processing.

Information processing analyses are not foreign to attitude researchers. One of the earliest attempts to provide a formal analysis of attitudes was advanced by Hovland et al. (1953). Their approach, which came to be known within the field of attitudes as an "information processing" analysis, argued that attitude change is mediated by three steps: *attention* to the communication, *comprehension* of the contents, and *yielding* to the comprehended elements. McGuire (1968) added two more steps (*retention* of the newly acquired attitude position and *action* based on the new position) to create a five-stage stochastic process, and subsequently expanded it to 12 steps (McGuire, 1985).

A modern cognitive approach to attitudes regards all of these steps as relevant to understanding attitudinal processes. However, despite the use of the term "information processing," this early approach was formulated at a time when little was known about cognitive dynamics. Even in McGuire's 12-stage version, the steps are little more than descriptive labels that guide intuitive analyses of the separate stages. Little or no research from cognitive psychology informed the understanding and usage of these labels by attitude researchers. This tactic was not unreasonable; at the time of the original formulation, little formal research in experimental psychology dealt with complex verbal stimuli, such as persuasive communications.

However, several attitude researchers and theorists have embraced the revolution in cognitive psychology, and have begun to explore the possible utility of these ideas for attitudes. On the theoretical side of the spectrum, Lingle and Ostrom (1981) reviewed several widely accepted principles of encoding, retrieval, and inference generation, arguing that attitudes could usefully be viewed as "thematic structures." Borrowing from a different area of study within cognitive psychology, Zanna and Rempel (1988) explored whether attitudes could be conceptualized in terms of the process of categorization; that is, according to these theorists, attitude formation represents the categorization of an attitude object along some evaluative dimension. Drawing from yet another area of cognition (Tulving's [1983] distinction between conceptual and episodic memory), Pratkanis (1989) argued that attitudes serve a heuristic function in conceptual memory and a schematic function in episodic memory.

On the empirical side of the spectrum, researchers turned to cognitive constructs in an attempt to better understand classic issues in the attitude literature. For example, consider the problem of attitude–behavior consistency. Researchers in the area of self-awareness had noted that enhancing people's awareness of their attitudes prior to behavior produced high attitude–behavior consistency (e.g., Snyder & Swann, 1976). Their conclusion was that heightening people's conscious awareness of their attitude made it more likely that the attitude would serve as a guide for behavior. Research by Wilson and his colleagues (see Wilson, Dunn, Kraft, & Lisle, 1989) challenged this conclusion by demonstrating that, sometimes, asking subjects to think about their attitudes paradoxically lowers attitude–behavior consistency.

By borrowing ideas about knowledge structures and about how information in those structures is accessed from cognitive psychology, attitude researchers have resolved this apparent paradox. These researchers assume that there is a richly elaborated cognitive structure that is associated with an attitude object, and under normal circumstances, highly accessible elements of that structure serve as the primary contributor to attitudes, and hence, to behavior. Asking people to think about their attitude brings less accessible elements of the structure into play. If these less accessible elements have differing implications for behavior than the more accessible elements, then the access and use of these less accessible elements may serve to temporarily change subjects' attitudes, and hence, to change subjects' behaviors as well.

Research by Millar and Tesser (1986, 1989) supports this idea. Millar and Tesser suggested that sometimes the implications of peoples' cognitions and their affective reactions toward an attitude object will be inconsistent with each other. Using manipulations designed to activate only cognitive or affective elements (not both), Millar and Tesser found that thinking reduced attitude–behavior consistency when the affective and cognitive elements were inconsistent; when these elements were consistent, no such reduction occurred. Further support for this notion was provided by Edwards (1990). Edwards found that, among subjects with affect-based attitudes, an affectively oriented message was more persuasive than a cognitively oriented appeal, but the reverse was true among subjects with cognition-based attitudes.

Another classic problem in the attitude literature concerns the effects of context on responses to attitude questions. It has often been noted that the order in which questions are asked on a questionnaire affects responses to the questions (for recent discussions, see Schwarz & Sudman, 1992). Researchers in this area have turned to the cognitive literature on priming and construct activation to help address this problem. Previous questions on a questionnaire, or contexts, can serve to prime concepts, making them more accessible. These accessible concepts are more likely to be used to process subsequent information. Hence, shifts in the processing of or interpretation of attitude-relevant information may be due to the activation of attitude constructs associated with the context or question primes. Extending this logic, Tourangeau, Rasinski, Bradburn, and D'Andrade (1989) suggested that priming effects due to judgmental contexts should be strongest in those for whom an attitude is important (so that the relevant beliefs are stored in memory) and in those whose feelings are conflicted (so that information about both sides is represented in the cognitive structure). In research looking at carry-over effects in surveys, Tourangeau et al. found support for their proposition.

Ideas about construct activation have helped us to better understand other phenomena associated with attitude assessment, as well. For example, it is often the case that attitude questionnaires assess the same construct repeatedly in several items spread throughout the questionnaire. Research by Knowles (1988) indicates that the consistency in peoples' responses to items assessing a particular construct increases as one proceeds through a questionnaire. This outcome makes sense if one assumes that each individual question assessing the construct has the potential to cause a different part of the cognitive representation of the construct to be accessed and used, so that as the number of construct-related items presented increases, the proportion of the cognitive structure that is included in the working conceptualization also increases. Thus, successive answers become increasingly stable because the standard used to evaluate the item (i.e., the conceptualization constructed in responding to the item) becomes more consistent.

Researchers have also turned to cognitive constructs in an attempt to better understand the cognitive structure of attitudes. For example, attitude theorists have often behaved as if attitudes were inherently bipolar: that is, both the positive and negative aspect of an attitude are inextricably intertwined. Although some data is supportive of this proposition (see Judd & Kulik, 1980), a surprising amount of work challenges this assumption. For example, extensive factor analytic research by Kerlinger (1984) suggests that some constructs that have typically been treated in a bipolar fashion, such as the concepts liberalism–conservatism, may be better thought of as separate concepts in the mental network (also see Pratkanis, 1989). In general, this work implies that liberalism is not the opposite of conservatism; rather, liberals and conservatives appear to have differing, not necessarily opposite, patterns of beliefs. In an investigation into attitudes toward abortion, Tourangeau, Rasinski, Bradburn, and D'Andrade (1991) came to much the same conclusion. Proabortion and antiabortion advocates did not hold opposing views on the same beliefs; rather, pro- and antiabortion attitudes appeared to be linked to very different belief systems.

In terms of both theory and research, one of the more comprehensive attempts to integrate modern cognitive constructs into the attitude domain comes from the work of Fazio (see Fazio, 1989, 1990). Fazio postulates that an attitude can be viewed as an association in memory between a given object and one's evaluation of that object. In Fazio's view, the "strength" of the attitude is determined by the strength of this linkage (also see Judd & Krosnick, 1989). Fazio also postulates that, in some cases, the linkage may be so strong that the attitude may be automatically activated when the individual encounters the attitude object.

Research by Fazio, Sabonmatsu, Powell, and Kardes (1986) supports this notion. Fazio et al. conducted a priming study in which subjects were presented with the name of an attitude object, then a positive or negative evaluative adjective. The subject's task was to indicate whether the adjective had a positive or negative evaluative content. Subjects' responses were facilitated when there was congruency between the evaluation of the attitude object and the target word. Hence, if a subject had a negative association to the attitude object "football," their response to the word "terrible" would be facilitated. However, this effect only occurred if there was a strong link between the attitude object and the evaluation; that is, to produce a facilitation, both evaluative congruency and a strong (i.e., frequently used) object-evaluation linkage needed to be present. Furthermore, this facilitation occurred only when a short amount of time passed between the prime and the target, but not when longer intervals were used. This effect is congruent with the rapid excitation decay that is thought to occur in spreading activation models.

In Fazio's view, these variations in attitude accessibility are of more than passing interest: attitude accessibility is thought to be an important moderator variable, potentially affecting both the subsequent processing of information and attitude-behavior relations, and research confirms these conjectures. For example, Houston and Fazio (1989) manipulated associative strength by asking some subjects to repeatedly express their attitudes toward the death penalty, while other subjects were not asked to do so. In a subsequent task, subjects who had repeatedly expressed their attitudes judged the empirical evidence in a manner that was more congruent with their attitudes than subjects who did not repeatedly state their attitudes. These findings support the conclusion that when attitudes are automatically activated, they serve to color the interpretation of incoming information.

A confirmation of the behavioral implications of accessibility comes from a study by Fazio and Williams (1986). In this study, rather than manipulating accessibility, Fazio and Williams assessed individual differences in attitude accessibility. Accessibility was strongly related to voting behavior in the high-accessibility group: attitudes toward Reagan accounted for 80% of the variance in voting behavior. However, in the low-accessibility group, those attitudes accounted for only 44% of the variance.

COGNITIVE CODES, STRUCTURES, AND PROCESSES: A NEW LOOK AT ATTITUDES

The foregoing sampler of the contemporary attitude and cognition literature makes it clear that cognitive concepts have not been ignored by researchers and theorists in the attitude area. Yet, we find it curious that the implications of these concepts for attitudes have not been more vigorously pursued. One possible reason for this lack of activity, curious in an area that has been so consistently "cognitive," is that there is not a wide recognition of the metatheoretic assumptions that early attitude theorists adopted, and of how the newer cognitive constructs might map onto those assumptions.

Furthermore, we note that with few, if any, exceptions, cognitively oriented attitude researchers do not begin with a full understanding of cognitive dynamics. Instead, they have adopted a minimalist strategy of selectively examining one or two cognitive constructs that provide insight into a specific classic issue in the attitude literature (e.g., the attitude–behavior relation, or biases in attitude measurement); that is, researchers and theorists began with relatively well-understood attitudinal properties and phenomena, and looked for relevant explanatory constructs that had been advanced by cognitive psychologists. This has proved to be useful, at least as an initial step, in that it illustrates how attitudes can be linked to a broader conceptual and empirical base. However, this approach has resulted in a rather fragmented "cognitivization" of attitudes, one that does not provide a comprehensive analysis of how attitudes might fit into the cognitive system.

In an attempt to rectify these problems, the balance of this chapter adopts a different strategy for investigating the interface between cognition and attitudes. Instead of starting with a list of known characteristics of attitudes, it reviews a broad array of constructs from cognitive psychology and asks how these notions might inform our understanding of attitudes. This provides an especially effective way of revealing the inadequacies of the traditional "point-on-a-continuum" presumption that continues to guide the work of many attitudes researchers.

Our discussion of these issues is subdivided into sections describing cognitive codes, cognitive structures, and cognitive processes. However, because the cognitive system operates as a holistic, quasi-integrated unit, these three subdivisions provide a somewhat arbitrary way of focusing on different features of the information processing system. As a consequence, our discussion of each of the three topics will necessarily draw upon issues and constructs from the other two.

Cognitive Codes

What is the nature of the irreducible "cognitive element" from which cognitive representations and structures are built? What are the basic "elements" that are stored in memory and what are the units of encoding and retrieval activity? To understand cognition, one must understand how information is coded, that is, the exact form taken by the information that is stored in memory. Cognitive psychologists have proposed many different types of coding. Below, we discuss several of these types and examine their implications for improving our understanding of attitudes.

Symbolic Nodes versus Distributed Networks

A recent theoretical debate in cognitive psychology has focused on two fundamentally different ways to represent cognitive codes. The first, and more traditional, form is a symbolic code. This is a generic form of code that would be familiar to most attitude researchers. For example, each unit of information or belief can be represented as a single node in a network of such nodes. Proponents of local symbolic coding (e.g., Anderson, 1983; Wyer & Srull, 1989) suggest that information is stored in symbolic form in restricted locations in memory. In contrast, theorists in the area of connectionist modeling (e.g., Rumelhart, McClelland, & the PDP Research Group, 1986) have suggested that conceptual knowledge is stored in a "distributed" fashion, that is, by a pattern of activity occurring throughout the neural system as a whole. Individual nodes in a network have no single meaning. For reasons of expository clarity, we shall delay discussion of distributed systems until a later section, and for now, shall concentrate on local symbolic codes.

Symbolic representations historically preceded distributed ones, and so there has been a considerable amount of work in differentiating among several subtypes. Four commonly discussed types of local symbolic representations are: (1) propositional representations, (2) analog representations, (3) episodic (as opposed to semantic) representations, and (4) production systems.

Propositional Units

Many psychologists have suggested that information is represented in propositional units such as "John went home." A proposition is the smallest unit of analysis that can stand as a separate assertion; that is, the smallest unit about which it makes sense to make the judgment "true or false" (e.g., Anderson, 1976). Furthermore, in propositional representations, information is stored in abstract, languagelike units. These units are useful for capturing the ideational content of the mind, irrespective of the original source of the information.

When discussing propositional units, it is important to keep in mind the notion that these are thought to be "languagelike." It is conventional to use linguistic concepts to describe these propositional units, but these propositional units need not be linguistic. Instead, they represent our ideas and abstractions about the world, and they do so in a form that is substantially different from the original thoughts and perceptions that contributed to that knowledge.

Propositional codes are the dominant form of code found in attitude theories. When attitude theorists speak of beliefs, they are referring to a statement linking an attribute to the attitude object. Examples of propositional codes in attitude toward a car might be "the car is reliable" and "the car has bald tires." Such beliefs are experienced as a unit. One does not need to decompose them into their constituent semantic components to understand them. This notion was explicitly described by Abelson and Rosenberg (1958) who argued that primitive "cognitive units" were made up of two cognitive elements (e.g., the attitude object and a feature of that object) linked by a cognitive relation (which could be positive, negative, null, or ambivalent, e.g., "Tom likes Mary").

Analog Representations

Part of the knowledge we may have about an attitude object, such as a person or a car, is its appearance. The sleek, racy appearance of a sports car or the shifty-eyed, insincere reply of a political candidate may be more evocatively stored as a visual image than as a simple proposition. Some cognitive theorists have suggested that this kind of knowledge involves a separate memory code: an analog code. In contrast to propositional units, analog representations (e.g., images, mental models) are thought to "conserve" many of the configural relationships that characterize real-world stimuli. For example, a television is an analog representation device that preserves many of the relationships that exist among real-world stimuli.

Analog theorists speculated that if these representations were close replicas of real-world stimuli, then mental operations on those representations should resemble the same operations as performed on real-world stimuli. This sometimes appears to be the case. When an object is rotated mentally, the rotation takes longer if the rotation is 160° than if the rotation is 30°. Similarly, the mental image of an elephant is bigger than the mental image of a fly (see Kosslyn, 1975; Shephard & Cooper, 1983). Although such analog representations are, perhaps, easiest to understand for visual stimuli, analog representations may exist for other sensory channels (see Paivio, 1986).

Attitude theorists have not incorporated analog codes into their theories.

Although there has been some speculation about the relevance of this code to attitudes (Breckler & Wiggins, 1989), formal empirical work has been negligible. This is surprising, because images intuitively play a strong role in attitudes. A mother's loving embrace of her child, the gaunt pleading eyes of a concentration camp victim, and the revolving door in the Willie Horton commercials opposing Michael Dukakis for president of the United States all make a vivid and enduring impact on the perceiver. The evocative power of these images suggests that a greater understanding of images is crucial in advancing our understanding of attitudes.

Episodic and Semantic Representations

The distinction between propositional and analog codes is similar to a distinction between semantic memory and episodic memory offered by Tulving (1972). In Tulving's view, semantic memory is the memory system that is used to verbally represent conceptual knowledge about the world, and is compatible with ideas about propositional codes. By comparison, according to Tulving, episodic memory reflects knowledge about specific events. Similar to the claims made by those favoring analog representations, episodic memories are thought to conserve aspects of the original stimulus event, in particular, information about time and context. The parallel between episodic and analog representation claims is also made stronger by Tulving's suggestion that sensory experiences are a primary source of episodic information. The differences between semantic and episodic memory systems can perhaps be made clearer by the following example: knowing that you hit a game-winning home run is a semantic memory, but remembering the actual experience of that event is an episodic memory.

This episodic/semantic distinction may have importance for our understanding of attitudes. It is certainly true that episodes are part of the knowledge base we have about attitude objects, especially familiar objects such as friends and possessions. Furthermore, attitude research suggests that these episodes may have important implications for attitudes. More specifically, attitudes that are based on direct experience seem to have somewhat different characteristics from attitudes that do not: they are more specific, are held more confidently, are more resistant to counterargument, and predict behaviors better than attitudes derived from indirect experience (e.g., Fazio & Zanna, 1978, 1981; Zanna & Fazio, 1982).

However, it is unclear if these effects are due to the episodic memory system. Conscious recall of the sensory features of episodic memories, along with their features of time and context, tends to fade over time. Often, only the gist of the episodic memory (which may take the form of a proposition) is retained. The experience itself may have had a strong effect on attitude toward the object at the time the event occurred, but the explicit memory for that experience may subsequently play a negligible role. Thus, it would seem that one relevant question for attitude research would be to investigate whether the relation between direct experience and attitudes can be attributed to the effects of episodic memory or semantic memory.

Production Systems

Propositional, analog, and episodic coding systems attempt to represent our knowledge about the world (otherwise known as declarative knowledge); production system representations attempt to represent actions or action systems (sometimes referred to as procedural knowledge). Several current theories of production systems use a modeling system consisting of condition–action (or "If–Then") rules (e.g., Newell & Simon, 1972; Smith, 1990). The "If" component of the rules specifies the conditions for action, and the "Then" component of the rules specifies the action to be completed. The conditions for performance of the action need not be simple, but can be compound in form, as in the following example: "*If* the goal is to write a paper *and* the deadline is one month away *and* one's collaborator is known to be a recalcitrant writer, *then* begin writing immediately." The If–Then modeling format can be applied to either general or specific action domains, and many If–Then statements can be compounded to account for a wide range of actions or cognitive products.

Attitudes can be involved in either the condition or action components of a production. When part of the "If" component, the attitude serves as a determinant of the consequent action. The effect of attitude on perceptions and behaviors can be illustrated as follows. "*If* an opposing basketball player elbows a member of my team *and* I have a negative attitude toward the opposing team, *then* conclude the foul was intentional *and* shout to the referee to call a technical foul." When an attitude is part of the "Then" component, the production refers to determinants of attitude change. For example, "*If* the communicator is trustworthy *and* new information is provided in the message, *then* change your attitude to be consistent with the new information."

Although some work in the realm of social judgment and inferences has been conducted with production codes (Smith, 1990), the field of attitudes has largely ignored this approach. However, it is not too hard to see the potential applicability. Consider the classic finding in attitude research indicating that, by increasing the situational specificity in an attitude question, one can produce a better match between responses to the question and attitude-relevant behavior (e.g., Fishbein & Ajzen, 1974). This finding can be reconceptualized as illustrating the importance of conditional specificity to productions. That is, one reason that one's expressed attitude and one's behavior may sometimes differ is that the attitude in question does not adequately capture the conditions that cause the production of a specific behavior.

Affect as a Code

One of the hallmarks of attitudes is that they have evaluative content; that is, attitudes involve feelings. In fact, many ideas and beliefs about others (Kim & Rosenberg, 1980), and about the world (Osgood, Suci, & Tannenbaum, 1957) produce affective reactions. The ubiquity of these affective reactions, and the propensity of affect to cut across domains of experience, led Fiske and Taylor (1991) to speculate that affect may constitute a separate memory code. As Fiske and Taylor note, the direct evidence for this proposition is scanty, but given that affect is so basic to human existence, an affective code may be necessary.

Several theorists have already attempted to describe the representation of affect in memory. For example, Gilligan and Bower (1984) argue that one affect-based construct, emotions, can be incorporated into associative propositional coding schemes. These theorists suggest that emotions can be regarded as units or nodes in a semantic network, with numerous connections to related ideas, to physiological systems, to events, and to muscular and expressive patterns. Borrowing an example from Wyer and Srull (1989), consider the likely cognitive structure for the emotion "angry." This structure would incorporate semantic elements (angry, furious), behaviors (swears loudly, slams door), muscular patterns (facial expressions), and physiological responses.

It is an easy leap from emotions to attitudes, and some theorists have suggested that attitudes can also be thought of as nodes in a network (e.g., Pratkanis, 1989). In these conceptions, an attitude node represents an evaluation of the attitude object. In some cases, this node may be a summary of the strengths and weaknesses of the object, and thus, might be linked to the nodes representing these individual strengths and weaknesses. In other cases, this evaluation might be directly derived from an emotional response, as might be developed through classical conditioning (e.g., Staats & Staats, 1958; Staats, 1968).

Attitudes are evaluations, and affective responses are obviously contributors to those evaluations. However, the affect associated with attitudes may be linked to attitudes in several ways. For example, affect may be incorporated into attitude representations by means of direct links between attitude objects and emotions (e.g., Christmas directly linked to happiness). Alternatively, affect may contribute to an attitude by means of indirect links between attitude objects and emotions (Christmas not directly linked to happiness, but linked to presents, which is linked to happiness). This suggests that, at least under some circumstances, there may be a conflict between evaluation of an attitude object from affect associated with the properties of that object (Christmas linked to going shopping, which in turn is linked to "Bah! Humbug!") and affect directly associated with the attitude object itself (Christmas linked to happiness).

One Code or Many?

There have been debates over whether there is one cognitive code or whether there are more than one. For example, some theorists have made concerted and innovative attempts to argue that, because the "visionlike" qualities of reconstructed images can be captured by propositional representations, analog codes are not necessary (e.g., Anderson, 1976; Pylyshyn, 1981). The "one code" position has also been supported by the failure of empirical attempts to conclusively establish a distinction between semantic and episodic memory systems (see Johnson & Hasher, 1987).

However, the current zeitgeist in cognitive psychology appears to favor the position that there are multiple forms of information coding. Several prominent theories explicitly make such an assumption (e.g., Anderson's ACT* model, 1983; Carlston's Associated Systems Theory, 1992; Paivio's Dual-Coding model, 1986).

The empirical evidence, though by no means conclusive, seems to be converging on the idea of multiple cognitive codes. For example, the results of an experiment by Santa (1977) indicated that the identification of a geometric figure array was facilitated when the figures were positioned in their original orientation, but this was not the case with a word array. Instead, recognition of verbal test arrays was facilitated by a "linear" ordering (as in a typical sentence). This result suggests that the information about the different types of arrays was coded differently. Studies of blood flow in the brain converge with this conclusion, suggesting that different parts of the brain are active in the processing of verbal and spatial information (Roland & Friberg, 1985). Studies of amnesiacs suggest that they may have a deficit in the ability to form new conscious memories (declarative knowledge), while their ability to learn new motor skills (procedural knowledge) is relatively intact (e.g., Cohen & Squire, 1980). Studies on the impact of making repeated trait judgments indicate that some of the facilitation observed is due to repeated access of the content of the items, but that there is additional facilitation that has been interpreted as illustrative of the effects of practice on procedural knowledge (Smith, 1990).

The possibility that there are multiple cognitive codes has numerous implications for attitude theory. For example, consider the possibility that cognitive structures simultaneously incorporate elements from several different cognitive codes: that is, analog, verbal, behavioral, and affective information, all included in a single attitude representation (see Carlston, 1992; Fazio, 1989; Hastie, 1986; Pratkanis, 1989). If one assumes that links in the representation can be lost (as in the cue dissociation hypothesis for the sleeper effect; see Gruder et al., 1978), or that only part of the attitude representation need be active at any one time (see Fazio, 1989), such multiple coding and organization can help to explain data suggesting that behaviors can become divorced from attitudes (e.g., Dishman, 1982), and that there is a degree of independence between attitude-relevant behaviors and attitudes (e.g., Mittal, 1988).

Even more generally, if one assumes that an individual's attitude reflects input from multiple memory sources, and if these multiple sources reflect different memory codes, then, in principle, attitude change may occur by attacking any of the possible contributors to the attitude. In fact, this has already occurred: research indicates (e.g., Ostrom, 1969) that attitudes can be changed by attacking peoples' thoughts or beliefs (i.e., propositions), by inducing people to change their behaviors (i.e., procedures), or by changing the affect associated with issue attributes. This perspective also suggests that to be maximally effective, attitude change techniques should attack several of these different representational systems. It may not be enough to simply change beliefs about an issue (often the goal of central route persuasion; see Petty & Cacioppo, 1986) if the associated affective, episodic, or behavioral aspects of the representation remain intact.

Alternative Codes for Attitude

The possibility that there are different cognitive codes leads to the question of how attitudes are coded. More specifically, one might speculate how the "point-on-a-continuum" conception that has long guided attitude research might map onto the alternative coding schemes.

One possibility is that an attitude could be represented as a simple *proposition,* as in "I like President Clinton." However, the term "like" is too vague for the strong form of the "point-on-a-continuum" assumption. The proposition would need to include a more precise numerical value, such as "My attitude toward President Clinton is +10." A second possibility is that the attitude could be cognitively represented in *analog* fashion, with the person storing the image of a continuous rating scale with an arrow marking the current location of the person's attitude. These two possibilities seem implausible.

A third, more reasonable, possibility is that the evaluative response to an object is associatively linked to the cognitive designation of that object (Fazio, 1989; Gilligan & Bower, 1984; Pratkanis, 1989). Accessing the code that represents the object activates an evaluative tag that indicates whether or not the attitude object has a positive or negative valence. Thus, the evaluative tag may operate in a manner similar to the belief (or plausibility) tag that is regarded to be an intrinsic part of propositional representations (Reder, 1982). Such tags may be intrinsic to all forms of cognitive code, not just to propositions.

It is widely believed that evaluative reactions to attitude objects vary not only in their valence (i.e., positive vs. negative), but also in strength or intensity. The question then arises regarding the code used to represent strength. The simplest possibility is that the evaluative tag itself varies in strength. This, however, is simply a restatement of the point-on-a-continuum approach.

An alternative approach is to assume that evaluative codes differ only in valance, that the code itself contains no information about intensity. For example, Fazio (1989, 1990) suggests that intensity may be derived from the strength of association between the attitude object and the evaluative code. Alternatively, tags may vary in their ability to arouse autonomic and visceral activity (Breckler & Wiggins, 1989) or to influence attributions and actions. When an attitude is part of the "condition" portion of a condition–action production, its ability to evoke the action may be exclusively dependent on the strength of the production.

Another way to accommodate differences in attitude strength derives from the view that an attitude object can be simultaneously represented by many codes. This is because an object can be denoted in many different ways. President Clinton, as an attitude object, could be denoted by a photograph, a video clip, his name, or phrases like "the President" and "Hillary's husband." The evaluative tag on each of these different codes could vary from positive to negative to none, despite the fact that they all denote the same object. Repeated presentation of one of the codes (repeated presentation is one of the ways that Fazio [see Fazio, 1989] manipulates the "strength" of the association between the object and the tag) may lead the respondent to transfer a well-formed evaluative tag from an alternative (but denotatively equivalent) code to the code currently being encountered.

In sum, the information processing perspective offers a potentially fruitful reanalysis of the fundamental code used to represent attitudes, affect, and beliefs. The analog nature of the traditional "point-on-a-continuum" perspective is but one of many potential forms of code representation, and on the face of it, it is the least plausible of the lot.

Cognitive Organization and Structure

The models of coding discussed in the preceding section are primarily concerned with the nature of the information units that are stored in peoples' cognitive representations of the world and operated on by the processing system. However, there is no organization that is necessarily inherent in these different coding schemes: different organizational models are, to some extent, independent of the exact units into which information is coded. Numerous organizational structures have been proposed by cognitive psychologists; we shall highlight several that have been more thoroughly explored or that seem especially applicable to attitudes.

Cognitive Categories

Early theoretical views of cognitive categories (e.g., Smith, Shoben, & Rips, 1974) represented categories as feature lists: an unstructured compendium of features that were either necessary or sufficient for category membership. For example, the attitude object designated as "professor" might have such features as "has PhD," "teaches college courses," "is smart," and "publishes research." However, this position frequently conflicted with empirical data (see Smith & Medin, 1981; Barsalou, 1992a, for excellent discussions), leading to the proposal of alternative types of categorical representations.

One major class of these alternative models suggests that information is stored in terms of exemplars: specific (e.g., episodic) memories about a concept (e.g., Nosofsky, 1984). Hence, according to these models, the categorical representation of the concept "women" might contain a collection of your memories about women you have met and the actions they have engaged in. Exemplar representations are less clear-cut when they are applied to abstract categories such as "democracy" or "communism." Abstract categories constitute an important class of attitude objects. Although such categories have not received much research attention in cognitive psychology, relevant exemplars might include persons, countries, actions, and slogans that convey philosophical premises.

A second major class of category models assumes that information is stored in terms of prototypes: a centralized representation that comes from summaries and abstractions that are derived from, and representative of, a category's exemplars (e.g., Cantor & Mischel, 1977; Reed, 1972). Hence, according to these models, the cognitive representation of the concept "women" would consist of the typical features or feature "packages" that are common to most women. It is less clear what a prototype of "communism" might be. Possibly there would be multiple, coexisting prototypes representing the different constituents, such as the prototypical communistic country, person, domestic policy, foreign policy, and the like. After empirical attempts to distinguish between the exemplar and prototype approaches, some recent theorizing (e.g., Barsalou's theory of mental frames, 1992b) suggests that both types of knowledge, prototypes and specific exemplars, can be stored in the same cognitive structure.

Associative Networks

One dominant approach to cognitive organization is the associative network model, which was one of the earliest explored in social cognition (e.g., Wyer & Carlston, 1979) and which has recently been applied to the conceptualization of attitudes (e.g., Fazio, 1989; Tourangeau & Rasinski, 1988). Network models assume that information is stored as nodes in memory, with pathways connecting to the nodes. In a simple attitude network, the evaluative tag may serve as one node; the code designating the attitude object may serve as a second node; and episodic memories, beliefs, and images may all have separate nodes, and these may be linked to the object node and to the attitude node (for example, see Hastie, 1986; Pratkanis, 1989).

One of the postulates of network models is that nodes can be in varying states of "readiness," and that the level of readiness affects the likelihood that a node will be used to guide processing (see Wyer & Carlston, 1979). A second postulate of network models is that there is a spread of excitation from an activated node to other closely associated nodes, and the effect of this spreading excitation is to increase the readiness of these associates to subsequent activation (see Sedikides & Skowronski, 1991, for a review of research on these ideas).

The research on the effects of accessibility (often referred to as "priming") on attitude phenomena is a direct consequence of these assumptions. In particular, the research program of Fazio and his associates (see Fazio, 1989, 1990) has served to demonstrate the breadth of applications involving networks and priming. This research has demonstrated that the attitudes of low self-monitors (those who are supposedly guided by their attitudes) are more accessible than the attitudes of high self-monitors (who are supposedly guided by perceived situational demands). Thus, individual differences in attitude accessibility can occur, and persist, because of frequent attitude reactivation and use. In addition, Fazio's research also indicates that highly accessible attitudes can apparently be activated automatically, thus serving as a guide to processing and to behavior with little cognitive effort.

The impact of primed material on subsequent processing was illustrated in a recent study by Sherman, Mackie, and Driscoll (1990). This study used a priming manipulation to heighten the accessibility of the foreign policy concept in some subjects or the economic concept in other subjects. In a subsequent task, political candidates were described in terms of information relevant to both concepts. Individuals' evaluations of the candidates tended to be more strongly influenced by information that was relevant to the primed concept.

Similar work by Judd, Drake, Downing, and Krosnick (1991) demonstrated that answering attitude questions about one political issue increased the accessibility of attitudes on related issues. Furthermore, building on Tesser's (1978) work showing that answering questions on one attitude issue tends to polarize attitudes, Judd et al. showed that answering questions on an attitude issue results in more extreme responses to questions about a related issue, as well. In theory, these effects occurred because of the spread of activation between attitudes that are closely linked in long-term memory.

Priming research can also help to understand attitude–behavior inconsistency. Consider the results of a study by Neuberg (1988). He used a priming manipulation to heighten the accessibility of constructs related to cooperation in some subjects, or to heighten the accessibility of constructs related to competition in other subjects. When asked to participate in a subsequent task allowing either cooperative or competitive behavior, subjects tended to perform in a manner that was consistent with the primed construct. Hence, people's behavior can be influenced by temporarily active cognitive constructs, causing them to engage in actions that may differ from those dictated by their own personal norms.

Working Memory

Some of the results of priming studies can, perhaps, be best understood when activation models are combined with the idea of a limited-capacity "working memory" system (Baddeley, 1986; also wee Wyer & Srull's [1989] discussion of the Work Space). Working memory is a temporary repository of information, and it is in working memory that information is reviewed and integrated in the process of making judgments.

Assume for the moment that many of the cognitive structures that surround attitudes are far too large to be wholly retrieved into working memory at any one time. Instead, perhaps only part of any attitude structure can be accommodated in working memory. Now, in this light, consider the results of the Tourangeau et al. (1989) work reported previously suggesting that priming effects occur primarily for important issues, and in those who have conflicted feelings. Given these assumptions, it is possible that this result occurs because: (1) important attitudes tend to produce large cognitive structures with contradictory elements (see Pratkanis, 1989), with the entire structure being too large to be accommodated in working memory, and (2) priming might activate only one part of the cognitive structure, facilitating review of only the activated information in the process of reporting an attitude judgment.

Given the long history of work in cognitive psychology suggesting that we must distinguish between long-term memory, with an unlimited capacity to store information, and a capacity-limited working memory system (earlier research used the term "short-term memory" to refer to this system), it might be surprising to note that this research conflicts with some of the early assumptions that attitude theorists made about memory and the role of memory in attitudes. For example, the early "information processing" conceptions of Hovland et al. (1953), and even the later elaboration by McGuire (1968), did not distinguish between different memory systems. Instead, this work treated memory as a unitary, undifferentiated system. Again, this difference highlights the need for attitude theory to incorporate more recent ideas about cognitive structure and processing.

One other possible aspect of working memory might be of interest to attitude researchers. Discussions of attitude activation seem to commonly imply that the activation process leaves the form of the attitude unchanged; that is, the process of transferring an attitude into working memory leaves the representation of the attitude essentially unchanged. This perspective is clearly consistent with those individuals who propose that working memory simply is that portion of memory that is activated for use.

However, this need not be the case. It is entirely possible that the representation of the attitude in working memory is fundamentally different from the passive representation that is stored in long-term memory. For example, in the analog/propositional debate, proponents of propositional coding account for imagery effects by suggesting that the information that is stored in long-term memory is propositional, but that this information is "decoded" to construct a working visual image. The same situation might apply to attitudes. Attitudes might be stored in one format, but that format might be substantially altered when the attitude-relevant information is entered into working memory.

There are a couple of important implications of this line of reasoning. First, investigations of attitude representations that use working memory might be misleading, for these would reveal the structure of attitudes as implemented in working memory, not necessarily as implemented in long-term memory. Research using implicit memory measures (see the section on Implicit and Explicit Memory later in this chapter) might be important in bypassing this possible deception. Alternatively, investigations that focus on the structure of attitudes in long-term memory might be a red herring, for it may be that the structure of attitudes as represented in working memory might be significantly more important to understanding such problems as the attitude–behavior relation and attitude change.

Structured Networks

At the most general level, network models specify that nodes making up the cognitive representations may be connected to other nodes, and they identify conditions affecting the strength and activation of those connections. These models do not, by themselves, imply that these networks have any a priori pattern to the links between nodes. Each person's idiosyncratic experiences determine which nodes become linked to which other nodes. However, research and theory addressing the structure of cognition has shown that, in some domains, well-formed structures do exist.

One form of structured cognitive representation exhibits a *hierarchical structure;* that is, more complex concepts subdivide into more specific concepts, and so forth, until one reaches concepts that cannot be further subdivided. Formal taxonomies illustrate one such form of structure. For example, living things can be divided into plants and animals, and animals can be subdivided into birds, fish, mammals, reptiles, and so on. Each of these can be further subdivided into classes and species. Another example of structured representations are partonomies (e.g., arms are parts of a human body, hands are parts of arms, fingers are parts of hands, etc.).

Hierarchical representations can also be used to represent social knowledge. An example of such a structure, one that includes both exemplars and prototypes, is depicted in Figure 1. In this figure, the concept of athlete contains three aspects (size, race, sport), different values on each of these aspects (e.g., for size, the aspects are tall, average, short), two prototypes (one prototype for a quarterback and a second prototype for black athlete),

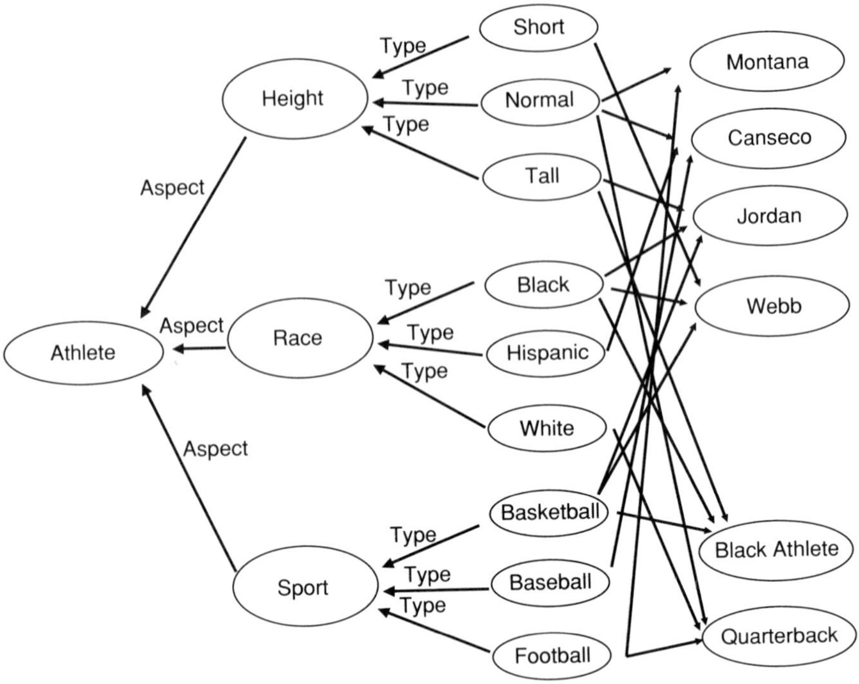

FIGURE 1.
Hypothetical hierarchical representation for the athlete concept.

and four separate exemplars (Michael Jordan, Jose Canseco, Joe Montana, Spud Webb).

The hypothetical structure depicted in Figure 1 is greatly simplified: representations of real-world categories and concepts are likely to be much more complex, and may include multiple subprototypes, each connected to different sets of exemplars. This complexity, along with the hierarchical nature of the representation, suggests that, depending on the portion of the representation that is activated by the construct, the working conceptualizations (i.e., the portion of the structure active in working memory) constructed for a category might vary significantly across time and across contexts. For example, the descriptions "To get the results of his course exam back, Don saw the psychologist" and "To help get out of his depression, Don saw the psychologist" may activate different subcategories (or working conceptualizations) for the category "psychologist."

Evidence from cognitive psychology (e.g., Barsalou & Billman, 1989; McCloskey & Glucksberg, 1978) suggests that this is the case. For example, McCloskey and Glucksberg (1978) presented subjects with various entities and asked them whether they belonged to particular categories. It was found that peoples' categorizations varied substantially across occasions, indicating that their conceptions of categories also varied across those occasions.

What implications might these theories and findings have for the concept of attitudes? Consider the vexing problem of attitude instability. One characteristic of peoples' attitudes is that these attitudes are sometimes relatively unstable across time. The research on cognitive categories provides one explanation for why this should be so: people may access different subrepresentations for a construct on different occasions. If these subrepresentations serve as standards of comparison in the process of making attitudinal judgments, then the judgments might differ because the judgment standards differ. Hence, on occasion 1, when Don is asked how much he likes psychologists, he may conceptualize psychologists in terms of the academic subtype, one that he likes; on occasion 2, when Don is asked how much he likes psychologists, he may conceptualize psychologists in terms of the clinical subtype, one that he dislikes.

The notion of a structured cognitive hierarchy has several additional implications for attitude research. For example, one of the hierarchy-related findings in the cognitive literature concerns peoples' supposed preference for categorizations at "basic levels." Basic-level categories are those categories in a hierarchy that represent the optimal trade-off between the principles of efficiency and informativeness (Rosch, Mervis, Gray, Johnson, & Boyes-Braem, 1976). In other words, the categories that we typically prefer to use are those at moderate levels of specificity (basic levels). This is because these midlevel categories (such as "politician") represent a reasonable trade-off between speed (as would be obtained from broad, superordinate categories, such as "person") and informativeness (as would be obtained from specific subordinate categories such as "state representative for my district").

This preference for basic-level categorizations may help to explain why some types of attitude judgments are more accessible than others. As indicated earlier, the research program of Fazio (see Fazio, 1990) has consistently noted that some attitude judgments are made faster than others, seemingly because those attitude judgments have been made more frequently than others, and hence, are at a higher level of activation and are more easily accessed. What determines the frequency of past use? Undoubtedly, many things, but one of the predictions derivable from the basic-level notion is that highly accessible judgments should tend to be basic-level judgments.

Ideas about hierarchical representations have begun to emerge in the attitudes domain. For example, Greenwald (1989) proposed a hierarchical structure for representing cognitive constructs, and applied that structure to attitudes. The lowest level consisted of perceptual features (e.g., sounds, shapes, and smells), the second level was objects (e.g., my dog Kacy), the third level was categories (e.g., dogs and doctors), the fourth level was propositions (e.g., Kacy bites people), and the fifth level was schema (e.g., the story of how Kacy bit the Polish doctor). This "levels-of-representation" system was developed so that units of one level are built from elements of the immediately subordinate level. In this system, attitudes applied to all elements in levels two through five. Greenwald's view is that attitude is an affective tag associated with any mental object His hierarchical system can be viewed as a way of classifying attitude objects; presumably, the effects of the affective tags operate in a similar manner at each of the levels.

Moving away from hierarchies, we now turn to another form of cognitive structure that has been little used in the attitude domain: *scripts*. A script is a cognitive structure, stored in long-term memory, that specifies the conditions and actions for achieving a goal (e.g., Schank & Abelson, 1977). Scripts have the quality of production systems, as were discussed earlier, in that they specify conditions and actions. But these conditions and actions are of a macro nature and are used to make sense of complex social events. For example, most of us have a script for attending a birthday party. Such a script consists of a number of standard activities: you arrive, hand over your gift, sing "Happy Birthday to You," the celebrant blows out the candles on the cake, everyone eats ice cream and birthday cake, and all go home.

The script does not specify a rigid series of events: instead, scripts contain information about a large number of considerations that might arise when trying to achieve a goal, and about how to handle those factors. This allows scripts to provide both structure and flexibility to relevant endeavors, such as one's own goal attainment efforts, or the processing of information relevant to others' attempts at goal attainment. Knowledge of event sequence is an integral part of a script structure. Blowing out the birthday cake candles precedes eating the cake. If singing the birthday song did not occur prior to cutting the cake, then the script dictates it should follow the cake cutting.

This script concept is relevant to attitudes in several ways. First, some attitudes might be formed or might change because of the execution of scripted behaviors. More specifically, scripted behaviors may have been the real cause of behaviors that the actor assumed were done by "free choice." Dissonance processes resulting from such behaviors can be a source of attitude formation and change (Aronson, 1969), but reminding people of the script that they followed in performing the behavior might be sufficient to remove the illusion of choice. Hence, there would be no attitude effects consequent to the behavior.

A second area in which the script concept might be useful is the area of attitude–behavior relations. One reason that behaviors might be inconsistent with attitudes is that different cognitive structures might be active when the attitude was measured than when the behavioral act was observed. During attitude assessment, the semantic construct defining the attitude might be active, but during performance, the behaviors might be part of a scripted action series. Hence, one might profess to be a fan of cooperation, but if the competition script is activated in the course of performing an activity, and if the script determines one's actions, one's behavior might be competitive or obstructive. Alternatively, the report of an attitude might itself be seen as part of a scripted activity. If the goal to be achieved is to present oneself in a positive light, then one's report of an attitude on sensitive topics (e.g., racism) may not reflect one's "true" attitude. Regardless of the time of its involvement, at attitude assessment or at attitude-relevant behavior, it seems clear that scripts can make a contribution to our understanding of attitudinal issues.

A third kind of cognitive structure is found in the *story model.* Researchers have suggested that we often elaborate incoming information online, and that these elaborations can often take the form of inferences or explanations (e.g., Hastie, 1984). Pennington and Hastie (1988, 1992) have suggested that, in some circumstances, these inferences might be interlinked to form a mental structure. These linked inferences (which Pennington & Hastie call a story or explanation) can then serve as the basis for later judgments about a person. For example, in the case of jury decision making, jurors may weave a story about the accused that includes the event sequences, motives, dispositions, and goals. Pennington and Hastie found that jurors construct explanatory stories based on incoming evidence, and those stories, rather than the evidence itself, serve as the basis for a subsequent decision about the proper verdict.

This model has direct relevance to attitudes. Indeed, concepts central to the model are not entirely foreign to the attitude literature: extensive research on cognitive response approaches to persuasion have frequently found that peoples' cognitive responses to a message are often more predictive of subjects' attitudes than the actual factual information contained in the message (see Petty, Ostrom, & Brock, 1981). The advance of the Pennington and Hastie story model is that it explicitly argues: (1) that some of these online cognitive responses are explanatory or causal, (2) that these responses are sometimes entered in the memory network as an explanatory story, and (3) that this story will be important to attitude responses when the story is accessed prior to an attitude judgment.

This model can help us to better understand attitude judgments in several ways. One of the continuing difficulties with attitude models that are based on the "averaging" of attributes (e.g., Anderson's [1981] information integration models) is that they allow differential weighting of attributes, but do not adequately specify the causes of these differential weights. The story model provides such an explanation: the importance of an attribute to an attitude judgment is, in part, a function of the importance or centrality of the attribute to the causal story. As a second example, witnesses in trials can vary in credibility, and this will affect the weight given the witness's testimony. This may occur because part of the story that jurors develop is whether or not any of the witnesses are motivated to lie. The texture of explanations covered by the story model provides the structure for determining what part of a witness's testimony is believed and what part is disbelieved.

Classic Views of Attitude Structure

With but few exceptions, the cognitive structures reviewed thus far have not been actively studied in connection with the attitude construct. However, attitude scholars have recognized that attitudes and their constituent beliefs do possess some form of structure (see McGuire, 1989, for an overview of this work). A number of approaches have been taken by these theorists to the study of structure. To illustrate the revisionist potential of the information processing approach, two of these will be examined here.

Attitude relevant beliefs have long been regarded as having a *dimensional* or *multidimensional* structure. For example, beliefs about capital punishment may cluster into subgroups relating to its effectiveness as a deterrent to crime, to the right of society to take a life, and as a way of restoring justice to the victim. Racial attitudes may include belief clusters relevant to perceived intelligence, job opportunity rights, open housing rights, and willingness to enter into close relationships. The identification of these separate clusters has been important in the study of attitudes because people often respond differently to the different clusters. One white person may be comfortable working with an African-American, but object to having African-Americans buying homes near his. Another might show the exact opposite pattern.

The predominant way in which these belief clusters have been identified has been through the use of factor analysis. This technique identifies belief clusters on the basis of patterns of agreement and disagreement. Two items will fall in the same cluster if peoples' response to one is highly correlated with their response to the other. Clusters differ to the extent that the items in one cluster correlate weakly with items in another cluster. The traditional view has been that the overall attitude can be decomposed into factor-specific attitudes. A person's attitude then becomes a point in multidimensional belief space. Each dimension in this space reflects a different belief cluster. This view inherently accepts the point-on-a-continuum conception of attitude, but extends it from a single continuum to multiple, coexisting dimensions.

The information processing approach has no use for this dimensional analysis of belief clusters. The dimensional metaphor has for too long masked fundamental questions about the nature of the cognitive system. Our concerns here should properly be with the nature of the codes and structures inherent in these belief clusters, and how the clusters give rise to attitudinal responses.

Beliefs, as they appear on attitude questionnaires, appear in the form of propositional units (e.g., "Capital punishment makes murderers think twice before pulling the trigger"). However, this is not the only code that is likely to be used when thinking about attitude objects. In most cases people will have stored both analog and episodic representations of the attitude object. In the case of concrete attitude objects such as commercial products and ethnic groups, peoples' encounters with these objects will yield such codes. In the case of more abstract attitude objects, such as democracy and cooperation, people will have experience reading about and discussing these issues, as well as contact with their symbols (e.g., flags waving in the breeze and hands clasped in solidarity). The traditional concept of "beliefs" must be expanded to include this wider array of mental codes.

The dimensional approach provides a way of identifying which beliefs cluster together, but it does not give us an answer to the question of why those particular clusters emerged. The answer to this question will come from an analysis of the cognitive structures used to organize those beliefs. One approach that has already received some attention is based on the premise that the beliefs are organized into an associative network. This approach views attitudes as possessing a schematic structure and has advanced our understanding of attitude influences on memory (Hymes, 1986; Judd & Kulik, 1980; Pratkanis, 1989), unipolar versus bipolar attitudes (Pratkanis, 1989), and order effects in attitude measurement (Tourangeau et al., 1989).

This schematic approach adopted a minimalist view of associative networks. The network terminology of nodes and pathways provided a basis for describing which beliefs were strongly associated and which were weakly associated. The advantage provided by the schematic model is that it provides a basis for predicting both memory and priming effects. Unfortunately, this does not take us far beyond the dimensional approach in providing an understanding of why some white persons may be content to work with an African-American but resist allowing African-Americans to move into their neighborhoods.

Knowing only which beliefs are closely associated does not provide an answer to the kinds of causal and explanatory structures that people build to bring meaning to their beliefs. For this kind of understanding, we will want to look at other structures people develop to organize their beliefs. The white, middle-class worker may have acquired direct experience with one or more African-American co-workers, and may have come to trust and respect their abilities and competence on the job. This set of responses is supported by job-related scripts and a job-specific person subcategory for which race plays no role.

This same person's reactions to the prospect of an African-American family moving into his neighborhood derives from different cognitive structures. This person may invoke their naïve economic theories about the effect of integration on property values, their naïve sociological theories regarding neighborhood crime, and their naïve theories of racial animosity regarding interfamily social relationships. The kinds of anticipated scripts and episodes generated by these knowledge structures will produce a different emotional reaction toward neighborhood integration than was shown by this person toward occupational integration.

The second kind of attitude structure we will discuss (and one of the oldest to be proposed, Fleming, 1967) is the *tripartite* approach. This view separates attitudinal responses into the three components of affect, cognition, and conation. An attitude can manifest itself, respectively, through feelings toward the attitude object, through the knowledge and beliefs one holds about the attitude object, and through the action plans and actual behaviors that characterize one's interactions with the attitude object. Past research has shown that these components tend to be discriminable from one another, yet positively correlated with one another (Breckler, 1984; Ostrom, 1969).

This conception of structures does not map well onto any of the forms of structure that have emerged from cognitive psychology. The problem is that the tripartite formulation is imprecise in two critical ways: (1) the constituents of each component are imperfectly specified, and (2) the structural relationship among the components is completely unspecified. Several scholars have recently revisited this conception of structure (Ajzen, 1989; Cacioppo, Petty, & Geen, 1989; McGuire, 1989) in an effort to better specify its character.

The cognitive concepts we have reviewed thus far are relevant in several ways to reconceptualizing the tripartite distinction. The three components almost certainly differ in terms of the cognitive code used to represent their contents. The cognitive component contains knowledge and beliefs represented in terms of propositions, analog units, and episodic units. These multiple codes may be organized within the cognitive component by means of any of the structures described in this section. It is difficult to see, however, how all the elements in the cognitive component would be organized into a single coherent unit.

The conative component would reasonably have "If–Then" production units as part of its code. It may also have scripts to guide more goal-oriented, planful, and large-scale molar actions. In addition, to the extent that memories of past actions are included in this component, then episodic memories also would be part of the conative representation. But like the cognitive component, it is difficult to imagine a single structure that would harbor all cognitive constituents of this component.

The affective component would refer to the evaluative tags along with their capacity to elicit physiological responses. The nature of those tags, as was discussed earlier, remains an open issue. On the other hand, several investigators have begun to explore the relation between evaluative responses and physiological responses (e.g., Cacioppo et al., 1989). The structure of the affective component remains largely unexplored. For example, we we need to ask if evaluative tags have a structure independent of the structure of the cognitions to which they are attached. At the physiological level, Zajonc and Markus (1984) distinguish between the arousal of autonomic and visceral activity on one hand (which is presumably triggered by activation of evaluative tags) and the muscle activity involved in the expression of emotion on the other. There are multiple opportunities for interaction among these several affective processes that require exploration.

The question of tripartite structure has traditionally referred to the relation among the three components rather than the structure within each of the separate components. For example, Ajzen (1989) proposed a hierarchical structure in which the three components were subordinate to the overall attitude. But his model was primarily for expository purposes. Accepting the point-on-a-continuum view of attitude, his model asserts that the latent variable of attitude is an influence on both verbal and nonverbal responses that fall within each of the three components. The associative properties of cognitive hierarchies, and the processes that strengthen and weaken those associations, played no role in his metaphorical use of the hierarchy concept.

The information processing approach offers a different route for understanding why the different components tend to correlate with one another. Since different codes and structures are involved in the different components, there appears to be no reason inherent in the cognitive system that requires evaluative consistency among those components. Predicting a correlation requires identifying what elements are activated in any particular measurement setting and appraising the evaluative tags associated with the activated elements. Consistency would be enhanced, for example, by ensuring that structures from one component have been activated (e.g., through priming) just prior to assessing responses from another component.

Cognitive Processes

In this chapter, we have partitioned information processing constructs into the categories of code, structure, and process. At the time we introduced these groupings, we added a cautionary comment that bears repeating here. It is impossible to completely disentangle the constructs from these categories. The information processing system simultaneously incorporates all three components; our understanding of each constituent of the system, whether it be from the subdivision of code, structure, or process, is dependent on the role that constituent plays in the functioning of the entire system.

We chose to place our discussion of cognitive processes as the last of these three categories. Processes need something to operate on, and so we found it difficult to discuss processes before introducing the reader to an array of codes and structures. Processes can be viewed as the engine that drives the structure. They determine the rules inherent in the dynamic functioning of the entire cognitive system over time. It is "processes" that tie together our understanding of both codes and structures.

Spreading Activation

One of the important processes to emerge from recent theory and research is the process of spreading activation. This process is often associated with semantic network models, and we will discuss this process in the context of those models. There are a number of different spreading activation models, and we will focus on assumptions and properties that are common to many of them.

Recall that associative network models are composed of "nodes and pathways." The nodes are simply thought to represent different types of information, from simple property detectors (e.g., horizontal lines in a letter array) to more abstract concepts (e.g., democracy). The pathways represent the associations formed between the nodes. As illustrated by the network depicted in Figure 1, nodes that are relevant to a concept are linked with that concept and, for that matter, may be linked with each other. The process of spreading activation uses the metaphor of a "spread of excitation." That is, when a concept is activated, that concept "radiates" excitation to other nodes that are closely linked to the concept.

Understanding how the pathways influence the spread of excitation is one key to the predictive power of these models. First, some pathways can be more efficient conductors of excitation than others. The efficiency of conduction is thought to be a direct function of the frequency with which two concepts have been associated. Thus, if the concepts *baseball* and *pitcher* have been frequently associated in a person's life, then there will be an efficient pathway linking those two concepts. If those two concepts have not been frequently associated, then the pathway will be less efficient. Using this principle, one can predict that response times, or decision times, will be faster for frequently linked than for infrequently linked concepts. This outcome has been often demonstrated in research. For example, Collins and Loftus (1975) found that verification times for the question "Is a robin a bird?" were faster than verification times for the question "Is a penguin a bird?" Their explanation for this effect focused on association frequency: the robin–bird pairing is more frequent than the penguin–bird pairing.

Second, the number of pathways associated with a node is also thought to affect the spread of excitation. That is, many network models assume that the available excitation is divided among all possible pathways, so that the more pathways available, the less likely it is that any one associated concept will be activated. This principle also can be translated into decision times: the more associates linked to an activated concept, the longer it will take to respond to any single associate of that concept. Research by Anderson (1983) demonstrates this principle quite nicely. In a laboratory experiment,

Anderson constructed stimulus sets so that concepts had differing numbers of linkages to other concepts. Anderson found that sentence recognition times were directly related to the number of linkages possessed by the concepts in the sentence: the more linkages possessed, the longer the recognition times. This outcome has become known as a *fan effect.*

A second general key to understanding network models lies in the properties of the nodes. Nodes can be at various states of "readiness," from a relatively "dormant" baseline level, to a moderately "intermediate" state of readiness, to a state of activation (in working memory). Thus, when excitation spreads along pathways from one node to another, the effect of this spread of excitation may simply be to heighten the readiness state of the associated node. This nodal excitation is thought to decay relatively quickly (see Wyer & Carlston, 1979).

One implication of a relatively rapid decay process is the importance of recency: constructs receiving excitation from another activated construct should be in a high state of readiness immediately after receiving this excitation, but the readiness level should decay relatively quickly. Alternatively, when a number of concepts are "primed," the most recently primed construct should be the one that tends to be used. These predictions have been confirmed by Higgins, Bargh, and Lombardi (1985).

As we noted earlier in this chapter (e.g., much of Fazio's [1990] research program; Judd et al., 1991), many of these principles have already been applied to the attitude domain. The results of these studies illustrate the possible utility of a spreading activation approach for enhancing our understanding of attitudes. However, spreading activation models have been criticized for a number of reasons, and the predictions of spreading activation models can also be generated by other theoretical approaches (e.g., see Ratcliff & McKoon, 1988). Nonetheless, activation models are attractive because they can potentially account for a number of phenomena: among them are bottom-up processing, top-down processing, typicality effects, interfeature correlations, and expectancy effects. Although some attitude researchers have used a spreading activation approach, the research applying this perspective to attitudes has investigated only a few of these implications.

Automatic and Controlled Processing

Cognitive psychologists have distinguished between automatic and controlled information processing (e.g., Shiffrin & Schneider, 1977; Bargh, 1989; Logan, 1989). Research indicates that information processing will sometimes occur automatically, without using cognitive capacity. However, on other occasions, information will be processed in a controlled fashion, a condition that requires considerable cognitive capacity.

Learning to drive a car provides a useful example of this distinction. In the early stages of learning, almost every activity is a controlled response. You actively need to decide when to turn the steering wheel to the right or the left, and you actively decide when to move your foot from the brake pedal to the accelerator. These decisions require your full thought and attention. After enough practice, however, these activities become automatic. You can perform these activities while musing about your plans for the day and while talking to your traveling companions. The required motor responses occur without the expenditure of much cognitive capacity.

This distinction between automatic and controlled processing, and the conditions under which each occurs, are of tremendous importance to the understanding of attitudes. For example, consider a recent program of research by Martin (e.g., Martin, 1986; Martin, Seta, & Crelia, 1990). Martin investigated people's judgments under two circumstances: when they had been exposed to blatant primes (i.e., a priming manipulation that was clumsy and relatively obvious) or to subtle primes (a priming manipulation that was not obvious). When the primes were subtle, Martin obtained "normal" priming effects: an ambiguously described target was perceived in terms of the construct activated by the primes. However, when the primes were blatant, Martin obtained the opposite result: subjects' judgments of the target were contrasted away from the activated construct.

These data can be understood in terms of a two-stage model of judgment in which the first stage is regulated largely by automatic processes and the second stage is governed by controlled processes (Devine, 1989; Gilbert & Osborne, 1989; Trope, 1989). The automatic processes, such as those instantiated by subtle primes, help to determine the concept that will be activated and used to process incoming information. Controlled processes, such as those instantiated by the blatant prime, govern any adjustments that are made to the initial inferences.

Several lines of evidence provide converging support for this idea. One line comes from research into the "anchor-and-adjust" heuristic, which demonstrates that presenting a randomly selected number before a frequency judgment task will bias the frequency judgments in the direction of the random number (Tversky & Kahneman, 1982). The anchor-and-adjust explanation for this effect is that the random number automatically "pops" into mind during the frequency task, thereby serving as an anchor. The final judgment is rendered by adjusting from that anchor.

A second line of evidence comes from studies looking at subjects' ability to make use of situational information in dispositional inferences (e.g., Gilbert, Pelham, & Krull, 1988). Results of these studies indicate that subjects under cognitive load draw equivalent inferences to no-load subjects when no situational explanations for an actor's behavior are provided, suggesting that this inferential process is relatively automatic. However, when situational explanations for behaviors were presented, only no-load subjects were able to use these to modify their ratings; subjects under cognitive load provided ratings similar to those provided when no situational explanations were presented. Hence, adjustments to judgments appear to require cognitive capacity.

A third line of evidence comes from the results of a study by Martin et al. (1990). In this study, subjects were exposed to a manipulation designed to affect their motivation to avoid errors in judgments. The results of this study indicated that, in blatant priming conditions, contrast effects occurred primarily in those subjects who were motivated to avoid the biasing effects of the blatant prime. This result again suggests that subjects make a conscious adjustment to the results of processing induced by an automatically activated construct.

These results suggest that knowing the activated construct being used to process information about an issue is not enough: to understand attitude judgments, one must discern exactly what cognitive products were automatically activated, and whether the person processing the information is both capable of and motivated to adjust the output of this automatic, first-stage processing. However, there appears to be even more complexity: to understand subjects' judgments when adjustments are made, it is also necessary to understand the nature of the adjustments subjects are likely to make.

Deliberative adjustments will depend on subjects' ideas about judgment biases. A recent study by Petty and Wegener (1993) gave subjects differing "cover stories" about the likely effects of a judgment context: subjects were told either that the context produced assimilation, or it produced contrast. In a subsequent judgment task, subjects' judgments demonstrated that they were attempting to correct for bias: assimilation was observed when subjects thought that the context produced contrast, and contrast was observed when subjects thought that the context produced assimilation.

Collectively, these data encourage several new lines of attitude research. For example, one of the classic problems in attitude measurement is that people do not always report their attitudes honestly. If one conceptualizes this problem in terms of conscious adjustment processes applied to automatically activated judgments, then it becomes apparent that a cognitive load task similar to that employed by Gilbert et al. (1988) might allow an exploration of subjects' automatically activated attitudes; that is, subjects might be presented with information that is ambiguous with respect to an attitude issue, and be placed under cognitive load while evaluating that information. The cognitive load manipulation might prevent adjustment processes from being invoked, so that subjects' evaluations will presumably reflect their automatically activated attitudes.

This logic should not be terribly foreign to the attitude domain: attitude researchers interested in cognitive responses have frequently distracted subjects (essentially a cognitive load manipulation) to prevent message counterarguing (Brock, 1967). The idea we have proposed extends this logic, using a cognitive load manipulation to bypass retrieval-based processing, and in doing so, assessing subjects' automatically activated attitudes. It also raises the question of which attitude is the "true" attitude.

Another key issue in this area concerns the coexistence of automatic and controlled processing in the same system. Both types of processing seem to occur, but little is known about when either predominates, and about how the types of processing might interact (Logan, 1989). A recent attempt at integrating automatic and controlled processes in attitudes has been made by Fazio (1990). Fazio's model (called the MODE model) is an explicit attempt to unite the research investigating the relatively automatic influences on attitudes (e.g., attitude accessibility work) with more controlled processing (e.g., Ajzen & Fishbein's theory of reasoned action, 1980).

This approach is relatively new, and largely untested. Nonetheless, it is Fazio's hope (and ours, too) that a focus on these processes, and in how and when they operate, will be able to propel attitude research beyond describing the variables known to affect attitudes, and will provide a theoretical integration that will serve as a useful framework for understanding the effects of these variables.

On-Line and Memory-Based Processing

One of the problems that has repeatedly vexed the literature on attitudes (e.g., Greenwald, 1968; Loken, 1984), as well as the impression formation literature (Anderson & Hubert, 1963; Dreben, Fiske, & Hastie, 1979) is the frequent finding that judgment and memory are uncorrelated; that is, there is often not a systematic relation between the judgments that one makes and the judgment-relevant information that one can recall.

A major breakthrough on this problem was provided by Hastie and Park (1986) who distinguished between on-line and memory-based modes of judgment. The assumption in on-line judgment tasks is that information recipients are performing judgment operations on information as the information is being received. This might occur, for example, when you meet a new person at a party. You are forming and modifying your impression of such persons continuously as you talk with them. Under these circumstances, when perceivers are processing information with the goal of forming or evaluating an inference, Hastie and Park argue that there is no reason to expect memory to be correlated with th results of the inferential processing.

Although this expectation might be counterintuitive, research on the incongruity effect supports this prediction. The incongruity effect refers to the finding that information that is incongruent with a person expectancy is often well remembered (for a review, see Stangor & McMillan, 1992). As a number of studies reveal, this incongruity effect emerges in on-line processing where the goal is to evaluate a target with respect to a trait expectancy. The effect does not emerge as powerfully (or even at all) when subjects do not have this processing goal (e.g., Srull, Lichtenstein, & Rothbart, 1985).

This incongruity effect is thought to emerge because perceivers attempt to reconcile the incongruent information with the expectancy and/or with other expectancy-congruent behaviors (Hastie, 1984; also see Wyer & Srull, 1989). If successfully explained away, the incongruent information will have little impact on judgments. However, the more extensive processing of the incongruent information will lead to heightened recall for the incongruent behaviors. Hence, under on-line conditions, there is no necessary correlation between memory and inference: inferences of equal extremity might be associated with relatively low levels of event recall (if the inference is unchallenged) or high levels of recall (if challenged by incongruity that is explained away).

The attitudes literature has also addressed the absence of memory–judgment correlations, but it has done so by focusing on the issue of cognitive responses. That is, a number of studies demonstrate that the cognitive responses that people have to a message are correlated with reported attitudes, even when recall for the specific information is not correlated with attitudes (Greenwald, 1968). This outcome is not inconsistent with the memory-based versus on-line distinction: these cognitive responses are generated on-line, and may often be formed in the process of counterarguing a message, a process that has some functional similarity to explaining away inconsistency.

The contribution that the on-line versus memory-based distinction can make to this area is that it can be used to specify conditions under which recall for facts is a determinant of reported attitudes. This should occur if "on-line" processing can be avoided at information reception, so that when asked to make a subsequent judgment, a respondent must do so by accessing and reviewing the information stored in memory (see Chaiken & Stangor, 1987).

Some would argue that the primacy of affective responding (e.g., Zajonc, 1980) may inevitably and unavoidably lead to on-line formation of evaluative tags. If this were true, it would not be possible for attitudes to be created in a retrieval-based manner. Nonetheless, it may be possible to devise processing goals that prevent or interfere with the spontaneous creation of on-line attitudes. If so, one would expect to find a correlation between attitude and memory-for-original-information (as opposed to memory-for-cognitive-responses) when attitude judgments are subsequently requested. A study by Mackie and Ascuncion (1990) obtained exactly this outcome. Subjects whose on-line judgment capability was reduced by presentation of cognitive load tasks (spelling and grammar checks) simultaneous with message presentation showed higher correlations between attitudes and recall than subjects who were not presented with the load manipulations.

Implicit and Explicit Memory

The on-line versus memory-based distinction, combined with the cognitive response approach, suggests that in order to understand memory–judgment relations, one must understand how information is processed at the time of encoding. The importance of this relation is emphasized by recent research into the differences between implicit and explicit memory processes. The term *implicit memory* refers to the fact that people frequently retrieve memories incidentally, without having the intention to do so. Moreover, they are not often aware of these retrievals, nor of their effects on subsequent processing. The term *explicit memory* refers to the fact that, sometimes, performance on a memory task requires conscious recollection of previous experiences.

In an extensive review of the implicit versus explicit distinction, Schacter (1987) notes that a number of areas of research seem to converge on the idea that at least some memory functions are implicit. First, Schacter points to research on the savings effect in relearning. The savings effect refers to the fact that prior learning (e.g., of a word list) facilitates subsequent learning, even when all of the old material has supposedly been "forgotten." Nelson (1978) provides direct evidence for the implicit nature of this effect, demonstrating that this savings effect occurs even for items in a list that are neither recalled nor recognized (also see Macleod, 1988; Carlston & Skowronski, in press).

A second area cited by Schacter as support for the implicit versus explicit distinction is the research demonstrating that subliminally presented stimuli can affect subsequent processing. For example, Bargh and Pietromonaco (1982) have found that subliminal exposure to words related to the concept of hostility affected subjects' later hostility judgments of a social target. This effect occurred despite the fact that recognition of the words as they were presented was at a chance level (also see Bargh, Bond, Lombardi, & Tota, 1986; Lewicki, 1985).

A third area cited by Schacter shows that learning and conditioning can proceed without conscious awareness of the rules or contingencies involved. For example, work on language learning by Reber (1976) suggests that, by the systematic presentation of letter strings organized around various rules, subjects can learn an unfamiliar, synthetic grammar. This occurred even when the subjects were not aware of the rules (also see Lewicki, 1986).

A fourth area cited by Schacter as support for the implicit versus explicit distinction are repetition priming effects. Work on this topic suggests that concepts that are activated, or "primed" by repeated exposure to a concept can affect subsequent processing. Priming effects have been demonstrated in a number of areas, ranging from lexical decision tasks (in which subjects have to make a decision about whether a string of characters is a word or not; Neely, 1977) to social inference tasks (in which exposure to a concept biases subsequent concept-relevant social information processing; e.g., Srull & Wyer, 1979). Furthermore, evidence suggests that, at least under some conditions, these priming effects occur implicitly, without subjects' awareness. For example, in the research looking at the effects of priming on social inferences, the assimilative effects of priming seem to partially depend on whether subjects' are explicitly aware of the priming manipulation (see Martin et al., 1990; Skowronski, Carlston, & Isham, 1993).

Finally, as support for the implicit versus explicit distinction, Schacter also cites research on amnesiacs, which suggests that amnesiacs can often learn skills. For example, early research by Milner (e.g., Milner, Corkin, & Teuber, 1968) on the amnesic patient H. M. demonstrated that practice could improve the performance of the patient on pursuit rotor and mirror tracing tasks. This improvement persisted despite the fact that H. M. could not explicitly remember having performed the task.

One of the important lessons from this work on implicit and explicit memory is that measures of memory are not interchangeable. That is, whether one obtains evidence that an individual "remembers" something is dependent on the match between the mental operations performed at learning and those required during the memory test (e.g., Blaxton, 1989). Researchers in the attitudes domain have tended to exclusively focus on measures of explicit memory, measures such as recognition and recall, and these may not always be appropriate. Depending on the aspect of memory that an attitudes investigator is interested in (e.g., visual memory, conceptual memory), implicit memory measures, such as perceptual identification or category accessibility, may sometimes be preferable.

A recent study by von Hippel and Baker (1993) demonstrates that implicit memory measures can be highly useful in domains that have traditionally used explicit measures. These researchers argued that the traditional recall measures used in incongruency studies (see Stangor & McMillan, 1992) were ill suited to testing models suggesting that subjects elaborated the incongruent information (e.g., Klein & Loftus, 1990). Instead, because conceptually driven implicit memory measures are sensitive to elaborative processing (Smith & Branscombe, 1988), von Hippel and Baker reasoned that if there was increased elaboration of incongruent items at encoding, then there should be better implicit memory for the incongruent than for the congruent information. More important, these researchers predicted a negative correlation between impressions and memory. Both of these predictions were confirmed.

These findings suggest that the well-documented finding of no correlation between attitude and information recall (e.g., Greenwald, 1968) may hold only when explicit memory is assessed. Because attitude researchers have often suggested that message recipients cognitively respond to messages (e.g., engage in elaborative processing) the implication of the von Hippel and Baker research is that a memory–judgment correlation may emerge when implicit memory measures are used (see Greenwald & Banaji, 1993, for a more thorough discussion of relations between attitudes and implicit memory).

Serial versus Parallel Processing

Another example of the applicability of cognitive process theories to the attitude domain comes from an examination of assumptions concerning how processing proceeds: in serial or in parallel form. When a baby is born, the proud parents and grandparents play the game of "Who does the newborn look like?" Often, a specific person will immediately come to mind. It is as if a parallel matching process was simultaneously conducted between the baby and all members on both sides of the family, and the best match leaps out. Other times this matching process is done in a serial manner, as might be the case when asked which of the two grandfathers the little boy most resembles.

Parallel processes have assumed increasing importance in cognitive psychology. For example, the early work on automatic search and identification processes seems to demonstrate that at least some processing tends to proceed in parallel. A serial process implies that as processing steps are added, the time it takes to complete processing should increase. However, experiments demonstrate that increasing the number of "noise" targets in a stimulus array does not apparently have a great impact on the time it takes to search the array for a target that substantially differs from the noise targets (Schneider & Shiffrin, 1977).

Parallel processing has also emerged in memory research. Many of the major models of memory assume parallel search, so that large portions of the long-term memory storage system can be assessed quickly (e.g., Anderson, 1983). Finally, many connectionist modelers also explicitly assume that neural elements in the neural network process information in parallel (McClelland, Rumelhart, & the PDP Research Group, 1986). This parallel processing, especially due to the presence of both excitatory and inhibitory elements in the neural network, allows the neural net models to rapidly "settle" on items in memory searches or in perceptual identification tasks (e.g., Rumelhart et al., 1986).

The idea that information can be processed in parallel can aid our understanding of several attitude-related issues. For example, there has been a long-standing debate over the processes used to report an evaluation once it has been formed and stored. In general, there are two possibilities: the evaluation can be recomputed from recall of the original information that went into the evaluation in the first place, or a previously formed evaluation can be retrieved and reported without any recomputation. Several studies (Lingle & Ostrom, 1979; Lingle, Geva, Ostrom, Leippe, & Baumgardner, 1979; Carlston, 1980) suggest that subjects retrieve and use the prior evaluation, although under some conditions, the original information may also be retrieved (Carlston & Skowronski, 1986; Lingle, Dukerich, & Ostrom, 1983).

Parallel search processes suggests a third possibility: that both the original information and the evaluation might be simultaneously accessed. In fact, the "computation" necessary to compute the attitude may occur simultaneous with (in fact, may be exactly the same as) activating the representation of the original evaluation.

A second implication of this parallel search process may help to solve one of the paradoxes of priming. One assumption of many models of attitudes is that attitude evaluations, especially for well-known attitude objects, are precomputed and stored in memory. Hence, to report an attitude for these objects, all one has to do is to reaccess that node and report a readout. However, this concept of a precomputed and stored evaluation is inconsistent with the idea that priming portions of a cognitive representation can alter reported attitudes. If the concept is precomputed and stored, why should this happen?

In fact, this result would be expected if the attitude that one reports is a result of parallel distributed processing that simultaneously accesses all attitude-relevant components. In this type of processing, the reported attitude may simply be a "readout" of a pattern of activation in the cognitive system representing an attitude. Change one aspect of the system (e.g., by priming), and the attitude may change. Thus, parallel distributed processing models offer one possible solution to the problem of attitude instability across time.

Classic Views of Attitude Process

Cognitive theories of attitude have dominated research in the field of the past thirty years. The early competitors to cognitive theories had been models derived from principles of classical and instrumental conditioning (Ostrom, 1968). Those competitors quickly lost the race; almost nothing appeared in the literature on those models after 1970. Cognitive theory became the near exclusive focus of research thereafter.

Over the last three decades attitude researchers have viewed themselves as studying "attitudinal processes." The term "processes" was used by these scholars to capture their interest in the dynamics of attitude formation and change. The concern addressed in this section is one of identifying the processes (as opposed to the codes and structures) that were inherent in their theories. We recognize that social psychologists have posited a number of psychological forces relevant to attitude formation, maintenance, and change. For example, McGuire (1985), has isolated sixteen "guiding-idea theories" that may be involved in the dynamics underlying attitudes. We have chosen to discuss only two of these process concerns. They are the ones that dominated attitude research from the 1960s into the 1980s: cognitive consistency and cognitive integration.

Research on *cognitive consistency* was one of the few theoretical efforts in the field of attitudes in which scholars explicitly tried to identify code, structure, and process. The theory employed an associative network metaphor that involved nodes and pathways. The typical network involved three nodes and pathways connecting all three to each other. For example, Heider's (1958) "*p-o-x*" system involved nodes for person (*p*), other (*o*), and attitude object (*x*). The pathways linking the nodes could either be positive

(+) or negative (−), and they could refer to either sentiment bonds (where + means "likes" and − means "dislikes") or unit formation bonds (where + means "associated with" and − means "disassociated from").

The dynamic process identified by balance theorists (e.g., Abelson et al., 1968; Festinger, 1957; Insko, 1981) was that these structures tended toward "balance." The more they became imbalanced, the greater the need to restore balance. Balance is a state of evaluative harmony in which two elements linked by a positive bond (e.g., *p* and *o* like each other) should share a common attitude toward an object (e.g., either they both like *x* or they both dislike *x*). So if two friends discover they have diametrically opposite attitudes about a new car or a political candidate, they experience pressure to develop a common attitude. Two persons who dislike each other will experience pressure to develop opposite attitudes toward a common object.

The principle of balance also applies to sets of beliefs held by one person. The person (*p*) can hold beliefs *x* and *y*. If beliefs *x* and *y* are positively linked (through either a unit or sentiment relation), then *p* should either accept both or reject both beliefs. In general, balance exists among three elements either if all three bonds are positive or if one bond is positive and two are negative. The remaining combinations produce an imbalanced state. The concept of balance also applies to systems containing more than three elements (Abelson & Rosenberg, 1958). In this case, the level of balance of the system is determined by the relative number of balanced to imbalanced triads in the system as a whole.

There are problems in trying to translate the construct of balance into contemporary information processing constructs. This is due both to a lack of precision in the concept of cognition used by balance theorists, and to inadequacies in the formal understanding of evaluative tags by cognitive psychologists. Heider defined balance as "a harmonious state in which the entities comprising the situation and the feelings about them fit together without stress" (p. 180). Balance theorists appropriately recognized the need to identify the constituent cognitive elements in the system and to recognize that these nodes could be arranged in an associative network (through unit bonds). The sentiment bond between *p* and other cognitive elements (*o* and *x*) translates into the code for the evaluative tag (i.e., the person likes or dislikes each cognitive object).

It is known that experiencing imbalance is unpleasant (Jordan, 1953; Newcomb, 1968) and that it can produce physiological arousal (Cooper & Fazio, 1984). But there is a problem of incorporating the concept of a "harmonious state" into the conceptual structure of the information processing approach. The balance concept was offered by Heider (1958) as a Gestalt-level description of the entire cognitive system. This was in contrast to defining it as a drive state from the perspective of classic learning theories (Jordan, 1968). A common approach in cognitive psychology has been to recast the concept of "drive" in terms of a cognitively stored "processing goal." Being hungry is nothing more than having a goal of consuming food. But arguing that people have a stored "goal" to maintain balanced structures seems to be a less than satisfactory solution to understanding the human tendency to achieve balanced structures.

The concept of balance describes the system as a whole. Such system-level constructs are not yet well developed in cognitive psychology, but recent research in dynamical systems (which we will address in greater detail later in the chapter) is moving in that direction. Future work on dynamical systems may provide a bridge between information processing constructs and the construct of balance.

There are two areas of past research that illustrate the links between balance processes and cognitive processes. One of the first topics of research in social cognition was an examination of whether balanced structures were stored as a schematic structure in long-term memory. Schematic structures have two properties relevant to our present concerns: (1) they are stored as a single unit and (2) they can be used to fill in missing information. Research has generally supported the idea that balanced structures are more schematic than unbalanced structures. Balanced structures are processed more rapidly (Sentis & Burnstein, 1979) and are learned more readily (Picek, Sherman, & Shiffrin, 1975) than unbalanced structures. Errors in learning pairwise bonds (Zajonc & Burnstein, 1965a,b) and errors in recall of entire structures (Picek et al., 1975) tend to be in the direction of establishing balance.

Other evaluation-based structures that do not involve principles of balance have also been explored by social cognition researchers. Both an "attraction effect" (in which triads containing positive *p* to *o* relation are more schematic than those with a negative *p* to *o* relation) and an "agreement effect" (in which triads that show agreement between the *p* to *x* bond and the *o* to *x* bond are more schematic than ones showing disagreement) have been empirically supported (Cacioppo & Petty, 1981; Cottrell, 1975; Insko, Songer, & McGarvey, 1974; Gollob, 1974). Unfortunately, as far as we know, the idea of cognitive structures being based on the pattern of evaluative tags has yet to be seriously considered by cognitive psychologists.

A second area of research bridging the processes of balance theory and cognitive psychology is the work described earlier on memory for incongruent information. When presented with both expectancy-congruent and expectancy-incongruent behaviors, people have better recall for the incongruent than for the congruent behaviors (Srull & Wyer, 1989; Stangor & McMillan, 1992). For example, the subject may learn that the stimulus person is generally kind. Then both kind and unkind behaviors of that person are described. From a balance theory perspective, the kind behaviors combine with the kind expectancy to form balanced triads and the unkind behaviors combine with the expectancy to form unbalanced triads.

The finding of superior memory for incongruent information is in apparent conflict with the research showing greater difficulty in learning unbalanced structures (Picek et al., 1975; Zajonc & Burnstein, 1965a,b). However, unlike work on memory for balanced versus unbalanced structures, the incongruency effect is studied in a context in which multiple items of information are sequentially presented about the actions of just one person or group. The role of balance schemas in this context is to focus cognitive effort on resolving the imbalanced triads. That is, attributional activity focuses on the incongruent behaviors to resolve their inconsistency with the expectation and with the congruent behaviors. It is presumably this greater processing time and the resulting additional links to other memory items that lead to better recall of the incongruent information. The concept of balance as an evaluative schema provides a conceptual basis for being able to understand why more cognitive effort is devoted to the incongruent behaviors than to the congruent behaviors in this setting.

The second of the two classic attitude processes is *cognitive integration*. It deals with the question of how people derive an overall attitudinal disposition from the array of knowledge and beliefs they hold about the attitude object. One of the best developed theoretical accounts of these issues is provided by Anderson's Information Integration Theory (Anderson, 1981). Other attitude theorists who have addressed this problem of information integration include Fishbein and Ajzen (1975) and Rosenberg (1956).

Anderson distinguishes between the cognitive operations of information valuation and information integration. *Valuation* refers to the process of determining the evaluative scale value and the weight assigned to each item of information that contributes to the attitudinal judgment. The scale value varies on a continuum from positive to negative and is considered to be unaffected by context and the nature of the other cognitive elements. From the information processing point of view, the scale value corresponds to the evaluative tag linked to the cognitive element. The information integration approach requires that this tag not be just two-valued (positive vs. negative), but that it be a value on a continuum that ranges from very positive to very negative.

The weight parameter reflects the functional influence of the cognitive element in determining the overall attitude. It can vary from zero to one, and its value will be influenced by context. There is no clear counterpart for this property within the information processing framework. It is true that the term "weight" is used to describe feature weighting mechanisms in categorization processes (e.g., Smith & Medin, 1981) and in models of similarity judgments (Vosniadou & Ortony, 1989). However, these so-called weight parameters actually correspond to Anderson's scale value parameter in that they refer to how much the feature does or does not relate to the category.

From an information processing perspective, information units exist as parts of structures (e.g., associative networks and scripts) and do not carry weight tags that indicate their separate contributions to determining responses. Of course, people may respond quite differently to structures that contain (vs. ones that do not contain) a particular cognitive element. However, this can occur without positing the existence of a weight tag associated with each element. For example, elements that are highly activated, or that are in working memory, will contribute more than other elements. In traditional attitude models, weight plays a central conceptual role. However, our present analysis indicates that the concept of weight is at best a summary label for the result of more fundamental cognitive mechanisms.

Integration refers to the process of combining the information units into an overall attitudinal judgment. Broadly speaking, it addresses the problem of the relationship between knowledge, beliefs, and inferences on one hand, and the overall evaluative judgment on the other.

In Anderson's information integration theory, the integration process is one of algebraically combining the weight and scale value parameters into a single judgment. The algebraic rule that appears to best describe evaluative judgments such as person impressions is averaging: the numerator contains the sum of the products of weight times scale value (across all cognitive elements) and the denominator is simply the sum of all the weights. Information integration theory allows for the possibility that other algebraic rules might be relevant to different judgment domains. For example, summation might describe the value of a stock portfolio (i.e., adding the scale value of each stock) and multiplication might describe evaluations of job performance (i.e., multiplying the scale value of ability times that of motivation).

A literal view of such algebraic "processes" would involve postulating a series of cognitive steps such as: (1) there exists a memory store in which weight and scale value parameters were stored for each cognition, (2) the parameters for each relevant cognition are retrieved (perhaps serially), (3) the requisite algebraic operations are performed on those parameters (perhaps in working memory), and (4) the resulting implicit evaluative response is used as the basis of the overt response.

Such an analysis raises a variety of questions. Where do the weights and scale values come from? How can there be a store large enough to contain all the weights and scale values for all cognitive elements, especially given that each cognitive element must have these two parameters for every possible judgment dimension a person could potentially encounter? If such a store did exist, what indexing mechanism would allow efficient retrieval of the relevant parameters? How accurate is the "synaptic calculator" that conducts the needed algebraic manipulations on the parameter values? Is the implicit judgment discarded upon overt response, or is a decision made whether or not to store it for future use?

The processes involved in information integration are only a subset of the broader set of cognitive activities potentially involved in producing attitudinal responses. There must be some instigating event that activates attitude generating processes. Often it is being in a context that requires an overt response toward the attitude object. Other times it is the need to respond to the question "What is your attitude?" Higgins and King (1981) have identified six factors that can lead to concept activation: goal relevance, situational salience, expectations, relation to other concepts, frequency of past use, and recency of past use. Many cognitive activities, of which information integration is only one, result from such instigating events.

One line of research relevant to this question examines the cognitive basis of question answering (e.g., Lehnert, 1978; Ostrom, 1987; Strack & Martin, 1987; Tourangeau & Rasinski, 1988). For example, Tourangeau and Rasinski (1988), viewing attitudes as being structures in long-term memory, suggest that four stages are involved in answering questions about one's attitude: (1) interpretation of the question, (2) retrieval of relevant knowledge and beliefs, (3) generation of an implicit attitudinal response, and (4) mapping the implicit response into the response options available in the instigating question. This analytic structure could easily be broadened to include other instigating events than just questions. Anderson's (and other attitude theorist's) concerns with cognitive integration pertain only to Stage Three of this process.

Not all attitudinal responses involve the algebraic integration of knowledge and beliefs about the attitude object. In the Tourangeau and Rasinski (1988) system some responses result directly from Stage Two activities and so never involve the Stage Three mechanisms. Some attitudinal judgments have been invoked frequently or recently enough that they can be directly retrieved (e.g., Lingle et al., 1983). Directly basing a response on the evaluative tag linked to the attitude object, as has been proposed by Fazio (1989), is also a Stage Two process.

Of course, many responses do involve Stage Three processes. But even here, the algebraic processes posited by the classical attitude theorists are not the only possible way to represent the cognitive events involved. One alternative, for example, is the random walk model (Stone, 1960). This model suggested that persons may randomly sample knowledge and beliefs about the attitude object, extracting the valence of the evaluative tag from each. A register keeps track of the net balance of positive and negative elements. A positive response is generated as soon as the register reaches a predetermined positive count (e.g., the number of positive elements exceed the number of negative elements by the preset parameter of, say, three). Similarly, a negative response is triggered should the register exceed the predetermined negative count. The first of these two thresholds that is reached will terminate the search and trigger the response. This is a different cognitive mechanism than that which has been proposed by the algebraic theorists, and yet it may provide a more satisfactory account of how attitudes are generated in retrieval-based contexts.

This section has argued that contemporary work in cognitive psychology offers a much more differentiated view of attitude process than that which was offered by the classic attitude theorists. It has also suggested, most notably in the case of balance schema, that cognitive psychology has to date overlooked evaluative processes that can guide cognitive functioning.

EMERGING CONCEPTIONS OF COGNITION

Thus far, this chapter has partitioned information processing issues into the topics of code, structure, and process. We have periodically cautioned the reader that this distinction has a fuzzy quality and that it is difficult to talk about one set of issues without touching on the other topics. Despite these difficulties, the distinction allowed us to highlight many of the information processing issues that bear on our understanding of attitudes.

In the present section, all attempts to maintain this three-way distinction are abandoned. Over the past decade new conceptions of cognition have appeared that inextricably blend code, structure, and process. These conceptions challenge the ideas outlined earlier in the chapter that cognitive elements can be represented as discrete, unitary nodes in a network, that associative structures exist as interrelations among concept nodes, and that spreading activation processes are responsible for patterns of node activation. Instead, these newer conceptions are founded upon three assumptions: (1) cognitive activity resides in patterns of neural activation, (2) system-level properties are most informative, and (3) understanding dynamic change over time is rudimentary to all explanations.

Parallel Distributed Processing Networks

The network models discussed earlier in this chapter are examples of a class of models referred to as local network models. This refers to the fact that information is stored "locally" (e.g., in "nodes") and is accessed as a single unit. More recent work has proposed an alternative conception of networks. Connectionist and neural network modeling (e.g., Rumelhart et al., 1986) has suggested that conceptual knowledge is not stored locally, but rather in a "distributed" fashion. That is, units of knowledge exist as a pattern of activity occurring throughout the network as a whole.

Fiske and Taylor (1991) provide a useful illustration of distributed memory by suggesting the analogy of an electronic display board composed of many separate individual bulbs. Each bulb, by itself, is meaningless: no single bulb represents a unique piece of information (as would be the case with local network models). Instead, meaningful patterns emerge when a bulb is lit in conjunction with selected other bulbs on the board. One pattern may display the word "Merry" and another pattern the word "Christmas." Of course, in actual neural networks the pattern of node activation cannot simply be read like a marquee. The main point to be made is that in such networks information is derived from the overall pattern of activity, with each node able to participate in the production of multiple patterns.

Although they share some similarities, there are important differences between distributed processing networks and associative networks. One key component of distributed models is that some connections are inhibitory; that is, some connections serve to make activation of a concept less likely. In fact, Rumelhart et al. (1986) suggest that, in memory searches, incompatible concepts might be mutually inhibitory, so that activating one concept inhibits activation of the other. This suggests the possible presence of "antipriming" effects, in which stimulation of a concept may inhibit the activation of an incompatible target concept, making the target concept less likely to be used in subsequent attitude judgments.

To explore this idea more concretely, consider a variation of the Sherman et al. (1990) study described earlier. Imagine exposing a subject to a priming manipulation that increases the accessibility of the construct "conciliatory." Subsequently, subjects are given information in which some of the information is ambiguous with respect to the target's hostility, and subjects are asked to report their attitude toward the target. If this inhibition exists, then repeated prior activation of the construct conciliatory will make it less likely that the ambiguously hostile behaviors will be interpreted in terms of hostility, and subjects will have a more positive attitude toward the target after such priming.

Parallel distributed processing models are also useful in explaining the recognition of imperfect stimulus patterns (i.e., patterns that don't exactly match an original template). The reason for this is straightforward: in some parallel distributed processing models, if a significant part of the pattern is activated, then the rest of the pattern becomes activated as well. This property might help to explain why we often have affective responses to entirely new objects—if the new object sufficiently resembles the old object, even in superficial ways, then the similarity might be sufficient enough to activate stored patterns, which might include affective responses that could contribute to an attitude.

One of the authors vividly remembers a time when this happened to him in the context of a search for a new car. He and his wife had done a thorough job of reviewing available reference material, and having established preferences based on that material, ventured onto dealership lots to actually look at cars. One model was high in their personal evaluative ratings—a Mazda GLC. However, in looking at the car, there were a couple of features that reminded them strongly of an old car that they had owned, one that was a real lemon. These features were basically irrelevant to the performance of both old and new cars. For example, especially prominent in both cars were large plastic rivets used to hold carpeting in place. Despite the fact that they otherwise liked the car's performance, price, and service record, and despite the fact that the car scored highly in the information integration decision scheme being used at the time, the car was down rated and eventually discarded from consideration, largely because of these superficial similarities. This might be an example of parallel distributed processing at work: the superficial similarities between the cars were significant enough to reactivate information and affective responses pertaining to the old car, and these affected the attitude response.

Dynamical Systems Approaches to Attitudes

A fundamental feature of the cognitive approach to attitudes is the appreciation that attitudes are not single entities, but rather are the product of a system composed of many interacting cognitive and emotional elements. The exact nature of these elements, and the form of the interactions among them, may be described differently by various cognitive theories. However, the idea that a mental representation is a system of multiply interacting elements is a fundamental assumption of all cognitive theories.

Traditional cognitive theories have taken a "building block" approach modeling cognitive systems: they assemble codes into structures, and posit possible forms of process that operate on the structure. Dynamical systems have a different starting point; they are more holistic in nature. Their primary focus is on (1) properties of the system as a whole (with less emphasis on the constituent elements) and (2) the temporal dynamics that characterize the system. These dynamical models place a premium on understanding the system as a whole, and on understanding how the dynamic forces inherent in the system will themselves shape changes in the system over time.

The Nature of Dynamical Systems

The theory of dynamical systems constitutes one of the most powerful paradigms of modern natural sciences. It has been developed in mathematics and physics to describe the behavior (specifically, the temporal evolution) and properties of systems of interacting elements. It is an advanced, precise mathematical theory in which the system's temporal evolution is modeled by a set of differential or difference equations (see Gleick 1987; Nowak & Lewenstein, in press; Schuster, 1984). Although the dynamical systems paradigm has been used to describe physical phenomena for quite a long time, recent developments in the area of nonlinear dynamical systems have led to revolutionary advances in the natural sciences. Such phrases as deterministic chaos, attractors, sensitivity to initial conditions, bifurcation, and fractals all refer to phenomena occurring in nonlinear dynamical systems. These constructs are appearing with increasing frequency in scientific journals, and even in magazines targeted to the educated lay public.

The basic property of a dynamical system is that its state at any given moment in time depends on its state in the previous instant. The classic example of a dynamical system is a pendulum, where its position and velocity at one moment determine its position and velocity at the next moment. The key characteristic of a dynamical system, then, is that the very parameters that govern the behavior of the system will shift dynamically over time.

This property is important, for it allows these systems to exhibit extremely "complex" behavior. In the case of cognitive systems, feedback channels allow the system to operate iteratively on the information and inferences they generate; the output of one iteration serves as part of the input for the next iteration. Thus, small energy flows through one part of the system can be amplified by the presence of these feedback channels, so that small changes in the value of a variable can ultimately have a large impact on the system. Alternatively, these systems may also settle into relatively stable states (or equilibria), so that even relatively large changes on a variable can have relatively little impact on the system.

In some nonlinear dynamical models, the behavior exhibited by the system can change radically, going from a relatively stable pattern to seeming randomness and back to seeming stability again. The ability of these models to account for a wide range of patterns of data, even patterns that seem to involve discontinuous shifts or seemingly random behavior, is one of the features that make these models attractive to psychologists. Such phenomena, which are often observed in the behavior of individual experimental subjects or clinical patients, are difficult to explain on the basis of conventional theories.

In the dynamical systems approach, all dissipative systems—that is, systems that, loosely speaking, are not perturbed by external influence—are said to follow one of several possible scenarios of temporal evolution. To better understand these scenarios, it is useful to use a spatial representation, called a phase space, to describe a system's dynamics. Phase space is a coordinate space where the axes in the coordinate space represent dynamical variables. Dynamical variables are parameters that continuously change as the system evolves in time.

A simple example of a dynamical system is the pendulum. Only two variables are needed to describe the behavior of the system: the angle of the pendulum at a given instant provides one dimension of the phase space, and the speed of the pendulum provides the other. As the system evolves, the changes in the system may be represented as a trajectory in such a space. After some time, the trajectory representing the system's evolution will be confined to a subset of the phase space, and will get progressively closer to elements within that subset. The subset to which the trajectory evolves is called an attractor.

Only four general types of attractors are possible. The simplest scenario is associated with the evolution toward a *point attractor,* where all the trajectories end in a limited number of points in a phase space. This scenario describes a situation where the changes in the system get smaller in time, until no more changes occur. When this occurs, the system is said to be resting in one of its equilibria.

A pendulum illustrates the point attractor. A phase space plot of the pendulum's movement involves the two coordinates of angle and speed. Plotting a point for each successive moment in time would yield an inward spiral, with the loop size gradually diminishing as the pendulum approached a resting state. This point attractor scenario characterizes many of the neural network models developed in cognitive psychology. For example, the stable equilibria of a family of neural networks called attractor neural networks (Hopfield, 1982) are interpreted as corresponding to memories stored in the network.

This fixed-point attractor scenario fits nicely with ideas that have already appeared in the attitude literature. For example, balance theories proposed that the elements of cognitive structures (the variables in the dynamical system) would evolve toward one of the possible balanced states (the fixed point attractors). The scenario of evolution toward a fixed point attractor also may describe the phenomenon of thought-induced polarization (Tesser, 1978), where the attractors of the system correspond to configurations associated with extreme evaluations (see Vallacher & Nowak, in press, for an expanded discussion and empirical data).

A second scenario in dynamical systems is associated with *periodic attractors*. With these attractors, the values of all the variables repeat in a periodic fashion. A perfect oscillator, in which the driving forces precisely and regularly oppose each other (think of a perfectly balanced, frictionless pendulum) is an example of a periodic attractor. When such a system is plotted in the phase space, the trajectory followed by these periodic attractors settles down into a closed loop: the same trajectory (i.e., the same combinations of dynamical variables) is repeated indefinitely.

Lewin's (1933) description of an approach–avoidance conflict would fit the periodic attractor pattern. In the classical description of this conflict, the avoidance component starts closer to the goal but grows faster than the approach component. The person oscillates at the point where the strength of the approach tendency matches the strength of the avoidance tendency. To get periodic oscillations in this model, one merely has to assume a tendency to overshoot: while approaching, the person gets a little bit closer than the point of equilibrium; when withdrawing, the person gets past the equilibrium point in the opposite direction. A related example of periodic evolution in attitudes is found in the concept of ambivalence. Under some conditions ambivalent attitudes may regularly oscillate between positive and negative evaluations of the attitude object (see Vallacher & Nowak, in press, for a more detailed discussion).

A third dynamical pattern is *quasi-periodic* evolution. This occurs when two or more variables in the system evolve periodically, but the respective periods of these variables are incommensurable, so that exact combinations of values do not repeat. For example, consider a moon circling a planet that circles a star. Both the revolutions of the moon around the planet and the planet around the star are periodic. Often these periods are incommensurate (i.e., a full orbit of the moon usually takes less time than a full orbit of the planet). A continuous plot of the evolution of the moon's position vis-à-vis the star in a phase space yields a torus (or doughnut) shape. However, although the trajectory never leaves the boundaries of the torus, it never exactly repeats itself within the torus. The exact position (i.e., the exact combination of dynamical variables) of each point traced by the trajectory is unique.

Application of this system to attitudes is speculative. However, assume for the moment that attitudes do have three separable components, a cognitive component, a behavioral component, and an emotional component. Assume further that each of these components would individually cause attitude oscillation, but each with a different periodicity. For example, assume that the emotional component of the attitude oscillates daily, that the behavioral component oscillates every pi days (roughly 3.1), and that the cognitive component oscillates every square root of two days (roughly 1.4). Because these periods are incommensurate (e.g., they are not integer multiples of a single quantity), the exact combination of the values of these three variables will never repeat. Hence, each variable of the system will experience full periodicity and full regularity, but within this regularity the system will never be in exactly the same state twice.

The fourth, and perhaps most fascinating, scenario in dynamical systems is chaos. Chaotic systems (examples are thought to be turbulence in a stream and the weather) are those in which the behavior of the system is seemingly random, but in fact, is totally prescribed by the determining variables. These systems can radically shift from relatively stable and periodic states to states where the behavior of the system appears wildly unpredictable, and then back to periods of relative stability.

Attractors of chaotic systems are called "strange attractors." They have a complex, self-similar structure, where part of the attractor looks similar to the whole attractor. In other words, the attractor looks similar under different scales of magnification. Such an attractor has an exceedingly fine structure, one that is described by chaos theorists in terms of fractal dimensions (see Peitgen & Souppe, 1988, for a discussion of fractals).

It is clear that the behavior of chaotic systems is not random, otherwise there could be no underlying order in the phase space plot. The plot shows that the possible values the system can take are constrained by the boundaries of the attractor. However, exact predictions are not possible. Even the smallest uncertainty in the initial state of the system will be amplified with the passage of time so that it becomes virtually impossible to predict where, within the attractor, the system will be at any given instant.

The most general consequence of the theory of dynamical systems is that there may be quite general laws connecting the behavior of systems that, at first glance, appear to be extremely diverse. In this theory, the behavior of any system simply depends on the rules of interaction among elements, as described by the differential or difference equations. Hence, the same basic laws may apply to such diverse phenomena as weather patterns, pulsation of lasers, interacting neurons, and biological rhythms. In the next section, we consider some empirical findings that have already resulted from applying this theory to the concept of attitude.

Intrapsychic Dynamical Attitudes Systems

Attitude is dynamic rather then static. Such a view of attitudes captures the intuitions underlying much classical attitude research (e.g., balance theory), which explicitly emphasized the "dynamics of attitude." Loosely speaking, dynamics refers to the process of change, and thus, is defined in terms of time. Not surprising, then, the notion of time is central to the description and understanding of dynamics in dynamical systems theory. The concept of time was practically lost, however, in the classic research concerning "attitude dynamics." Traditionally, in attitude research many measurements are averaged to arrive at the central tendency of the distribution of the measurement values, which is regarded as the best representation of the true attitude value. In this process, all the information concerning the possible temporal patterns of change is lost.

The notion of the intrinsic dynamics of judgment was introduced by Vallacher and Nowak (in press) to convey the idea that even in the absence of external stimuli, evaluative judgments may show meaningful patterns of change. A mouse paradigm was developed to investigate this idea. In this paradigm, subjects express their moment-to-moment feelings regarding a target of judgment by means of a computer mouse that controls the position of the cursor on a computer screen. In the center of the computer screen is a small circle representing the attitude object. Subjects are instructed to adjust the cursor (arrow) displayed on the screen by moving the computer mouse in such a way that the arrow's position in respect to the circle reflects their moment-to-moment feelings toward the object. The position of the arrow is recorded several times a second over a 2- to 3-minute judgment interval.

Preliminary research utilizing this procedure has shown that subjects produce identifiable patterns of movement during the judgment period. For example, in response to univalent objects (i.e., consistently positive or consistently negative targets), subjects began by moving the mouse a great deal with respect to the circle, and did so relatively rapidly. However, over time the movements slowed down and became more-or-less stable. For a univalently positive target, the movements converged to a relatively small distance from the target, whereas for the univalently negative target, the movements converged to a relatively large distance from the target. Hence, subjects' movements tended to become polarized over time, as though they were, in dynamical systems terminology, converging on different fixed point attractors.

The observed patterns were different for other attitude objects. For example, when confronted with mixed-valence descriptions, subjects moved the mouse large distances during the judgment period, and the distance from the target did not converge on a single point as time passed. Instead, some of the observed patterns of movement were chaotic, whereas others were periodic. It is important to reiterate that these movements are not random. For example, certain features of the mouse movements were related to self-report criteria of judgment. Speed and acceleration, in particular, were greater for targets that were evaluated negatively than for those that were evaluated positively. The movement was also more dynamic (i.e., higher speed and more acceleration) when subjects were relatively uncertain of their self-reported judgments.

The important feature of this research is to demonstrate that patterns of change in time reflect important features of mental dynamics, rather than measurement error or random variation. Note that such characteristics of attitude change as speed or acceleration make no sense in the traditional approach treating attitudes as stable points on a dimension. However, internally generated dynamics, such as those demonstrated within the mouse paradigm, are to be expected from a dynamical systems perspective.

Consideration of attitudes in terms of dynamical systems yields several important insights. For example, it follows from the dynamical conception of attitudes that an attitude is not a passive object and that attitude change is not a passive process. An attitude not only reacts to environmental pressures and incoming information, but also, the cognitive and affective components contributing to an attitude interact with each other: attitudes will sometimes change solely on the basis of interactions among their components. Most traditional theories of attitudes are silent on the question of how attitudes might change in absence of external influences.

The dynamical approach goes beyond an emphasis on change in the absence of external pressures; it provides a taxonomy of attractors that allows identification of when and how attitudes can be changed. In some cases locating the stable, existing equilibria in a system will be a useful and informative way of describing that system. For example, if an attitude is described by a point attractor, when it reaches a stable equilibrium point the attitude might be resistant to change. However, points of equilibria may themselves vary in the degree of their stability. Some may be quite stable, so that even after a strong perturbation the system will return to the same stable equilibrium point. Some equilibria may be unstable, so that even after the slightest perturbation the system will go to a different equilibrium.

Another implication of this approach concerns the relation between the information given and the final attitude that emerges. Typical attitude models, such as information integration models, lead to the conclusion that people who are given similar inputs (assuming equivalent valuations and weights) should evince similar attitudinal evaluations. However, dynamical systems can be characterized by multiple attractors, and the boundaries between the different attractors may have a complex shape (Peitgen & Souppe, 1988). In some dynamical systems (especially chaotic ones) small changes in the value of one variable can lead to different equilibria. Hence, a dynamical systems approach to attitudes suggests that it is easily possible for people to develop different attitudes on the basis of similar information.

Interpersonal Dynamical Attitude Systems

The discussion so far has focused on applying dynamical systems to intraindividual attitudes. However, a dynamical systems approach can also be used to describe attitudes and attitude change at a group level. For example, let us suppose that a new attitude issue is individually presented to members of a group, and everyone develops some initial opinion about the topic. Further, suppose that the group members are subsequently brought together, and they begin communicating. Dynamical systems modeling can be used to describe the pattern of attitude change that might occur as a result of this communication.

One way to do this is to assume that each individual's attitude is partly a function of the attitudes held by other members of the group. In their model of attitude change, Nowak, Szamrej, and Latané (1990) assumed exactly this. The model was a simple nonlinear, binary influence model that assumed that those individuals who predominantly interacted with others who had differing opinions switched to that opinion, while those who interacted predominantly with like-minded people stayed with their original attitude.

The results of the simulations run by Nowak et al. were enlightening (also see Nowak & Latané, in press). Under some circumstances, social interaction among group members produced coherent "clusters" of minority opinion groups within the larger majority field. A number of model parameters could be altered to change the pattern of influence, and under most model assumptions, the pattern of attitudes ended in a stable equilibrium, so that all changes ultimately ceased. This outcome is reminiscent of some of the majority/minority influence literature suggesting that interaction between majority and minority group members sometimes tends to freeze, or even polarize, existing attitudes. However, in some circumstances (most notably when the model assumes that it is easier to persuade somebody to change their opinion than to stay with the currently held opinion) a periodic oscillation was observed. That is, the opinion of some individuals located on the border between the majority and minority groups oscillated between the two attitudinal positions.

Although one can derive dynamical systems models that may be useful in describing the temporal evolution of attitudes, a skeptic might wonder whether these models are not simply "pie in the sky" conceptions with no basis in physical reality. After all, how do these abstract mathematical conceptions relate to "the mind"? There is an obvious link. Parallel distributed processing networks, concerned with the linkage between the structure of connections and rules of propagation in a network and evolution of the network across time, can essentially be thought of as programmable dynamical systems (Hopfield, 1982). Hence, the abstract mathematical conceptions of dynamical systems theory may indeed have a physical basis in the mental network. Exactly how other cognitive constructs, such as semantic memory or episodic memory, will fit into this scheme is unclear. Nonetheless, the success of dynamical systems models in other domains, combined with the promise of parallel distributed processing models in psychology, should encourage attitudes researchers to vigorously pursue this form of modeling.

FINAL THOUGHTS

This chapter has not been as comprehensive in its coverage of information processing constructs, or in its tying of those constructs to traditional issues in attitudes, as will ultimately be necessary for a thorough understanding of attitudes. For example, constructs from the areas of attention, visual and auditory perception, and text comprehension are essential for modeling attitudinal responses to persuasive communications. We earlier referred to efforts of Hovland et al. (1953) and McGuire (1985) to identify the information processing stages involved in communication and persuasion. These previous attempts to identify the relevant information processing stages drew minimally on work in cognitive psychology. However, the stages developed by these scholars do provide important guidelines to cognitively oriented attitude researchers.

This earlier information processing framework advanced our understanding in several ways. First, it showed that there are multiple processes operating at the cognitive level that influence the acquisition and change of attitudes. This makes the complexity of the analytic and scientific task vividly apparent. Second, the effort provided a focus to cognitively oriented researchers as to which realms of cognitive principles should be of most use in understanding attitudes. Third, it helped us better understand that different principles will be involved in different persuasion settings. For example, passive reception of a message engages different cognitive structures and resources than does engaging in a spirited discussion about gun control with a roommate or a spouse.

In this chapter, we have identified many of the contemporary linkages between social cognition and attitude research, and have speculated about some of the cognitive and social cognitive ideas that have yet to become a target for attitude research. We wish to make it clear, however, that these attempts do not reflect implicit criticism of current attitude research. Indeed, given the continuing flood of research (e.g., McGuire, 1985, estimated that over 1000 new attitude studies appear in the literature each year) and the increasing tendency to draw upon conceptions from cognitive psychology, it appears that as an area of research, attitudes are in energetic and capable hands. Instead, we hope that we have made attitude researchers more aware of the importance of understanding issues of coding, structure, and process, and that we have stimulated creative thinking about the potential application of these constructs to attitudes.

In fact, we hope that this chapter leads to an outcome similar to that obtained in *It's a Wonderful Life*. George's guardian angel got his wings (as indicated by the ringing of a bell) as a result of having opened George's eyes. George, from his new perspective, realized that his life had actually been quite fruitful, and that a number of people valued him. George's feelings were confirmed when, at the end of the film, his friends contributed money to keep his bank afloat, all the while indicting their positive feelings toward George.

The attitude construct has many friends in the form of principles and methods in cognitive psychology. Those friends have supported the attitude construct in the past, and will doubtlessly be increasing that support in the future. All the skeptical attitude researcher need do is walk among these friends with open and receptive eyes. As for us, the authors of this chapter, we hope some day to hear the ringing of a bell!

ACKNOWLEDGMENTS

We thank all those who provided us substantive feedback on portions of, or all of, this chapter. In particular, we thank Trish Devine, Tony Greenwald, Dave Hamilton, Rich Petty, and Bill von Hippel for their thoughtful commentaries.

REFERENCES

Abelson, R. P., & Rosenberg, M. J. (1958). Symbolic psycho-logic: A model of attitude cognition. *Behavioral Science, 3*, 1–13.

Abelson, R. P., Aronson, E., McGuire, W. J., Newcomb, T. M., Rosenberg, M. J., & Tannenbaum, P. H. (Eds.). (1968). *Theories of cognitive consistency: A sourcebook*. Chicago: Rand McNally.

Ajzen, I. (1989). Attitude structure and behavior. In A. Pratkanis, S. Breckler, & A. Greenwald (Eds.), *Attitude structure and function* (pp. 241–274). Hillsdale, NJ: Erlbaum.

Ajzen, I., & Fishbein, M. (1980). *Understanding attitudes and predicting social behavior*. Englewood Cliffs, NJ: Prentice-Hall.

Allport, G. W. (1935). Attitudes. In C. Murchison (Ed.), *Handbook of social psychology* (Vol. 2, pp. 798–844). Worcester, MA: Clark University Press.

Anderson, J. R. (1976). *Language, memory and thought*. Hillsdale, NJ: Erlbaum.

Anderson, J. R. (1983). *The architecture of cognition*. Cambridge, MA: Harvard University Press.

Anderson, N. H. (1974). Cognitive algebra: Integration theory applied to social attribution. In

L. Berkowitz (Ed.), *Advances in experimental social psychology* (Vol. 7, pp. 1–101). New York: Academic Press.

Anderson, H. H. (1981). *Foundations of information integration theory.* New York: Academic Press.

Anderson, N. H., & Hubert, S. (1963). Effects of concomitant verbal recall on order effects in personality impression formation. *Journal of Verbal Learning and Verbal Behavior, 2,* 379–391.

Aronson, E. (1969). The theory of cognitive dissonance: A current perspective. In L. Berkowitz (Ed.), *Advances in experimental social psychology* (Vol. 4, pp. 1–34). New York: Academic Press.

Baddeley, A. D. (1986). *Working memory.* Oxford: Oxford University Press.

Bargh, J. A. (1989). Conditional automaticity: Varieties of automatic influence in social perception and cognition. In J. S. Uleman & J. A. Bargh (Eds.), *Unintended thought* (pp. 3–51). New York: Guilford.

Bargh, J. A., & Pietromonaco, P. (1982). Automatic information processing and social perception: The influence of trait information presented outside of conscious awareness on impression formation. *Journal of Personality and Social Psychology, 43,* 437–449.

Bargh, J. A., Bond, R. N., Lombardi, W. J., & Tota, M.E. (1986). The additive nature of chronic and temporary sources of construct accessibility. *Journal of Personality and Social Psychology, 50,* 869–878.

Barsalou, L. W. (1992a). *Cognitive psychology: An overview for cognitive scientists.* Hillsdale, NJ: Erlbaum.

Barsalou, L. W. (1992b). Frames, concepts and conceptual fields. In E. Kittay & A. Lehrer (Eds.), *Frames, fields and contrasts: New essays in semantic and lexical organization* (pp. 21–74). Hillsdale, NJ: Erlbaum.

Barsalou, L. W., & Billman, D. (1989). Systematicity and semantic ambiguity. In D. Gorfein (Ed.), *Resolving semantic ambiguity* (pp. 146–203). New York: Springer-Verlag.

Blaxton, T. A. (1989). Investigating dissociations among memory measures: Support for a transfer-appropriate processing framework. *Journal of Experimental Psychology: Learning, Memory and Cognition, 15,* 657–668.

Breckler, S. J. (1984). Empirical validation of affect, behavior, and cognition as distinct components of attitude. *Journal of Personality and Social Psychology, 47,* 1191–1205.

Breckler, S. J., & Wiggins, E. C. (1989). On defining attitude and attitude theory: Once more, with feeling. In A. R. Pratkanis, S. J. Breckler, & A. G. Greenwald (Eds.), *Attitude structure and function* (pp. 407–428). Hillsdale, NJ: Erlbaum.

Brock, T. C. (1967). Communication discrepancy and intent to persuade as determinants of counterargument production. *Journal of Experimental Social Psychology, 3,* 269–309.

Cacioppo, J. T., & Petty, R. E. (1981). Effects of extent of thought on the pleasantness ratings of P-O-X triads: Evidence for three judgment tendencies in evaluating social situations. *Journal of Personality and Social Psychology, 40,* 1000–1009.

Cacioppo, J. T., Petty, R. E., & Geen, T. R. (1989). Attitude structure and function: From the tripartite to the homeostasis model of attitudes. In A. Pratkanis, S. Breckler, & A. Greenwald (Eds.), *Attitude structure and function* (pp. 275–309). Hillsdale, NJ: Erlbaum.

Cantor, N., & Mischel, W. (1977). Traits as prototypes: Effects on recognition memory. *Journal of Personality and Social Psychology, 35,* 38–48.

Carlston, D. E. (1980). The recall and use of traits and events in social inference processes. *Journal of Experimental Social Psychology, 16,* 303–328.

Carlston, D. E. (1992). Impression formation and the modular mind. In L. Martin & A. Tesser (Eds.), *Construction of social judgments* (pp. 301–341). Hillsdale, NJ: Erlbaum.

Carlston, D. E., & Skowronski, J. J. (1986). Trait memory and behavior memory: The effects of alternative pathways on impression judgment response times. *Journal of Personality and Social Psychology, 50,* 5–13.

Carlston, D. E., & Skowronski, J. J. (in press). Savings in the relearning of trait information as evidence for spontaneous inference generation. *Journal of Personality and Social Psychology.*

Chaiken, S., & Stangor, C. (1987). Attitudes and attitude change. *Annual Review of Psychology, 38,* 575–630.

Cohen, N. J., & Squire, L. R. (1980). Preserved learning and retention of pattern-analyzing skill in amnesia using perceptual learning. *Cortex, 17,* 273–278.

Collins, A. M., & Loftus, E. F. (1975). A spreading activation theory of semantic memory. *Psychological Review, 82,* 407–428.

Cooper, J., & Fazio, R. H. (1984). A new look at dissonance theory. In L. Berkowitz (Ed.), *Advances in experimental social psychology* (Vol. 17, pp. 229–266). New York: Academic Press.

Cottrell, N. B. (1975). Heider's structural balance principle as a conceptual rule. *Journal of Personality and Social Psychology, 31,* 713–720.

Devine, P. G. (1989). Stereotypes and prejudice: Their automatic and controlled components. *Journal of Personality and Social Psychology, 56,* 5–18.

Devine, P. G., & Ostrom, T. M. (1988). Dimensional versus information-processing approaches to social knowledge: The case of inconsistency management. In D. Bar-Tal & A.Kruglanski (Eds.), *The social psychology of knowledge* (pp. 231–260). Cambridge: Cambridge University Press.

Dishman, R. K. (1982). Compliance/adherence in health-related exercise. *Health Psychology, 3,* 237–267.

Dreben, E. K., Fiske, S. T., & Hastie, R. (1979). The independence of evaluative and item information: Impression and order recall effects in impression formation. *Journal of Personality and Social Psychology, 37,* 1758–1768.

Edwards, K. (1990). The interplay of affect and cognition in attitude formation and change. *Journal of Personality and Social Psychology, 59,* 212–216.

Fazio, R. H. (1989). On the power and functionality of attitudes: The role of attitude accessibility. In A. R. Pratkanis, S. J. Breckler, & A. G. Greenwald (Eds.), *Attitude structure and function* (pp. 153–179). Hillsdale, NJ: Erlbaum.

Fazio, R. H. (1990). Multiple processes by which attitudes guide behavior: The MODE model in an integrative framework. In M. P. Zanna (Ed.), *Advances in experimental social psychology* (Vol. 23, pp. 75–109). New York: Academic Press.

Fazio, R. H., & Williams, C. J. (1986). Attitude accessibility as a moderator of the attitude-perception and attitude-behavior relations: An investigation of the 1984 presidential election. *Journal of Personality and Social Psychology, 51,* 505–514.

Fazio, R. H., & Zanna, M. P. (1978). Attitudinal qualities relating to the strength of the attitude-behavior relationship. *Journal of Experimental Social Psychology, 14,* 398–408.

Fazio, R. H., & Zanna, M. P. (1981). Direct experience and attitude-behavior consistency. In L. Berkowitz (Ed.), *Advances in experimental social psychology* (Vol. 14, pp. 162–203). New York: Academic Press.

Fazio, R. H., Sabonmatsu, D. M., Powell, M. C., & Kardes, F. R. (1986). On the automatic activation of attitudes. *Journal of Personality and Social Psychology, 50,* 229–238.

Festinger, L. (1957). *A theory of cognitive dissonance.* Palo Alto, CA: Stanford University Press.

Fishbein, M., & Ajzen, I. (1974). Attitudes toward objects as predictors of single and multiple behavioral criteria. *Psychological Review, 81,* 59–74.

Fishbein, M., & Ajzen, I. (1975). *Belief, attitude, intention and behavior: An introduction to theory and research.* Reading, MA: Addison-Wesley.

Fiske, S. T., & Taylor, S. E. (1991). *Social Cognition* (2nd ed.). New York: McGraw-Hill.

Fleming, D. (1967). Attitude: The history of a concept. *Perspectives in American History, 1,* 287–365.

Gilbert, D. T., & Osborne, R. E. (1989). Thinking backward: Some curable and incurable consequences of cognitive busyness. *Journal of Personality and Social Psychology, 57,* 940–949.

Gilbert, D. T., Pelham, B. W., & Krull, D. S. (1988). On cognitive busyness: When person perceivers meet persons perceived. *Journal of Personality and Social Psychology, 54,* 733–740.

Gilligan, S. G., & Bower, G. H. (1984). Cognitive consequences of emotional arousal. In C. E. Izard, J. Kagan, & R. B. Zajonc (Eds.), *Emotions, cognition and behavior* (pp. 547–588). Cambridge: Cambridge University Press.

Gleick, J. (1987). *Chaos: The making of a new science.* New York: Viking-Penguin.

Gollob, H. F. (1974). The subject-verb-object approach to social cognition. *Psychological Review, 81,* 286–321.

Greenwald, A. G. (1968). Cognitive learning, cognitive response to persuasion and attitude change. In A. G. Greenwald, T. C. Brock, & T. M. Ostrom (Eds.), *Psychological foundations of attitudes* (pp. 147–170). New York: Academic Press.

Greenwald, A. G. (1989). Why attitudes are important: Defining attitude and attitude theory 20 years later. In A. Pratkanis, S. Breckler, & A. Greenwald (Eds.), *Attitude structure and function* (pp. 429–440). Hillsdale, NJ: Erlbaum.

Greenwald, A. G., & Banaji, M. (1993). *Implicit social cognition.* Manuscript under review.

Gruder, C. L., Cook, T. O., Hennigan, K. M., Flay, B. R., Alessi, C., & Halamaj, J. (1978). Empirical tests of the absolute sleeper effect predicted from the discounting cue hypothesis. *Journal of Personality and Social Psychology, 36,* 1061–1074.

Hastie, R. (1984). Causes and effects of causal attribution. *Journal of Personality and Social Psychology, 46,* 44–56.

Hastie, R. (1986). A primer of information processing theory for the political scientist. In R. R. Lau & D. O. Sears (Eds.), *Political cognition* (pp. 11–39). Hillsdale, NJ: Erlbaum.

Hastie, R., & Park, B. (1986). The relationship between memory and judgment depends on whether the judgment task is memory-based or on-line. *Psychological Review, 93,* 258–268.

Heider, F. (1958). *The psychology of interpersonal relations.* New York: Wiley.

Higgins, E. T., & King, G. A. (1981). Accessibility of social constructs: Information-processing consequences of individual and contextual variability. In N. Cantor & J. F. Kihlstrom (Eds.), *Personality, cognition, and social interaction* (pp. 69–122). Hillsdale, NJ: Erlbaum.

Higgins, E. T., Bargh, J. A., & Lombardi, W. (1985). Nature of priming effects on categorization. *Journal of Experimental Psychology: Learning, Memory and Cognition, 11,* 59–69.

Hopfield, J. J. (1982). Neural networks and physical systems with emergent collective computational abilities. *Proceedings of the National Academy of Sciences, 79,* 2554–2558.

Houston, D. A., & Fazio, R. H. (1989). Biased processing as a function of attitude accessibility: Making objective judgments subjectively. *Social Cognition, 7,* 51–56.

Hovland, C. I., Janis, I. L., & Kelley, J. J. (1953). *Communication and persuasion.* New Haven: Yale University Press.

Hymes, R. W. (1986). Political attitudes as social categories: A new look at selective memory. *Journal of Personality and Social Psychology, 51,* 233–241.

Insko, C. A. (1981). Balance theory and phenomenology. In R. E. Petty, T. M. Ostrom, & T. C. Brock (Eds.), *Cognitive responses in persuasion* (pp. 309–338). Hillsdale, NJ: Erlbaum.

Insko, C. A., Songer, E., & McGarvey, W. (1974). Balance, positivity, and agreement in the Jordan paradigm: A defence of balance theory. *Journal of Experimental Social Psychology, 10,* 53–83.

Johnson, M. K., & Hasher, L. (1987). Human learning and memory. *Annual Review of Psychology, 38,* 631–668.

Jordan, N. (1953). Behavioral forces that are a function of attitudes and of cognitive organization. *Human Relations, 6,* 273–287.

Jordan, N. (1968). Cognitive balance as an aspect of Heider's cognitive psychology. In R. P. Abelson, E. Aronson, W. J. McGuire, T. M. Newcomb, M. J. Rosenberg, & P. H. Tannenbaum (Eds.), *Theories of cognitive consistency: A sourcebook.* Chicago: Rand McNally.

Judd, C. M., & Krosnick, J. A. (1989). The structural bases of consistency among political attitudes: Effects of political expertise and attitude importance. In A. R. Pratkanis, S. J. Breckler, & A. G. Greenwald (Eds.), *Attitude structure and function* (pp. 99–128). Hillsdale, NJ: Erlbaum.

Judd, C. M., & Kulik, J. A. (1980). Schematic effects of social attitudes on information processing and recall. *Journal of Personality and Social Psychology, 38,* 569–578.

Judd, C.M., Drake, R. A., Downing, J. W., & Krosnick, J. A. (1991). Some dynamic properties of attitude structures: Context-induced response facilitation and polarization. *Journal of Personality and Social Psychology, 60,* 193–202.

Kerlinger, F. N. (1984). *Liberalism and conservatism: The nature and structure of social attitudes.* Hillsdale, NJ: Erlbaum.

Kim, M. P., & Rosenberg, S. (1980). Comparison of two structural models of implicit personality theory. *Journal of Personality and Social Psychology, 38,* 375–389.

Knowles, E. S. (1988). Item context effects on personality scales: Measuring changes the measure. *Journal of Personality and Social Psychology, 55,* 312–320.

Klein, S., & Loftus, J. (1990). Rethinking the role of organization in person memory: An independent trace storage model. *Journal of Personality and Social Psychology, 59,* 400–410.

Kosslyn, S. M. (1975). Information representation in visual images. *Cognitive Psychology, 7,* 341–370.

Lachman, R., Lachman, J. L., & Butterfield, E. C. (1979). *Cognitive psychology and information processing: An introduction.* Hillsdale, NJ: Erlbaum.

Latané, B., & Nowak, A. (in press). Attitudes as catastrophes: From dimensions to categories with increasing involvement. In R. Vallacher & A. Nowak (Eds.), *Dynamical systems in social psychology.* San Francisco: Academic Press.

Lehnert, W. G. (1978). *The process of question answering: A computer simulation of cognition.* Hillsdale, NJ: Erlbaum.

Lewicki, P. (1985). Nonconscious biasing effects of single instances on subsequent judgments. *Journal of Personality and Social Psychology, 48,* 563–574.

Lewicki, P. (1986). Processing information about covariations that cannot be articulated. *Journal of Experimental Psychology: Learning, Memory and Cognition, 12,* 135–146.

Lewin, K. (1933). Environmental forces. In C. Murchison (Ed.), *A handbook of child psychology* (2nd ed.). Worcester, MA: Clark University Press.

Lingle, J. H., & Ostrom, T. M. (1979). Retrieval selectivity in memory-based impression judgments. *Journal of Personality and Social Psychology, 37,* 180–194.

Lingle, J. H., & Ostrom, T. M. (1981). Principles of memory and cognition in attitude formation. In R. E. Petty, T. M. Ostrom, & T. C. Brock (Eds.), *Cognitive responses in persuasion* (pp. 399–420). Hillsdale, NJ: Erlbaum.

Lingle, J. H., Dukerich, J. M., & Ostrom, T. M. (1983). Accessing information in memory-based impression judgments: Incongruity vs. negativity in retrieval selectivity. *Journal of Personality and Social Psychology, 44,* 262–272.

Lingle, J. H., Geva, N., Ostrom, T. M., Leippe, M. R., & Baumgardner, M. H. (1979). Thematic effects of person judgments on impression formation. *Journal of Personality and Social Psychology, 37,* 674–687.

Logan, G. (1989). Automaticity and cognitive control. In J. S.Uleman & J. A. Bargh (Eds.), *Unintended thought* (pp. 52–74). New York: Guilford.

Loken, B. A. (1984). Attitude processing strategies. *Journal of Experimental Social Psychology, 20,* 272–296.

McClelland, J. L., Rumelhart, D. E., & the PDP Research Group (Eds.). (1986). *Parallel distributed processing: Explorations in the microstructure of cognition, Vol. 2., Psychological and biological models.* Cambridge, MA: MIT Press.

McCloskey, M. E., & Glucksberg, S. (1978). Natural categories: Well-defined or fuzzy sets. *Memory and Cognition, 6,* 462–472.

McGuire, W. J. (1968). Personality and attitude change: An information-processing theory. In A. G. Greenwald, T. C. Brock, & T. M. Ostrom (Eds.), *Psychological foundations of attitudes* (pp. 171–196). New York: Academic Press.

McGuire, W. J. (1985). Attitudes and attitude change. In G. Lindsey & E. Aronson (Eds.), *Handbook of social psychology* (Vol. 2, pp. 233–346). New York: Random House.

McGuire, W. J. (1989). The structure of individual attitudes and attitude systems. In A. R. Pratkanis, S. J. Breckler, & A. G. Greenwald (Eds.), *Attitude structure and function* (pp. 37–69). Hillsdale, NJ: Erlbaum.

Mackie, D. M., & Asuncion, A. G. (1990). On-line and memory-based modification of attitudes: Determinants of message recall–attitude change correspondence. *Journal of Personality and Social Psychology, 59,* 5–16.

Macleod, C. M. (1988). Forgotten but not gone: Savings for pictures and words in long-term memory. *Journal of Experimental Psychology: Learning, Memory and Cognition, 14,* 195–212.

Martin, L. L. (1986). Set/reset: The use and disuse of concepts in impression formation. *Journal of Personality and Social Psychology, 51,* 493–504.

Martin, L. L., Seta, J. J., & Crelia, R. A. (1990). Assimilation and contrast as a function of people's willingness to expend effort in forming an impression. *Journal of Personality and Social Psychology, 59,* 27–37.

Millar, M. G., & Tesser, A. (1986). Effects of cognitive and affective focus on the attitude-behavior relation. *Journal of Personality and Social Psychology, 51,* 270–276.

Millar, M. G., & Tesser, A. (1989). The effects of affective-cognitive consistency and thought on the attitude-behavior relation. *Journal of Experimental Social Psychology, 25,* 189–202.

Milner, B., Corkin, S., & Teuber, H. L. (1968). Further analysis of the hippocampal amnesiac syndrome: 14 year follow-up study of H. M. *Neuropsychologica, 6,* 215–234.

Mittal, B. (1988). Achieving higher seat belt usage: The role of habit in bridging the attitude-behavior gap. *Journal of Applied Social Psychology, 18,* 993–1016.

Neely, J. H. (1977). Semantic priming and retrieval from lexical memory: Roles of inhibitionless spreading activation and limited-capacity attention. *Journal of Experimental Psychology: General, 106,* 226–254.

Nelson, T. O. (1978). Detecting small amounts of information in memory: Savings for non-recognized items. *Journal of Experimental Psychology: Human Learning and Memory, 4,* 453–468.

Neuberg, S. L. (1988). Behavioral implications of information presented outside of conscious awareness: The effects of subliminal presentation of trait information on behavior in the Prisoner's Dilemma Game. *Social Cognition, 6,* 207–230.

Newcomb, T. M. (1961). *The acquaintance process.* New York: Holt, Rinehart & Winston.

Newcomb, T. M. (1968). Interpersonal balance. In R. P. Abelson, E. Aronson, W. J. McGuire, T. M. Newcomb, M. J. Rosenberg, & P. H. Tannenbaum (Eds.), *Theories of cognitive consistency: A sourcebook* (pp. 28–51). Chicago: Rand McNally.

Newell, A., & Simon, H. A. (1972). *Human problem solving.* Englewood Cliffs, NJ: Prentice-Hall.

Nosofsky, R. M. (1984). Choice, similarity, and the context theory of classification. *Journal of Experimental Psychology: Learning, Memory and Cognition, 10,* 104–114.

Nowak, A., & Latané, B. (in press). In R. Vallacher & A. Nowak (Eds.), *Dynamical systems in social psychology.* San Francisco: Academic Press.

Nowak, A., & Lewenstein, M. (in press). Dynamical systems: A tool for social psychology? In R. Vallacher & A. Nowak (Eds.), *Dynamical systems in social psychology.* San Francisco: Academic Press.

Nowak, A., Szamrej, J., & Latané, B. (1990). From private attitude to public opinion: A dynamic theory of social impact. *Psychological Review, 97,* 362–376.

Osgood, C. E., & Tannenbaum, P. H. (1955). The principle of congruity in the prediction of attitude change. *Psychological Review, 62,* 42–55.

Osgood, C. E., Suci, G. J., & Tannenbaum, P. H. (1957). *The measurement of meaning.* Urbana, IL: University of Illinois Press.

Ostrom, T. M. (1968). The emergence of attitude theory: 1930–1950. In A. G. Greenwald, T. C. Brock, & T. M. Ostrom (Eds.), *Psychological foundations of attitudes* (pp. 1–32). New York: Academic Press.

Ostrom, T. M. (1969). The relationship between the affective, behavioral and cognitive components of attitude. *Journal of Experimental Social Psychology, 5,* 12–30.

Ostrom, T. M. (1981). Attribution theory: Whence and whither? In J. Harvey, W. Ickes, & R. Kidd (Eds.), *New directions in attribution theory* (Vol. 3, pp. 421–424). Hillsdale, NJ: Erlbaum.

Ostrom, T. M. (1987). Bipolar survey items: An information processing perspective. In H. Hippler, N. Schwarz, & S. Sudman (Eds.), *Social information processing and survey methodology* (pp. 71–85). New York: Springer-Verlag.

Ostrom, T. M. (1988). Dimensional versus information processing conceptions of social judgment. *Wissenshaftliche Zeitschrift der Friedrich-Schiller-Universitaet, 6,* 629–638.

Ostrom, T. M. (1989). Interdependence of attitude theory and measurement. In A. R. Pratkanis, S. J. Breckler, & A. G. Greenwald (Eds.), *Attitude structure and function* (pp. 11–36). Hillsdale, NJ: Erlbaum.

Paivio, A. (1986). *Mental representations: A dual coding approach.* Oxford: Oxford University Press.

Peitgen, H-O., & Souppe, D. (Eds.). (1988). *The science of fractal images.* New York: Springer.

Pennington, N., & Hastie, R. (1988). Explanation-based decision making: Effects of memory structure on judgment. *Journal of Experimental Psychology: Learning, Memory and Cognition, 14,* 521–533.

Pennington, N., & Hastie, R. (1992). Explaining the evidence: Tests of the story model for juror decision making. *Journal of Personality and Social Psychology, 62,* 189–207.

Petty, R. E., & Cacioppo, J. T. (1986). *Communication and persuasion: Central and peripheral routes to attitude change.* New York: Springer-Verlag.

Petty, R. E., & Wegener, D. T. (1993). Flexible correction processes in social judgment: Correcting for context-induced contrast. *Journal of Experimental Social Psychology, 29,* 137–165.

Petty, R. E., Ostrom, T. M., & Brock, T. C. (Eds.). (1981). *Cognitive responses in persuasion.* Hillsdale, NJ: Erlbaum.

Petty, R. E., Priester, J. R., & Wegener, D. T. (in press). Cognitive processes in attitude change. In R. S. Wyer, Jr., & T. K. Srull (Eds.), *Handbook of social cognition* (2nd ed.). Hillsdale, NJ: Erlbaum.

Picek, J. S., Sherman, S. J., & Shiffrin, R. M. (1975). Cognitive organization and coding of social structures. *Journal of Personality and Social Psychology, 31,* 758–768.

Pratkanis, A. R. (1989). The cognitive representation of attitudes. In A. R. Pratkanis, S. J. Breckler, & A. G. Greenwald (Eds.), *Attitude structure and function* (pp. 71–98). Hillsdale, NJ: Erlbaum.

Pylyshyn, Z. (1981). The imagery debate: Analogue media versus tacit knowledge. *Psychological Review, 88,* 16–45.

Ratcliff, R., & McKoon, G. (1988). A retrieval theory of priming. *Psychological Review, 95,* 385–408.

Reber, A. S. (1976). Implicit learning of synthetic languages: The role of instructional set. *Journal of Experimental Psychology: Human Learning and Memory, 2,* 88–94.

Reder, L. M. (1982). Plausibility judgment versus fact retrieval: Alternative strategies for sentence verification. *Psychological Review, 89,* 250–280.

Reed, S. K. (1972). Pattern recognition and categorization. *Cognitive Psychology, 3,* 382–407.

Roland, P. E., & Friberg, L. (1985). Localization of cortical areas activated by thinking. *Journal of Neurophysiology, 53,* 1219–1243.

Rosch, E, Mervis, C. B., Gray, W., Johnson, D., & Boyes-Braem, P. (1976). Basic objects in natural categories. *Cognitive Psychology, 8,* 382–439.

Rosenberg, M. J. (1956). Cognitive structure and attitudinal affect. *Journal of Abnormal and Social Psychology, 53*, 367–372.
Rumelhart, D. E., McClelland, J. L., & the PDP Research Group (Eds.). (1986). *Parallel distributed processing: Explorations in the microstructure of cognition, Vol. 1, Foundations*. Cambridge, MA: Cambridge University Press.
Santa, J. L. (1977). Spatial transformations of words and pictures. *Journal of Experimental Psychology: Learning, Memory and Cognition, 3*, 418–427.
Schacter, D. L. (1987). Implicit memory: History and current status. *Journal of Experimental Psychology: Learning, Memory and Cognition, 13*, 501–508.
Schank, R. C., & Abelson, R. (1977). *Scripts, plans, goals and understanding*. Hillsdale, NJ: Erlbaum.
Schneider, W., & Shiffrin, R. M. (1977). Controlled and automatic information processing I: Detection, search, and attention. *Psychological Review, 84*, 1–66.
Schuster, H. G. (1984). *Deterministic chaos*. Weinheim, Germany: Physik Verlag.
Schwarz, N., & Sudman, S. (Eds.). (1992). *Context effects in social and psychological research*. New York: Springer-Verlag.
Sedikides, C., & Skowronski, J. J. (1991). The law of cognitive structure activation. *Psychological Inquiry, 2*, 169–184.
Sentis, K. P., & Burnstein, E. (1979). Remembering schema-consistent information: Effects of balance schema on recognition memory. *Journal of Personality and Social Psychology, 37*, 2200–2211.
Shepard, R. N., & Cooper, L. A. (1983). *Mental images and their transformations*. Cambridge, MA: MIT Press.
Sherif, M., & Hovland, C. I. (1961). *Social judgement: Assimilation and contrast effects in communication and attitude change*. New Haven: Yale University Press.
Sherif, C. W., Sherif, M., & Nebergall, R. E. (1965). *Attitude and attitude change: The social judgment-involvement approach*. Philadelphia: W. B. Saunders.
Sherman, S. J., Mackie, D. M., & Driscoll, D. M. (1990). Priming and the differential use of dimensions in evaluation. *Personality and Social Psychology Bulletin, 16*, 405–418.
Shiffrin, R. M., & Schneider, W. (1977). Controlled and automatic information processing II: Perceptual learning, automatic attending, and a general theory. *Psychological Review, 84*, 127–190.
Skowronski, J. J., Carlston, D. E., & Isham, J. (1993). Implicit versus explicit impression formation: The differing effects of overt labeling and covert priming on memory and impressions. *Journal of Experimental Social Psychology, 29*, 17–41.
Smith, E. E., & Medin, D. L. (1981). *Concepts and categories*. Cambridge, MA: Harvard University Press.
Smith, E. E., Shoben, E. J., & Rips, L. J. (1974). Structure and process in semantic memory: A featural model for semantic decisions. *Psychological Review, 81*, 214–241.
Smith, E. R. (1990). Content and process specificity in the effects of prior experience. In T. K. Srull & R. S. Wyer, Jr. (Eds.), *Advances in social cognition* (Vol. 3, pp. 1–60). Hillsdale, NJ: Erlbaum.
Smith, E. R., & Branscombe, N. R. (1988). Category accessibility as implicit memory. *Journal of Experimental Social Psychology, 24*, 490–504.
Snyder, M., & Swann, W. B. (1976). When actions reflect attitudes: The politics of impression management. *Journal of Personality and Social Psychology, 34*, 1034–1042.
Srull, T. K., & Wyer, Jr., R. S. (1979). The role of category accessibility in the interpretation of information about persons: Some determinants and implications. *Journal of Personality and Social Psychology, 37*, 1660–1672.
Srull, T. K., & Wyer, Jr., R.S. (1989). Person memory and judgment. *Psychological Review, 96*, 58–83.
Srull, T. K., Lichtenstein, M., & Rothbart, M. (1985). Associative storage and retrieval processes in person memory. *Journal of Experimental Psychology: Learning, Memory and Cognition, 11*, 316–345.

Staats, A. W. (1968). Social behaviorism and human motivation: Principles of the attitude-reinforcer-discriminative system. In A. G. Greenwald, T. C. Brock, & T. M. Ostrom (Eds.), *Psychological foundations of attitudes* (pp. 33–66). New York: Academic Press.

Staats, C. K., & Staats, A. W. (1958). Attitudes established by classical conditioning. *Journal of Abnormal and Social Psychology, 57,* 37–40.

Stangor, C., & McMillan, D. (1992). Memory for expectancy-congruent and expectancy-incongruent social information: A Meta-Analytic review of the social psychological and social developmental literatures. *Psychological Bulletin, 111,* 42–61.

Stevens, S. S. (1946). On the theory of scales of measurement. *Science, 103,* 677–680.

Stone, M. (1960). Models for choice reaction time. *Psychometrica, 25,* 251–260.

Strack, F., & Martin, L. L. (1987). Thinking, judging, and communicating: A process account of context effects in attitude surveys. In H. J. Hippler, N. Schwarz, & S. Sudman (Eds.), *Social information processing and survey methodology* (pp. 123–148). New York: Springer-Verlag.

Tesser, A. (1978). Self-generated attitude change. In L. Berkowitz (Ed.), *Advances in experimental social psychology* (Vol. 11, pp. 289–338). New York: Academic Press.

Thomas, W. I., & Znaniecki, F. (1918). *The Polish peasant in Europe and America* (Vol. 1). Boston: Badger.

Thurstone, L. L. (1928). Attitudes can be measured. *American Journal of Sociology, 33,* 529–554.

Tourangeau, R., & Rasinski, K. A. (1988). Cognitive processes underlying context effects in attitude measurement. *Psychological Bulletin, 103,* 299–314.

Tourangeau, R., Rasinski, K. A., Bradburn, N., & D'Andrade, R. (1989). Belief accessibility and context effects in attitude measurement. *Journal of Experimental Social Psychology, 25,* 401–421.

Tourangeau, R., Rasinski, K. A., Bradburn, N., & D'Andrade, R. (1991). Attitude structure and belief accessibility. *Journal of Experimental Social Psychology, 27,* 48–75.

Trope, Y. (1989). The multiple roles of context in dispositional judgment. In J. Bassilli (Ed.), *On-line cognition in person perception* (pp. 123–140). Hillsdale, NJ: Erlbaum.

Tulving, E. (1972). Episodic and semantic memory. In E. Tulving & E. Donaldson (Eds.), *Organization and memory* (pp. 381–403). New York: Academic Press.

Tulving, E. (1983). *Elements of episodic memory.* New York: Oxford University Press.

Tversky, A., & Kahneman, D. (1982). Judgment under uncertainty: Heuristics and biases. In D. Kahneman, P. Slovic, & A. Tversky (Eds.), *Judgment under uncertainty: Heuristics and biases* (pp. 3–20). New York: Cambridge University Press.

Vallacher, R., & Nowak, A. (in press). The stream of consciousness in social judgment. In R. Vallacher & A. Nowak (Eds.), *Dynamical systems in social psychology.* San Francisco: Academic Press.

von Hippel, W., & Baker, S. (1993). Implicit memory for incongruent information: The role of effortful encoding in stereotype maintenance. Unpublished manuscript.

Vosniadou, S., & Ortony, A. (Eds.). (1989). *Similarity and analogical reasoning.* New York: Cambridge University Press.

Wilson, T. D., Dunn, D. S., Kraft, D., & Lisle, D. J. (1989). Introspection, attitude change and attitude-behavior consistency: The disruptive effects of explaining why we feel the way we do. In L. Berkowitz (Ed.), *Advances in experimental social psychology* (Vol. 22, pp. 287–343). San Diego, CA: Academic Press.

Wyer, Jr., R.S., & Carlston, D. E. (1979). *Social cognition, social inference and attribution.* Hillsdale, NJ: Erlbaum.

Wyer, Jr., R. S., & Srull, T. K. (1989). *Memory and cognition in its social context.* Hillsdale, NJ: Erlbaum.

Zajonc, R. B. (1980). Feeling and thinking: Preferences need no inferences. *American Psychologist, 35,* 151–175.

Zajonc, R. B., & Burnstein, E. (1965a). The learning of balanced and unbalanced social structures. *Journal of Personality and Social Psychology, 33,* 153–163.

Zajonc, R. B., & Burnstein, E. (1965b). Structural balance, reciprocity, and positivity as sources of cognitive bias. *Journal of Personality and Social Psychology, 33*, 570–583.

Zajonc, R. B., & Markus, H. (1984). Affect and cognition: The hard interface. In C. E. Izard, J. Kagan, & R. B. Zajonc (Eds.), *Emotions, cognition, and behavior* (pp. 73–102). Cambridge, England: Cambridge University Press.

Zanna, M. P., & Fazio, R. H. (1982). The attitude-behavior relation: Moving toward a third generation of research. In M. P. Zanna, E. T. Higgins, & C. P. Herman (Eds.), *Consistency in social behavior: The Ontario Symposium* (Vol. 2, pp. 283–302). Hillsdale, NJ: Erlbaum.

Zanna, M. P., & Rempel, J. K. (1988). Attitudes: A new look at an old concept. In D. Bar-Tal & A. W. Kruglanski (Eds.), *The social psychology of knowledge* (pp. 315–334). Cambridge, England: Cambridge University Press.

8

The Social Cognition Analysis of Social Influence: Contributions to the Understanding of Persuasion and Conformity

Diane M. Mackie
John J. Skelly

INTRODUCTION

The chapters in this volume attest to the impact that the theories and methods of social cognition have had on many of social psychology's central research problems. As their content documents, a concern with the way social knowledge is represented in memory and with the processes by which such knowledge is developed, used, and modified has contributed dramatically to our understanding of many aspects of social behavior. In this chapter, we deal with some of the most pervasive and indispensable of human social behaviors: our mutual attempts to convince, cajole, beguile, and beseech one another into thinking, feeling, and doing what we want.

The study of social influence has been at the core of the social psychological scientific endeavor since the inception of the discipline (Jones, 1985). For almost as long, the investigation of social influence phenomena has been split between two research domains with very different concerns. Persuasion research, with its emphasis on argumentation, has been primarily concerned with influence that depends on "direct" evidence about the attitude object—

whether it is good, desirable, valuable, useful, and so on. In contrast, conformity research takes as critical the role of "socially mediated" evidence—what other people think about the attitude object, who those other people are, how many there are of them, and the extent of their agreement. Largely because of these different emphases, research on persuasion and research on conformity have existed as markedly disparate areas of inquiry, each with its own theories and methods. This division between persuasion and conformity research is reflected in the structure and organization of this chapter: the impact of social cognition principles and practices has been quite different in each of these domains, and dictates that we begin by dealing with persuasion and conformity research separately.

We turn first to the impact that social cognition approaches have had on the investigation and understanding of persuasion. Because persuasion researchers have long been interested in how and why persuasive information is accepted, neither the process models nor measurement techniques inspired by social cognition approaches triggered qualitative changes in persuasion research. And yet as processing models themselves have developed, so too has our knowledge of the nature and function of attitude structures and of the processes that help develop, maintain, or change those structures. In the second part of the chapter, we document the progress made by, and some of the problems that remain for, a social cognition analysis of persuasion.

In the third section of the chapter, we turn our attention to conformity. Compared to the study of persuasion, the investigation of conformity has remained relatively untouched by the principles and practices of social cognition. As a casual glance at most introductory textbooks reveals, treatments of conformity and group influence are still largely uninformed by the themes that so dominate their companion chapters on attitude change and persuasion. Why have social cognition concerns influenced conformity research so little? Perhaps because conformity has long been considered a purely "motivational" or "social interactional" phenomenon, it has seemed inappropriate to subject it to information processing analysis. However, recent theoretical developments and empirical evidence, discussed in the third section of the chapter, have demonstrated that many benefits accrue from a more thorough analysis of conformity phenomena in cognitive terms.

After considering the extent to which social cognition approaches have affected persuasion and conformity separately, we focus in the fourth section of the chapter on trying to bring them together. We do so by suggesting that both the cognitive processes advanced by persuasion research and the social processes studied in conformity research work together to confer validity on attitude-relevant information. We see this mutual interaction as providing an avenue for further integration of persuasion and conformity research within a social cognition framework.

PERSUASION

Since the late 1970s, a social cognition perspective has dominated the study of persuasion (Chaiken & Stangor, 1987; Eagly & Chaiken, 1984; Tesser & Shaffer, 1990). But such concern for the cognition mediators of attitude change constituted evolution rather than revolution in the study of persuasion (Krech & Crutchfield, 1948; Landman & Manis, 1983; Zajonc, 1980). The idea that successful persuasion depended on the processes of attention, comprehension, yielding, and retention had been made familiar by Hovland and his colleagues (Hovland, Janis, & Kelley, 1953), and was extended and formalized by McGuire (1969). Perceptual approaches to persuasion set stock in communicative meaning (Asch, 1948) and were largely focused on issues of selective attention and contextual framing (Sherif & Cantril, 1945, 1946). Even the motivational concerns of consistency theories were built on strong cognitive foundations (Abelson et al., 1968; Festinger, 1957). Long before the social cognition approach began to have mainstream acceptance, the idea that persuasion was cognitively mediated was axiomatic to attitude change theories (McGuire, 1969).

Nor were techniques designed to assess mediating processes entirely new to persuasion research. Many such techniques had a lengthy history of use in persuasion research (Petty, Ostrom, & Brock, 1981). Recall, of course, was one of the most important dependent measures used by message learning theorists. Although by no means as systematically used as they are today, subjective reactions to message content—now called cognitive responses or elaborations—were also gauged prior to the current interest in their mediational role (Brock, 1967; Festinger & Maccoby, 1964; Hovland et al., 1953; Hovland, Lumsdaine, & Sheffield, 1949; Smith, Bruner, & White, 1956). Even response latencies were featured in some early studies (e.g., Cartwright, 1941). In addition, the general strategy of investigating the impact of distal variables (source, message, media, and audience characteristics) on recipients' processing and acceptance of presented information has hardly changed since the Hovlandian program became mainstream (Eagly & Chaiken, 1993; Fiske & Taylor, 1991).

Social Cognition Contributions to Classic Issues in Persuasion

How, then, does the social cognition approach to persuasion research differ from its many predecessors? Although it built on some of the assumptions common in older information processing models, current social cognition thinking about persuasion differs quite markedly from them. These changes reflect a developing understanding of the dynamic nature of the cognitive system itself. Current thinking about the nature and functioning of attitudes has been transformed by conceiving of them as mental representations in which various types and items of information are organized to varying degrees by associations of differing strength (see Pratkanis, Breckler, & Greenwald, 1989; Fazio, 1986). Such approaches confer tremendous flexibility because they distinguish the *availability* of information both from its *accessibility* and from its actual *use*. At the same time, greater knowledge of various cognitive operations has resulted in more specific and fine-grained analyses of the many complementary *processes* underlying persuasion, and in more attention to the recipient's active role in allocating processing resources in persuasion contexts. In the following pages, we document how these changes in how attitude structures and attitude processes are viewed have contributed to our understanding of some of the most central and critical issues in the study of persuasion (for social cognition's contributions to understanding attitude structures, see Chapter 7, this volume; Pratkanis et al., 1989; Zanna & Rempel, 1988).

The Functions of Attitude Formation and Change

In the original functional formulations, attitudes were seen as meeting important psychological needs (Katz, 1960; Smith, Bruner, & White, 1956). These usually included a utilitarian or knowledge function that steered attitude holders toward positive outcomes and away from negative ones, a knowledge function that ensured a stable organized view of the world, an ego-defensive or externalization function that protected attitude holders from psychological conflicts, a value-expressive function that acknowledged needs for self-expression and personal growth, and a social adjustment function that mediated a person's relationships with others.

As Shavitt (1989) points out, the theory of attitude functions was often cited but seldom tested, primarily because functions could never be adequately defined or measured (Himmelfarb & Eagly, 1974; Insko, 1967). This proved to be a major stumbling block to further theoretical development as well, a situation that has only recently changed. Indeed, the recent progress in understanding attitude functions is largely due to the infusion of concepts and techniques from social cognition paradigms (Eagly & Chaiken, 1993; Shavitt, 1989; Tesser & Shaffer, 1990). From the social cognition point of view, attitude functions operate through the activation of particular goal strategies that direct processing in particular ways (see Shavitt, 1989, for a review). This framework offers the promise of correcting the traditional sources of weakness: while suggesting workable operationalizations of functions, it also provides the means for assessing antecedents and consequences of attitude functions. For example, Fazio and his colleagues (1986) have defined and assessed the knowledge function of attitudes using the concept of category accessibility, whereas Shavitt (1985) and Herek (1987) have used cognitive response methodology to evaluate the presence of utilitarian, social identity, and self-esteem functions of attitudes.

The current view of functions as accessible categories activating particular procedures has shifted the emphasis of recent functional theories. Although chronic individual differences continue to play an important role (Tesser & Shaffer, 1990; Herek, 1987), it is now clear that different functions may be acutely accessible in different individuals at different times. All attitudes are thought to serve a knowledge function, organizing beliefs pertaining to an appraisal of reality (Fazio, 1986; Greenwald, 1989). At the same time, however, current thinking is that attitudes might support several functions. For example, some attitudes also serve ego-defensive and value expressive functions, which may activate different concerns and direct processing in different ways. The particular function activated will depend on the particular aspects of the attitude object made salient in a particular context (Chaiken, Liberman, & Eagly, 1989; Johnson & Eagly, 1989; Shavitt, 1989). On a cold day a UCSB sweatshirt may activate utilitarian concerns, whereas at a basketball game the same sweatshirt may serve a value-expressive or identification function. Matching particular arguments to accessible functions increases persuasion (Snyder & DeBono, 1989; Shavitt, 1989).

The discussion of attitude functions leads naturally to a consideration of what motivates attitude formation and change. Although social cognition approaches have often been charged with ignoring motivational concerns, such an accusation can hardly be taken seriously in the persuasion domain. Its important role in regulating sufficient attention for elaborative processing has made motivation a central feature of most current theories of attitude change (e.g., in the systematic-heuristic model, Chaiken et al., 1989, and in the elaboration likelihood model, Petty & Cacioppo, 1986a,b).

From the social cognition point of view, the apparent effects of motives (like functions) can be understood in terms of the activation of structures that influence processing. Activation of goal structures that define desired end points determines many of the effects commonly associated with "motivational states". For example, activation of an attitude itself makes it more likely that new information will be perceived as attitude consistent (Lord, Lepper, & Ross, 1979; Houston & Fazio, 1989; Wood, 1982; Wood, Kallgren & Preisler, 1985), producing the same result as an attitude-defensive or protective motive. Activation of the self-concept during the processing of self-relevant or involving information may make it more likely that attitudes congruent with that concept (e.g., ones that are consistent with views of the self as beneficent; Greenwald, 1980) are formed and maintained (McGuire, 1985; Tesser & Shaffer, 1990; Shavitt, 1989). Preferences for balanced structures, rather than reflecting motivation alone, may reflect the ease of processing information that is consistent with activated structures.

The mechanisms by which a recipient's motivation to retain or revise a currently held opinion influence the nature and extent of message processing are easily incorporated into the social cognition framework. Answers to the perhaps more intriguing question—What are the motive or motives for attitude formation and change?—have not been made explicit, however.

Two basic motivations have long been posited as central to persuasion contexts producing private acceptance: the desire to hold a correct and valid opinion (accuracy motivation) and the desire to protect oneself (defense motivation). In the more traditional view, these are distinguished because under accuracy motivation the recipient is assumed to be openly seeking the "truth," whereas under defense motivation the recipient knows that he or she holds an incorrect answer but seeks to confirm it anyway. We suspect that such a distinction does not exist in the heads of the recipients of persuasive communications. If, for example, the recipient apparently engaged in defensive processing knows that he or she is selectively biasing the information, the strategy has failed. In some sense, the self cannot be well defended if one knows one had to fight hard to defend it. Attitudes that others may see as defensively motivated no doubt "feel" subjectively valid to their holders.

A perhaps more defensible distinction can be made between cases in which the perceiver has no expectation about the outcome of processing, and cases in which a particular outcome is expected (as in the case of a need for specific structure, e.g., Kruglanski, 1989). In each case, attaining subjective validity for some opinion is the overarching goal. The cases differ, however, both in which structures are activated and in the expectations of the likely outcome of processing. Such expectations are no doubt a reflection of the confidence with which a current attitude is held, how confident one is that processing will result in acquiring useful information, and the confidence level needed to attain subjective validity. Recently, Chaiken (Chaiken et al., 1989) has proposed that motivational concerns can be operationalized by appeal to the idea of judgmental confidence. Judgmental confidence influences processing motivation in two ways.

First, any given attitude requires a certain level of judgmental confidence before it is reconfirmed or changed. Chaiken describes this as a sufficiency threshold—the point at which the recipient is confident that further processing is unnecessary. Sufficiency thresholds are affected by the size and certainty of an attitude's current informational base, how important the attitude is (perhaps because of its personal and identity consequences) and the perceived validity of the available information. The second aspect of judgmental confidence is the actual level of confidence in one's current attitude. For example, receiving information with conflicting implications for an attitude would decrease actual confidence.

Many of the effects attributed to consistency striving in producing attitude change may be understood in terms of confidence reduction and reestablishment. Awareness of inconsistent information about oneself (as conveyed by inconsistency between one's beliefs and actions in dissonance situations, e.g.,) many decrease confidence in the validity of attitudes or self-views and increase biased processing to restore it, suggesting a new perspective on understanding dissonance motivation (cf. Cooper & Fazio, 1984).

The effects of actual and expected confidence combine to influence processing, because processing increases whenever actual confidence drops below the sufficiency threshold. In the case of attitudes held with extreme confidence, nothing might lower actual confidence and thus little processing would occur (suggesting a possible explanation of the resistance of ego-involving attitudes; Sherif & Sherif, 1967). Completely irrelevant attitudes also trigger little processing, but in this case because the sufficiency threshold itself was low.

The notion that structural activation and judgmental confidence set-points together guide the nature and extent of processing holds considerable promise for integrating motivational concerns with cognitive analyses of persuasion. Activation and expectancy effects may account for biases in processing, whereas perceptions of subjective validity guide the extent of processing. Importantly, such an approach allows the goals of processing to be considered independently of the extent of processing. Increases in motivation might increase or decrease processing and might produce either biased or objective evaluation of information (see Johnson & Eagly, 1989; Petty & Cacioppo, 1986b; Tesser & Shaffer, 1990).

Effective Persuasion: Understanding Persuasion Processes

From the social cognition perspective, attitude change can be modeled as one aspect of a processing sequence that culminates in an attitudinal judgment (Tourangeau & Rasinski, 1988). Attitudinal judgments reflect the classification of the attitude object into an evaluative category or along an evaluative dimension (Devine & Ostrom, 1988; Zanna & Rempel, 1988). Such judgments are based on some varying subset of information that the perceiver deems sufficient under the circumstances for making the judgment at hand. This information may include the content of activated relevant structures, and the results of initial encoding and comprehension of the semantic and evaluative aspects of presented information. Such information may also be further evaluated, elaborated, and integrated, both with other aspects of the presented information and with retrieved material. A summary evaluative judgment is then formed, an appropriate response chosen, and some subset of the presented or derived information re-stored (for more detailed overviews see Eagly & Chaiken, 1984; Lingle & Ostrom, 1981; McGuire, 1985; Petty & Cacioppo, 1986b; Sherman, 1987; Tourangeau & Rasinski, 1988; Wyer & Carlston, 1979).

Compared to earlier approaches, the effects of resource allocation during every substage of information processing is accorded much more emphasis in a social cognition analysis. Attention is no longer considered a discrete processing stage (as it was, e.g., in message learning theory). Instead, attention refers to the interplay of both conscious and nonconscious allocation of processing capacity (Bargh, 1984, 1989; Logan, 1988, 1989; Shiffrin & Schneider, 1977). Some processing prerequisites to attitude change may be completed with little conscious investment of resources. For example, initial processing of information in the persuasive context may be automatically achieved (Bargh, 1989; Sherman, 1987). Initial categorization of an object (with its semantic and evaluative concomitants) determines the informational base for later processing (Fazio, 1986; Ratcliff & McKoon, 1989; Tourangeau & Rasinski, 1988; van der Pligt & Eiser, 1984), and thus some aspects of persuasion may already be determined by this early, largely nonconscious processing step. Categorizing abortion as an act of murder, rather than as act expressing constitutional freedoms, seems certain to constrain the nature of later elaboration.

Whereas superficial comprehension and encoding of presented material may proceed with relatively little effort, the active contribution of the recipient necessary for elaboration demands capacity investment and increased processing effort. Elaboration generally refers to the evaluation, extension, and integration of information (Petty & Cacioppo, 1986b). The realization that elaboration is differentially vulnerable to attentional constraints (produced by either capacity or motivational deficits) has become the cornerstone of major contemporary models of persuasion. This idea is central, for example, to both the elaboration likelihood model (Petty & Cacioppo, 1986a,b) and the heuristic-systematic model of persuasion (Chaiken, 1980, 1987; Chaiken et al., 1989).

It is difficult to overestimate the role that elaboration plays in contemporary thinking about effective persuasion. On one hand, the concept of active elaboration has provided the bridge between the comprehension of information and its acceptance (Greenwald, 1968; Petty, Ostrom, & Brock, 1981). On the other hand, the fact that elaboration is particularly susceptible to cognitive constraints has produced a renewed concern with alternative, less resource-intensive routes to persuasion. We discuss each of these developments in turn.

For Hovland et al. (1953; and later Rosenberg, Hovland, McGuire, Abelson; & Brehm, 1960) the processes preceding message acceptance were the passive acceptance, accurate reproduction, and rehearsal of message content. Learning theories similarly attached importance to the repetition and retention of a presented association. And yet it became obvious that, in many circumstances, the persuasive impact of a particular communication was unrelated to how much of its content was recalled (Greenwald, 1968). The passive, reproductive process of rehearsal was apparently insufficient to explain many instances of persuasion. (Of course, one problem with tests of these earlier models may have been that recall is not the best measure of what has been attended, comprehended, or received: see Chaiken & Stangor, 1987; Eagly & Chaiken, 1984; Mackie & Asuncion, 1990, for further discussion.)

Social cognition analyses accord the recipient's active generation of evaluative elaborations an important role in mediating acceptance (Chaiken, 1987; Chaiken et al., 1989; Greenwald, 1968; Petty & Cacioppo, 1986a,b).

The idiosyncratic thoughts or elaborations that subjects generate in response to a persuasive communication extend and transform presented information. Arguments that produce favorable elaborations produce attitude change, whereas material that produces negative evaluations is ignored, or worse, produces an extremization of attitudes in the opposite direction. The centrality of evaluative elaboration distinguishes recent views from earlier theory on two counts: the recipient is an active rather than passive processor of information, and external factors are reduced in importance as direct explanations of acceptance.

No sooner had active elaboration been assigned the role of primary mediator in persuasion, however, than its vulnerability to resource constraints became apparent. Persuasion cannot occur through the extensive cognitive processing discussed by either the Yale theorists or by dissonance proponents if the recipient is incapable or unwilling to allocate required resources (see Chaiken et al., 1989; Petty & Cacioppo, 1986b, for reviews). Indeed, outside the laboratory, elaborative processing may be the exception rather than the rule. Recent models that feature the activation and use of rule-based judgments of validity (Chaiken et al., 1989; Schwarz & Clore, 1983), as well as other non-argument-based routes to persuasion (Petty & Cacioppo, 1986b), reflect an appreciation of the impossibility—and undesirability—of consciously processing all available information extensively. In addition, persuasion cannot occur through elaborative processing when the features of an attitude object are processed with little awareness (as in the mere exposure effect, Zajonc, 1968; or associationism, Zanna, Kiesler, & Pilkonis, 1970). Explorations of the extent to which at least some aspects of attitude-relevant information can be processed outside of conscious awareness have resurrected in a much more scientifically useful context issues such as selective attention and the possibility of subliminal or unattended persuasion (Frey, 1986; McGuire, 1969; Spielman, Pratto, & Bargh, 1988). Indeed, it is possible that processes operating outside of conscious awareness have potentially greater persuasive impact than conscious processes.

Although most recent research has focused on processing mediators of persuasion, interest in the structural determinants of persuasion is now increasing (see Pratkanis, 1989, for examples). The fact that activated structures direct and facilitate the processing of relevant information implies that matching message content to the content of already-present attitude structures might be particularly effective (Edwards, 1990; Cacioppo, Petty, & Sidera, 1982; Snyder & DeBono, 1987). Persuasive effectiveness could also be increased by temporarily activating structures other than the attitude itself. Activation of related concepts, for example, might promote more extensive processing of yet-to-be presented information (Sherman, Mackie, & Driscoll, 1990).

Social cognition's differentiation of representation and processes allows a fine-grained analysis of how the latter impact the former (McGuire, 1968).

Traditionally, investigation of attitude representations has been rather isolated from research on attitude change, despite some calls for their integration (Ajzen, 1989; Capella & Street, 1989; Fishbein & Ajzen, 1981; Greenwald, 1968; Ostrom, 1981). Attempts to track the impact of inclusion of new information, exclusion of old (especially inconsistent) information, and the modification and reorganization of content would do well to build on the sophisticated structural approach taken to attitude change by Peak (1955, 1958). Kitayama and Burnstein (1989) have demonstrated the benefits of developing her concepts of associative density (the extent to which stored arguments are associated with one another) and structural centrality (the extent to which arguments are associated with the attitude judgment) for understanding the relationship between message recall and attitude change: similar benefits are sure to derive from application of similar models to other substantive questions of persuasive effectiveness.

Attitude Longevity and Resistance

The interplay of structural and processing properties emphasized by the social cognition approach has provided new insights into the issues of attitude retention and resistance (Greenwald, 1981). The most widely accepted view of attitude resistance has long been inoculation theory (McGuire, 1964). Providing people with the opportunity to produce counterarguments against attacks on their views increased the resistance of those views to later stronger assault. Cognitively, inoculation worked because people had the opportunity to gather information defending their views and undermining alternatives. Approaches to resistance from the perspective of balance theory also involved promoting counterargumentation (Tannenbaum, 1967). However, other theories of resistance were almost purely motivational in nature: reactance theory (whereby information might be resisted because it threatened perceived freedom, Brehm, 1966) and ego-defensive or dogmatic resistance (whereby information was rejected because it threatened cherished views of the self, Katz, 1960; Rokeach, 1956).

These earlier views have been almost completely subsumed within contemporary thinking about the issues of persistence and resistance. From the social cognitive point of view, a longlasting attitude is one that can be retrieved in response to attitude inquires (and therefore in response to attitude-relevant situations) over time. The retrieval of a previously stored structure depends on the number and strength of associative pathways leading to it, that is, on its accessibility. To the extent that elaborative processes increase the number of pathways to any resultant attitude, attitude change processes that involve extensive evaluation, elaboration, and integration of attitude-relevant material—for whatever reason—are likely to produce long-lasting attitudes. It is no surprise, therefore, that attitudes formed via systematic or central route processing are comparatively long lived (Chaiken, 1980; Haugtvedt & Petty, 1992).

For many of the same reasons, attitudes formed on the basis of extensive processing are probably more resistant to further attempts to change them. First, such attitudes are more likely to be accessed whenever attitude-relevant information is encountered. Second, this ready activation of the attitude makes accessible other information and goal structures that bias information processing in favor of attitude maintenance (as discussed earlier; see also Houston & Fazio, 1989; Petty & Cacioppo, 1977, 1986a,b; Wood, 1982; Wu & Shaffer, 1987). Third, extensive processing makes information more accessible, and any resultant perceived ease of retrieval might in turn confer a subjective aura of validity on prior, as opposed to new, material. Having a subjectively valid opinion may lead to an increased motivation and/or ability to counterargue subsequent persuasive attempts (see Chaiken et al., 1989; Eagly & Chaiken, 1993, chap. 12; Petty & Cacioppo, 1986b, for reviews).

Although elaboration increases the number of possible retrieval routes, there are other determinants of strength of association and thus of attitude retrieval. Attitudes might become firmly anchored to another structure—like the self—simultaneously activated in the persuasive situation. Whenever that structure is activated, the attitude might also become spontaneously active, maintaining the attitude at least in the presence of the cue (Kruglanski, 1989; Mackie, 1987; Weber, 1972). Although attitudes formed on the basis of heuristic processing have been found to produce relatively ephemeral attitude change, the repeated presence of the cue, or the ubiquitous activation of a structure to which the attitude was tightly linked, might well produce longevity. For example, tight linkage of an attitude to a central structure such as the self (Abelson, 1988; Greenwald, 1981) or an important group membership (Kelman, 1961) would aid retention, providing a structural basis for attitudinal conviction.

Attitude–Behavior Relations

The relation of attitudes to behavior has been an enduring source of both fascination and frustration to social psychologists (Corey, 1937; LaPiere, 1934; Wicker, 1969). Early conceptual frameworks, which considered attitudes to comprise, at least in part, behavioral tendencies, allowed no possibility for disjunctions between cognitive or affective expressions of attitudes and behavior (see Eagly & Chaiken, 1993). No wonder, then, that results showing behavior to be quite often inconsistent with attitudes prompted many to suggest that the attitude concept be abandoned altogether (Wicker, 1969). Changes in our understanding of attitude activation and accessibility have, however, provided a new perspective on the issue (Fazio, 1986; Fazio & Zanna, 1981).

From the social cognition point of view, action is a consequence of a judgment about what to do (Kruglanski, 1989), and an attitude is only one of the many factors that might influence that decision. To influence such a decision, however, a relevant attitude must not merely be available, but also be activated (see Fazio, 1986, 1989, for reviews; Millar & Tesser, 1986, 1989). Thus the potential for attitudes to influence behavior depends on factors that increase or decrease the accessibility and thus activation of attitudes relevant to the behavior at hand. At one extreme, a mismatch between an attitude object and an apparently related attitude structure may mean that a relevant attitude is not activated, and thus cannot influence later behavior (Fishbein & Ajzen, 1975; Lord, Lepper, & Mackie, 1984). At the other extreme, an object may automatically activate its associated attitude, so that the attitude is chronically implicated in behavior toward the object (Fazio, 1990; Bargh, Chaiken, Govender, & Pratto, 1992). If automatic activation does not occur, attitude activation by more conscious and deliberate means becomes critical.

An understanding of attitude activation opens new possibilities for understanding and dealing with cases of maladaptive behavior and habit control. On one hand, habits can be viewed as action patterns triggered by environmental stimuli without relevant attitudes being activated (Ronis, Yates, & Kirscht, 1989). Remedial action would thus consist of efforts to deliberatively make appropriate attitudes accessible. On the other hand, habits might in fact be driven by chronically activated attitudes. Remedial action, here, might consist of trying to interfere with the chronic activation, or to activate attitudes (or norms) with conflicting behavioral implications. In both cases, conscious activation of appropriate attitudes in situations of behavioral choice may be thought of as an analog of self-control, and thus provides further means of integrating basic attitude change research and areas of applied and clinical concern.

Social Cognition Approaches to Persuasion: Accomplishments and Unresolved Issues

Much of the power of social cognition lies in its integrative capacity—the ability to explain an array of fragmented and sometimes inconsistent research findings using a set of common principles governing the nature and operation of structures and processes. At one level, this approach means that persuasion researchers can benefit from research in many different areas. Attitude structures may be compared with any and all other mental representations, and attitude processes with those used in forming impressions, changing stereotypes, and making decisions, for example. Much can be learned from ascertaining the commonalities and differences among structures and principles in different domains (Schneider, 1991, Sherman, Judd, & Park, 1989).

This unifying power also brings coherence to attitude research on another level. From the social cognition perspective, any and every distal factor can be studied as influencing persuasion via the same means. The impact of an affective state and the impact of an expert source, the number of arguments presented and whether or not conclusions are drawn, exposure to a pro- or counterattitudinal advocacy, can all be modeled and compared as they affect attitudinal structures, processes, or both.

At yet another level, cognitive mediation is offered as a parsimonious explanation of persuasion that integrates many of the previously suggested theories of attitude change. Learning theory, for example, can be seen as attempting to directly produce and strengthen associations between particular cognitive elements, with consequent implications for accessibility, activation, and use. Many of the results produced by studies in the perceptual tradition of persuasion can be viewed as due to interpretational effects of simultaneous category activation. The activation of information in one category provides a context for (and primes) particular interpretations of presented information (Kahneman & Miller, 1986; Yi, 1990). The perceptual selectivity of social judgment theory, the preference for functionally relevant information, and persuasion produced by consistency seeking can all be understood in terms of the impact of activated goal categories on the nature and direction of information processing. Persuasion, like other social judgments, is a function of the structures activated and the processes performed on them.

Has a social cognition approach succeeded in solving all the interesting questions in the study of attitudes and attitude changes? Obviously not. Perhaps the most commonly heard criticism of social cognition approaches in general is that motivation has been ignored. We believe our review of progress made in understanding classic issues refutes the idea that social cognition practitioners, at least in the attitude domain, are uninterested in motivational—or functional or affective—concerns. We wish instead to focus on an issue we believe to be central to understanding persuasion, yet neglected in social cognition analyses of persuasion. This issue is the nature of validity, and in particular how a sense of subjective validity is gained from the processing of information.

Only the processing of information perceived to be valid produces persuasion. But what makes some information strong and compelling, while some arguments seem weak and specious? Traditional approaches in the disciplines of communication and rhetoric taught the formal qualities of persuasive argumentation, with little appeal to why such forms were effective. Social cognition theories of persuasion are even less informative on the topic: they have not dealt explicitly with the idea of how validity is conferred, and thus they fall short of providing a complete theory of persuasion (Eagly & Chaiken, 1984). Two possibilities for thinking about validity, both largely unexplored, seem implicit in current social cognition approaches.

First, validity could be a consequence of processing itself, regardless of *what* is processed; that is, some kinds of processing might themselves confer validity. Imagine, for example, that ease of accessibility functions as a cue to the possible validity of information, just as it serves as a cue to frequency

(Kahneman & Tversky, 1973). If so, any processing that confers accessibility on material would also confer validity on it. Having dealt with the information previously might produce the impression that it is now easy to deal with, consistent with other material, and familiar—all of which might affect perceived validity (Arkes, Boehm, & Xu, 1991).

Second, validity might arise as a consequence of processing because processing allows the validity inherent in certain information to be recognized. This possibility is implicit in ideas about elaboration producing differential reactions to strong and weak arguments—the relative strength or weakness of the information is discovered through processing. This idea is also compatible with the activation and use of heuristic cues in persuasion contexts. Activation of information associated with the cue makes the recipient aware of the probable validity of some aspects of the information. And as noted above, information that is consistent with activated structures may also be perceived as more valid. Although processing is necessary to allow the validity of information to be recognized in these cases, validity appears to reside in some aspect or quality of the information itself.

Neither of these possible mediators of validity has received extensive research attention. Nor has a third possibility, one that is even further removed from current social cognition theories of persuasion. The possibility that social processes, particularly those of agreement and dissent, might confer validity on particular kinds of persuasive information has been largely ignored in current thinking about persuasion. Of course, there are some traditional distal variables—credibility, and likeability, for example—that convey information about the relations between source and recipient. Social cognition work has demonstrated, in fact, that awareness of a source's social status or credentials can influence the care with which such a source's information is processed (see Hass, 1981, for a review). Despite such findings, there has been no systematic attempt within persuasion work to assess the role of social processes in conferring validity. Although neglected in persuasion research, the importance of social factors in attitude and behavior change is, of course, central to conformity research.

CONFORMITY

For much of the first half century of its history, social psychology *was* the study of social influence, as reflected in the classic studies: LeBon (1897), Sherif (1936), Asch (1956), Milgram (1974), Newcomb (1953), and Festinger (1950, 1954). These studies were concerned not so much with the presentation of evidence about reality (although it was sometimes present), as with information about other people's reactions to that reality. Ironically, the theoretical legacy of these studies encouraged a bifurcation in thinking about social influence that increasingly isolated conformity research from persuasion research. While persuasion research continued at an ever-increasing pace during the 1970s and 1980s, conformity research went into a general decline. As a result, conformity research has remained largely untouched by the inroads social cognition approaches have made in other, crucially related, areas of study. Why has the study of conformity remained so separate from these developments?

Assumed Differences between Conformity and Persuasion Contexts

One reason is that conformity was often considered as arising from normative and social pressures, which produced outward compliance but no true attitude change. Despite Sherif's (1936) demonstration that group norms were internalized, the compliant nature of conformity was stressed in Allport's (1968) concern with "submission" to the group, Festinger's concept of group locomotion (1950), and Deutsch and Gerard's (1955) stress on normative influence in group settings. Although Asch (1956) in fact argued that face-to-face group pressure alone did not explain conformity, his results were widely interpreted as showing that the individual renounced reality when confronted by group consensus. To the extent that conformity was attributed to social pressures that ignored evidence about reality, it was regarded as beyond the pale of informational explanations.

Even when information about others' opinions was acknowledged as producing some privately accepted change, persuasion and conformity research were kept apart because of the radically different ways in which they viewed information. Persuasion research is concerned primarily with "arguments" or "evidence" about attitude objects and their material or psychological benefits. In contrast, conformity situations mainly convey information about the positions of other social actors: in these situations and in the theories derived from them, information resides in the knowledge that others agree or disagree, either with one's own view, or among themselves.

Direct evidence about attitude objects—the type of information usually presented in persuasion settings—has long been assumed to be more valid than social mediated information. In modern theories of attitude change, explicit assumptions about the superiority of direct evidence of physical reality can be traced back to Festinger (1954). Festinger asserted the priority of physical reality testing: only if direct tests of reality were impossible, or failed to yield unambiguous data, would socially mediated information become useful. The same assumption is reflected in Kelman's (1961) distinction of true internalization from mere identification, and in the assignment of group influence factors to the peripheral rather than the central route in the elaboration likelihood model (Petty & Cacioppo, 1986b). Knowledge of others' positions was not regarded as "good" evidence about reality, and situations that involved little exchange of direct evidence about reality received little attention from social cognition practitioners.

Information Processing Analyses of Conformity Situations

Only two aspects of conformity research have been subjected to extensive information processing analyses: the phenomenon of group polarization, and the case of minority influence. In both cases, these analyses occurred only after the influence situations in which they were studied were broadened to include the interchange of arguments, rather than of positions alone.

Risky shift (Stoner, 1961) research, for example, initially focused on the exchange of personal responses to choice dilemmas, and the effect of this exchange on extremizing a group's final response. Early explanations of the effect—social comparison, diffusion of responsibility, and social release—reflected the importance of exchanging *positional,* rather than *evidential,* information (see Turner, 1987, for a review). This situation changed when group discussion was demonstrated to also polarize attitudes in the direction initially favored by the group (Moscovici & Zavalloni, 1969), and it became much more common to study group polarization in contexts where arguments, rather than just choices, were exchanged.

This exchange of evidence opened the way for an information processing analysis of group polarization. According to the "persuasive arguments" explanation of group polarization (Burnstein & Vinokur, 1973, 1977; Burnstein, Vinokur, & Trope, 1973; Hinsz & Davis, 1984), most members' opinions polarize to the group's initial tendency because a majority of novel and compelling arguments supporting that tendency are presented. A debate soon raged between those who believed the effect was due to comparison with the positions of others in the group and those who argued that biases in the availability of particular arguments during discussion explained the findings. Detailed analyses of this debate are beyond the scope of this chapter, but we wish to make two points important to our later discussion. First, it is clear that influence targets provided with arguments are also being provided with positional information, and vice versa. Presenting people with arguments allows them to easily infer the position that such arguments support. At the same time, people can easily generate arguments that support a particular position. Thus, the distinction between physical and social evidence blurs considerably. Second, and not surprising, recent reviews suggest that both evidential and positional factors contribute to the polarization phenomenon, and that neither is single-handedly adequate for a complete explanation of group polarization (Isenberg, 1986; Kaplan & Miller, 1987; Turner, 1987).

A similar situation has developed much more recently in studies of majority and minority influence. The investigation of minority rather than majority influence owes its vitality to the assertion that majorities and minorities exert influence via qualitatively different processes (Nemeth, 1976; Moscovici, 1980). According to Moscovici, opposition from a majority (the classic conformity situation) produces compliance, but minorities produce true attitude change, or conversion. Originally, these ideas were the subject of innovative but controversial experiments using Asch-like situations featuring only the exchange of views about perceptual stimuli (Moscovici & Personnaz, 1980; Personnaz, 1981). Again, it was not until the paradigm was broadened to involve the exchange of information that the application of process tracing techniques from social cognition allowed Moscovici's assertions to be adequately evaluated (see Maass, West, & Cialdini, 1987; Kruglanski & Mackie, 1989, for reviews). Measures of attention, recall, and cognitive responding continue to be essential in identifying possible differences in the ways majority and minority sources exert their influence (Campbell, Tesser, & Fairey, 1986; Maass & Clark, 1983, 1984; Mackie, 1987; Nemeth, 1986; Nemeth, Mayseless, Sherman, & Brown, 1990; Tesser, Campbell, & Mickler, 1983). The emerging picture of majority and minority influence situations that produce private acceptance is important for our later discussion in a number of respects. First, it is again clear that positional and evidential information combine to produce the reported effects. Second, independent of majority and minority influence, consensus counts. The majority has a decided advantage because of its greater consensus. It is worth noting in this regard that majorities in juries and in laboratory simulations of juries where accuracy is paramount have far greater influence than minorities (Kassin & Wrightsman, 1987). In addition, a minority does not begin to have real influence until it gathers a consensus (Asch, 1956).

Social Cognition Approaches to Conformity: Benefits and Unresolved Issues

Recent research on both group polarization and minority influence thus provide examples of the benefits of integrating conformity and persuasion phenomena. First, a social cognition analysis of attitude change, generality, and longevity makes clear that conformity situations like polarization and majority influence can involve the exchange of evidence that produces internalization. Second, it is equally clear that the recipient's recognition of the social relationships present in the conformity setting (including majority or minority standing), like any other variable known to influence attitude change, can be thought of as activating various mental representations and processes by which available information is evaluated, elaborated, distorted, or discarded. Group membership representations include evaluative, cognitive, motivational, and affective information and activate cognitive, affective, and goal-directed processes. For example, the recognition of shared group membership (between the target and the source) can activate knowledge about issues and positions associated with such membership, enhancing processing of relevant messages. Activation of group membership concerns may act as a call for attention to available information, influencing which aspects of a message are attended and increasing message recall and argument differentiation (Mackie, Worth, & Asuncion, 1990; Mackie, Gastardo-Conaco, & Skelly, 1992). Group membership might also activate relevant heuristic cues, reminding us that agreement with others like ourselves is likely to result in correct attitudes, increasing persuasion without extensive message processing (Kelman, 1961; Mackie et al., 1990, 1992). Group membership factors operate to increase, decrease, and direct the extent of message processing, just as other source factors have been shown to do.

Where social cognition analyses have had an impact on conformity research, they have done so by emphasizing the exchange of evidential information and reasserting its persuasive superiority over socially mediated information. This assumed superiority comes under particular fire from Moscovici (1980). He points out, for example, that it is social conflict, not informational ambiguity, that provokes uncertainty and produces influence in Asch's classic study. Thus, social factors appear to play a crucial role in influence. In addition, Moscovici (see also Turner, 1985, 1987) argues that all information about reality is socially mediated. Even apparently direct interactions with physical reality—measuring a table with a ruler, for example—reflect social conventions. A ruler is a social convention that conveys information about a socially defined unit of a socially agreed-upon concept, length.

Such arguments undermine the assumed superiority of apparently asocial interactions with reality as inherently more valid or correct. They point out, together with decades of conformity research, the apparently powerful role that social conflict and consensus play in promoting influence. They suggest that conflict and consensus—the agreement and disagreement of others as conveyed in information about positions—as well as cognitive processes, may be intimately involved in conferring validity on particular pieces of information. How can social processes, and particularly social consensus, contribute to the perception of validity?

First, perceivers assess as accurate, objective, or valid whatever information appears to be demanded and determined by the nature of reality. In short, information about which external attributions are made appears valid (Asch, 1952; Kelly, 1967; Festinger, 1950; Turner, 1985). As most clearly asserted by Kelley, the basic mechanism for achieving such externality is social consensus. Consensus or agreement about a response leads to the external attribution of that response to the object or entity in question. Imagine that you prepare both peach pie and apple pie for a family gathering. Everyone comes back for seconds on the peach pie but leaves the apple untouched. Faced with such consensus, the likely attribution is that the peach pie was particularly good. That is, the shared reaction (*everyone* goes back for seconds) leads naturally to the attribution of the response to the entity itself (*the pie* was good). Consensus suggests that what is agreed upon reflects reality.

Ironically, the very certainty produced by social agreement appears to be external to those producing the agreement. It is possible, for example, that the popularity of the peach pie is due to the fact that your family are all peach lovers. Yet consensus always appears to indicate something about reality, not about the conveyors of the consensus (Asch, 1956; Allen, 1965, 1975). This is no doubt because consensus usually operates to nullify bias. One person may have a personal idiosyncratic love of peaches—but consensus provides converging evidence for the correctness of the response by seeming to eliminate the possibility that everyone could be wrong in the same way. Consensus, then, confers correctness. Informational validity depends, at least in part, on the formation of social consensus.

Integrating Informational and Social Indicators of Validity

Exploring the role of social consensus and dissent in ascertaining validity thus suggests an avenue for the reintegration of persuasion and conformity research. If social consensus also functions to confer validity on information, it may complement the role that cognitive processing of evidence plays in producing social influence. Both social and individual cognitive processes may contribute to particular information being deemed valid and thus becoming persuasive. If so, there should be evidence of social processes influencing the kinds of processes associated with cognitive accounts of attitude change. At the same time, social processes such as consensus formation and conformity should display information processing principles.

Social Aspects of Information Processing

Evidence for the powerful effect of explicit consensus information abounds (for reviews see Allen, 1965; Asch, 1956; Axsom, Yates, & Chaiken, 1987; Kruglanski & Mackie, 1989; Turner, 1991). However, consensus may also operate implicitly in many situations. First, in the absence of explicit information, people routinely assume the existence of a consensus (as suggested by the false consensus effect; Ross, Greene, & House, 1977). Second, the existence of consensus can often be inferred from the (apparently asocial) content of information itself. For example, statistical evidence may be persuasive because recipients assume it represents multiple replicable responses. Testimony by experts may be compelling because it is seen as representing or embodying a collective wisdom.

Third, arguments that further the attainment of consensually held goals, values, and experiences are typically seen as valid and compelling. For example, arguments that support the side that "wins" a group discussion are seen as more valid and compelling than the same arguments presented as representing the minority view (McLachlan, 1986). Shared or consensual information is much more likely to be aired during discussion than is individually unique information (Stasser & Titus, 1985). Arguments attributed to a majority are more persuasive than the same arguments attributed to a minority

(Mackie, 1987). In typical procedures used to operationalize argument quality in persuasion experiments, strong arguments are defined as ones that members of the subject population agree to be strong, and weak ones are arguments that others agree to be weak (Petty & Cacioppo, 1986b). The quality of the information that is later recognized during content-focused processing has already been established by consensus.

The fact that validity is thus socially defined (one group's strong arguments may not be another's) appears to undermine one of the advantages of consensus: that it eliminates possible biases. After all, agreement among those who share similar attributes might merely reflect shared biases produced by those shared attributes. In fact, it appears than consensus is expected among those who share the attributes relevant to making the judgment at hand (Turner, 1985; Sherman, Chassin, Presson, & Agostinelli, 1984; Gorenflo & Crano, 1989; Goethals & Nelson, 1973): we are almost always more powerfully persuaded by in-groups than by out-group members (Kelley, 1952; Kelman, 1961; Mackie et al., 1990, 1992). How can the validity of information that is a product of social processes be maintained?

Cognitive Aspects of Consensus Formation

One answer lies in *how* consensus is achieved or reaffirmed. If consensus is to be successful in eliminating biases, the process by which consensus is achieved is crucial: consensus must be established through the convergence of independent, rather than dependent, views. Consensus may be accepted as reflecting valid information about the state of the world only to the extent that any (and every relevant) other individual (including oneself) can process information independently to reach the same conclusion. When this independence of processing fails, the persuasiveness of its conclusions is undermined. Individuals classified as a group are less persuasive than individuals not so classified in their independence is questioned (Wilder, 1977; Harkins & Petty, 1987). Similar attributional analyses of the effects of shared biases have been shown to undermine the persuasive effectiveness of groups that have both a different opinion and some readily identifiable distinguishing feature (Maass & Clark, 1984).

The importance of independence in reaching consensus suggests three additional areas in which social cognition concerns could usefully be applied to an understanding of consensus. First, identification of contamination requires attributional analysis (Eagly, Chaiken, & Wood, 1981). Extending attributional accounts made in persuasive contexts to conformity situations seems promising. Second, social consensus information about validity may be accepted only when an individual can arrive at the same outcome through his or her independent processing. The social consensus becomes individual reality by the individual's replication of the consensual outcome in the cognitive processes long studied in persuasion research. Finally, the cognitive processes involved in perceptions of the source of persuasive messages may be particularly important. Consider, for example, the fact that in-groups are more persuasive than out-groups, even though the potential of other in-group members to contaminate our views must be more obvious. Why? The key appears to be in how different groups—and more importantly, their persuasive messages—are represented in memory (Wilder, 1990; see Messick & Mackie, 1989, for a review). Arguments presented by in-group members are perceived and stored in memory as independent entities, each associated with the particular individual presenting the argument. Consensus among the in-group is more powerful, not only because there are more individuals agreeing, but because in-group consensus appears to reflect convergence among separate independent processors. In contrast, out-group arguments are "lumped together"—the same old out-group "party line." There may appear to be less of a consensus (since fewer "units" contribute to it), and any apparent consensus is clearly associated with out-group-defining shared sources of possible bias. As a consequence of these representational differences, in-group messages seem much more persuasive than out-group messages (Wilder, 1990).

Both social and individual processes thus may contribute to particular information being deemed valid. Social consensus might be validated by individual cognitive processing and consensual agreement might be used to check the validity of the outcome of individual processes (Turner, 1985, 1991). The issue of whether these processes operate independently, or whether information about validity from one source biases processing about validity from the other remains to be investigated. Exploring the possibility that validity depends on the outcomes of both the social process of consensual validation and the individual process of cognitive validation is a promising and potentially powerful means of integrating social and cognitive processes in the study of conformity and persuasion.

CONCLUDING REMARKS

The research reviewed here reflects the substantial progress made by a social cognition analysis of social influence and provides evidence of the continuing vitality of a research area close to the heart of social psychology. Research on influence within the social cognition framework reflects a profound increase in the theoretical sophistication with which we think about the mediation of distal factors in the influence context. Such research is marked by a particular concern with understanding the interplay of structure and process in human information processing and providing experimental evidence of the processes underlying this interplay.

These developments produced the concern with delineating the microprocesses of influence and their mutual interactions. They focused attention on the chasm between comprehension and acceptance, and offered the individual's idiosyncratic responses as one viable bridge across the gap. They led to a deeper understanding of the interplay of processes requiring active allocation of attention on the recipient's part, and those that occur without the recipient consciously investing resources. Such progress has in turn expanded our understanding of the dynamics of attitude formation, modification, retention, and resistance. It has given us new insight into the conditions under which attitudes may be expected to influence other judgments, such as the decision to act. It has also rekindled interest in and provided a means for investigating the ways in which motivational, functional, and affective factors are mediated by available structures and active procedures.

Similar benefits are beginning to accrue from social cognition analyses of conformity phenomena. Specifically, such analyses indicate the basic similarities between conformity and persuasion, and suggest implications from one area that might benefit research in the other. First, social cognition analyses highlight the extent to which conformity produces true attitude change. Social processes can produce private acceptance and not just compliance. Second, the approach details the processing consequences of group membership that produce the powerful effects that in-groups have on our thoughts, feelings, and behaviors. Third, arguments and evidence can be important in conformity situations, just as they are in persuasion research. At the same time, consensus information can be as important in persuasion research as it is in conformity research. Such developments dismantle the artificial barriers that previously impeded the integration of persuasion and conformity into a more general approach to social influence phenomena. We suggest this integration could be furthered by considering the ways in which both cognitive and social processes depend on one another to produce validity (Turner, 1991).

Such an approach promises benefits in other areas of social influence research as well. We have been concerned in this chapter with influence that aims at or culminates in private acceptance. Social cognition analyses of compliance phenomena and of norm-driven behavior are also beginning to appear. From the social cognition perspective, compliance, rather than being derogated as "lack of sincerity" in attitude expression, can be seen as an answer to the question of what to do (Kruglanski, 1989), rather than what to think, allowing for a more systematic analysis of when and why behavior might deviate from attitudes. Turner (1991) discusses a cognitively mediated model of self-presentational concerns, and Cialdini (1984, 1987) has provided a heuristic analysis of influence techniques based on liking, reciprocity, obedience, and similarity.

There are many who claim that the vigorous and widespread application of social cognition thinking to social phenomena is merely a passing fad. Those looking forward to its imminent demise interpret the continual broadening and blurring of the borders of the enterprise as a sign of its rapid fading. We believe just the opposite to be true. The diffusion of social cognition into the diverse areas of social psychology demonstrates a widespread recognition of its power to integrate, the appeal of its analysis of diverse phenomena in simple and few principles, its provision of basic scaffolding on which to build, and its flexibility to both accommodate and assimilate. Where foundations have already been laid by an earlier concentration on information processing, its growth is rapid. However, even where no former structures stood, it provides easily adapted blueprints, so the work does not start from scratch. As they become familiar, social cognition principles and practices no longer appear novel and different. Such familiarity—and the many contributions documented in this and other chapters—demonstrates the extent to which the social cognition approach has become "normal" science in many different areas of social psychological research.

ACKNOWLEDGMENTS

Preparation of this chapter was aided by Grant MH 43041 to Diane Mackie. We acknowledge the extremely helpful comments of Steven J. Sherman, David L. Hamilton, and Thomas M. Ostrom.

REFERENCES

Abelson, R. P. (1988). Conviction. *American Psychologist, 43,* 267–275.

Abelson, R. P., Aronson, E., McGuire, W. J., Newcomb, T. M., Rosenberg, M. J., & Tannenbaum, P. H. (Eds.). (1968). *Theories of cognitive consistency: A source book.* Chicago: Rand McNally.

Ajzen, I. (1989). Attitude structure and behavior. In A. R. Pratkanis, S. J. Breckler, & A. G. Greenwald (Eds.), *Attitude structure and function* (pp. 241–274) Hillsdale, NJ: Erlbaum.

Allen, V. L. (1965). Situational factors in conformity. In L. Berkowitz (Ed.), *Advances in experimental social psychology* (Vol. 2, pp. 133–175). New York: Academic Press.

Allen, V. L. (1975). Social support for nonconformity. In L. Berkowitz (Ed.), *Advances in experimental social psychology* (Vol. 8, pp. 2–43). New York: Academic Press.

Allport, G. W. (1968). The historical background of modern social psychology. In G. Lindsey & E. Aronson (Eds.), *The handbook of social psychology* (2nd ed.) (Vol. 1, pp. 1–80). New York: Random House.

Arkes, H. R., Boehm, L. E., & Xu, G. (1991). Determinants of judged validity. *Journal of Experimental Psychology, 27,* 576–605.

Asch, S. E. (1948). The doctrine of suggestion, prestige, and imitation in social psychology. *Psychological Review, 55,* 250–276.

Asch, S. E. (1952). *Social psychology.* New York: Prentice-Hall.

Asch, S. E. (1956). Studies of independence and conformity: A minority of one against a unanimous majority. *Psychological Monographs, 70,* (9, no. 416).

Axsom, D., Yates, D., & Chaiken, S. (1987). Audience responses as a heuristic cue in persuasion. *Journal of Personality and Social Psychology, 53,* 30–40.

Barge, J. A. (1984). Automatic and conscious processing of social information. In R. S. Wyer & T. K., Srull (Eds.), *Handbook of social cognition* (Vol 3, pp. 1–43). Hillsdale NJ: Erlbaum.

Bargh, J. A. (1989). Conditional automaticity: Varieties of automatic influence in social perception and cognition. In J. S. Uleman & J. A. Bargh (Eds.), *Unintended thought* (pp. 3–51). New York: Guilford.

Bargh, J. A., Chaiken, S., Govender, R., & Pratto, F. (1992). The generality of the automatic attitude activation effect. *Journal of Personality and Social Psychology, 62,* 893–912.

Brehm, J. W. (1966). *A theory of psychological reactance.* San Diego, CA: Academic Press.

Brock, T. C. (1967). Communication discrepancy and intent to persuade as determinants of counterargument production. *Journal of Experimental Social Psychology, 3,* 296–309.

Burnstein, E., & Vinokur, A. (1973). Testing two classes of theories about group-induced shifts in individual choice. *Journal of Experimental Social Psychology, 9,* 123–137.

Burnstein, E., & Vinokur, A. (1977). Persuasive argumentation and social comparison as determinants of attitude polarization. *Journal of Experimental Social Psychology, 13,* 315–332.

Burnstein, E., Vinokur, A., & Trope, V. (1973). Interpersonal comparison versus argumentation. *Journal of Experimental Social Psychology, 9,* 236–245.

Cacioppo, J. T., Petty, R. E., & Sidera, J. (1982). The effects of a salient self-schema on the evaluation of proattitudinal editorials: Top-down versus bottom-up message processing. *Journal of Experimental Social Psychology, 18,* 324–338.

Campbell, J. D., Tesser, A., & Fairey, P. J. (1986). Conformity and attention to the stimulus: Some temporal and contextual dynamics. *Journal of Personality and Social Psychology, 51,* 315–324.

Cappella, J. N., & Street, R. L. (1989). Message effects: Theory and research on mental models of messages. In J. J. Bradac (Ed.), *Message effects in communication science,* (pp. 24–51). Newbury Park, NJ: Sage.

Cartwright, D. (1941). Relation of decision-time to the categories of response. *American Journal of Psychology, 54,* 174–196.

Chaiken, S. (1980). Heuristic versus systematic information processing and the use of source versus message cues in persuasion. *Journal of Personality and Social Psychology, 39,* 752–766.

Chaiken, S. (1987). The heuristic model of persuasion. In M. P. Zanna, J. M. Olson, & C. P. Herman (Eds.), *Social influence: The Ontario Symposium,* (Vol. 5, pp. 3–39). Hillsdale, NJ: Erlbaum.

Chaiken, S., & Stangor, C. (1987). Attitudes and attitude change. *Annual Review of Psychology, 38,* 575–630.

Chaiken, S., Liberman, A., & Eagly, A. H. (1989). Heuristic & systematic processing within and beyond the persuasion context. In J. S. Uleman & J. A. Bargh (Eds.), *Unintended thought* (pp. 212–252). New York: Guilford.

Cialdini, R. B. (1984). Principles of automatic influence. In J. Jacoby & C. S. Craig (Eds.), *Personal selling: Theory, research and practice.* Lexington, MA: D. C. Heath and Company.

Cialdini, R. B. (1987). Compliance principles of compliance professionals: Psychologists of necessity. In M. P. Zanna, J. M. Olson, & C. P. Herman (Eds.), *Social influence: The Ontario Symposium* (Vol. 5, pp. 165–184). Hillsdale, NJ: Erlbaum.

Cialdini, R. B. (1988). *Influence: Science and practice.* (2nd ed.) Glenview, IL: Scott, Foresman.

Cooper, J., & Fazio, R. H. (1984). A new look at dissonance theory. In L. Berkowitz (Ed.), *Advances in experimental social psychology* (Vol. 17, pp. 229–266). New York: Academic Press.

Corey, S. M. (1937). Professed attitudes and actual behavior. *Journal of Educational Psychology, 28,* 271–280.

Deutsch, M., & Gerard, H. B. (1955). A study of normative and informational social influences upon individual judgment. *Journal of Abnormal and Social Psychology, 51,* 629–636.

Devine, P. G., & Ostrom, T. M. (1988). Dimensional versus information-processing approaches to social knowledge: The case of inconsistency management. In D. Bar-Tal & A. W. Kruglanski (Ed.), *The social psychology of knowledge* (pp. 231–261). Cambridge: Cambridge University Press.

Eagly, A. H., & Chaiken, S. (1984). Cognitive theories of persuasion. In L. Berkowitz (Ed.), *Advances in experimental social psychology* (Vol. 17, pp. 268–359). New York: Academic Press.

Eagly, A. H., & Chaiken, S. (1993). *The psychology of attitudes.* Fort Worth, TX: Harcourt Brace Jovanovich.

Eagly, A. H., Chaiken, S., & Wood, W. (1981). An attributional analysis of persuasion. In J. H. Harvey, W. J. Ickes, & R. F. Kidd (Eds.), *New directions in attribution research* (Vol. 3, pp. 37–62). Hillsdale, NJ: Erlbaum.

Edwards, K. (1990). The interplay of affect and cognition in attitude formation and change. *Journal of Personality and Social Psychology, 59,* 421–433.

Fazio, R. H. (1986). How do attitudes guide behavior? In R. M. Sorrentino & E. T. Higgins (Eds.), *The handbook of motivation and cognition: Foundations of motivation and behavior* (Vol. 1, pp. 204–243). New York: Guilford.

Fazio, R. H. (1989). On the power and functionality of attitudes: The role of attitude accessibility. In A. R. Pratkanis, S. J. Breckler, & A. G. Greenwald (Eds.), *Attitude structure and function* (pp. 153–180). Hillsdale, NJ: Erlbaum.

Fazio, R. H. (1990). Multiple processes by which attitudes guide behavior: The MODE model as an integrative framework. In M. P. Zanna (Ed.), *Advances in experimental social psychology* (Vol. 23, pp. 75–109). San Diego, CA: Academic Press.

Fazio, R. H., & Zanna, M. P. (1981). Direct experience and attitude-behavior consistency. In L. Berkowitz (Ed.), *Advances in experimental social psychology* (Vol. 14, pp. 161–202). New York: Academic Press.

Fazio, R. H., Sanbonmatsu, D. M., Powell, M. C., & Kardes, F. R. (1986). On the automatic activation of attitudes. *Journal of Personality and Social Psychology, 50,* 229–328.

Festinger, L. (1950). Informal social communication. *Psychological Review, 57,* 271–282.

Festinger, L. (1954). A theory of social comparison processes. *Human Relations, 7,* 117–140.

Festinger, L. (1957). *A theory of cognitive dissonance.* Stanford, CA: Stanford University Press.

Festinger, L., & Maccoby, N. (1964). On resistance to persuasive communications. *Journal of Abnormal and Social Psychology, 68,* 359–366.

Fishbein, M., & Ajzen, I. (1975). *Belief, attitude, intention, and behavior: An introduction to theory and research.* Reading, MA: Addison-Wesley.

Fishbein, M., & Ajzen, I. (1981). Acceptance, yielding and impact: Cognitive processes in persuasion. In R. E. Petty, T. M. Ostrom, & T. C. Brock (Eds.), *Cognitive responses in persuasion* (pp. 339–359). Hillsdale, NJ: Erlbaum.

Fiske, S. T., & Taylor, S. E. (1991). *Social cognition* (2nd ed.). New York: McGraw-Hill.

Frey, D. (1986). Recent research on selective exposure to information. In L. Berkowitz (Ed.), *Advances in experimental social psychology* (Vol. 19, pp. 41–80). New York: Academic Press.

Goethals, G. R., & Nelson, R. (1973). Similarity in the influence process: The belief-value distinction. *Journal of Personality and Social Psychology, 25,* 117–122.

Gorenflo, D. W., & Crano, W. D. (1989). Judgmental subjectivity/objectivity and locus of choice in social comparison. *Journal of Personality and Social Psychology, 57,* 605–614.

Greenwald, A. G. (1968). Cognitive learning, cognitive response to persuasion, and attitude change. In A. G. Greenwald, T. C. Brock, & T. M. Ostrom (Eds.), *Psychological foundations of attitudes* (pp. 147–170). New York: Academic Press.

Greenwald, A. G. (1980). The totalitarian ego: Fabrication and revision of personal history. *American Psychologist, 35,* 603–618.

Greenwald, A. G. (1981). Cognitive response analysis: An appraisal. In R. E. Petty, T. M. Ostrom, & T. C. Brock (Eds.), *Cognitive responses in persuasion* (pp. 399–420). Hillsdale, NJ: Erlbaum.

Greenwald, A. G. (1989). Why are attitudes important? In A. R. Pratkanis, S. J. Breckler, & A. G. Greenwald (Eds.), *Attitude structure and function* (pp. 1–10). Hillsdale, NJ: Erlbaum.

Greenwald, A. G., Brock, T. C., & Ostrom, T. M. (Eds.). (1968). *Psychological foundations of attitudes.* New York: Academic Press.
Harkins, S. G., & Petty, R. E. (1987). Information utility and the multiple source effect. *Journal of Personality and Social Psychology, 52,* 260–268.
Hass, R. G. (1981). Effects of source characteristics on cognitive responses and persuasion. In R. E. Petty, T. M. Ostrom, & T. C. Brock (Eds.), *Cognitive responses in persuasion* (pp. 399–402). Hillsdale, NJ: Erlbaum.
Haugtvedt, C., & Petty, R. E. (1992). Personality and persuasion: Need for cognition moderates the persistence and resistance to attitude changes. *Journal of Personality and Social Psychology, 63,* 308–319.
Herek, G. M. (1987). Can functions be measured? A new perspective on the functional approach to attitudes. *Social Psychology Quarterly, 50,* 285–303.
Himmelfarb, S., & Eagly, A. H. (1974). Orientations to the study of attitudes and their change. In S. Himmelfarb & A. H. Eagly (Eds.), *Readings in attitude change* (pp. 2–49). New York: Wiley.
Hinsz, V. B., & Davis, J. H. (1984). Persuasive arguments theory, group polarization, and choice shifts. *Personality and Social Psychology Bulletin, 10,* 260–268.
Houston, D. A., & Fazio, R. H. (1989). Biased processing as a function of attitude accessibility: Making objective judgments subjectively. *Social Cognition, 7,* 51–66.
Hovland, C. I., Lumsdaine, A. A., & Sheffield, F. D. (1949). *Experiments on mass communication.* Princeton, NJ: Princeton University Press.
Hovland, C. I., Janis, I. L., & Kelley, H. H. (1953). *Communication and persuasion.* New Haven: Yale University Press.
Insko, C. A. (1967). *Theories of attitude change.* New York: Appleton-Century-Crofts.
Isenberg, D. J. (1986). Group polarization: A critical review and meta-analysis. *Journal of Personality and Social Psychology, 42,* 1141–1151.
Janis, I., Hovland, C., Field, P., Linton, H., Graham, E., Cohen, A., Rife, D., Abelson, R., Lesser, G., & King, B. (1959). *Personality and persuasibility.* New Haven: Yale University Press.
Johnson, B. T., & Eagly, A. H. (1989). Effects of involvement on persuasion: A meta-analysis. *Psychological Bulletin, 106,* 290–314.
Jones, E. E. (1985). Major developments in social psychology in the last five decades. In G. Lindsey & E. Aronson (Eds.), *The handbook of social psychology* (3rd ed.) (Vol. 2, pp. 47–108). New York: Random House.
Kahneman, D., & Miller, D. T. (1986). Norm theory: Comparing reality to its alternatives. *Psychological Review, 93,* 136–153.
Kahneman, D., & Tversky, A. (1973). On the psychology of prediction. *Psychological Review, 80,* 237–251.
Kaplan, M. T., & Miller, C. E. (1987). Group decision-making and normative versus informational influence: Effects of type of issue and assigned decision rule. *Journal of Personality and Social Psychology, 53,* 306–313.
Kassin, S. M., & Wrightsman, L. W. (1987). *The American jury on trial: Psychological perspectives.* New York: Hemisphere.
Katz, D. (1960). The functional approach to the study of attitudes. *Public Opinion Quarterly, 24,* 163–204.
Kelley, H. H. (1952). Two functions of reference groups. In G. E. Swanson, T. M. Newcomb, & E. L. Hartley (Eds.), *Readings in social psychology* (2nd Ed.) (pp. 410–414). New York: Holt.
Kelley, H. H. (1967). Attribution theory in social psychology. In D. Levine (Ed.), *Nebraska symposium on motivation* (Vol. 15, pp. 192–240). Lincoln: University of Nebraska Press.
Kelman, H. C. (1961). Processes of opinion change. *Public Opinion Quarterly, 46,* 57–78.
Kiesler, C. A., & Kiesler, S. B. (1969). *Conformity.* Reading, MA: Addison-Wesley.
Kitayama, S., & Burnstein, E. (1989). The relation between opinion and memory: Distinguish-

ing between associative density and structural centrality. In J. N. Bassili (Ed.), *On-line cognition in person perception* (pp. 91–123). Hillsdale, NJ: Erlbaum.

Krech, D., & Crutchfield, R. (1948). *Theory and problems of social psychology.* New York: McGraw-Hill.

Kruglanski, A. W. (1989). *The cognitive-motivational bases of human knowledge: A theory of lay epistemics.* New York: Plenum.

Kruglanski, A., & Mackie, D. M. (1989). Majority and minority influence: A judgmental process analysis. In W. Stroebe, M. Hewstone (Eds.), *European Review of Social Psychology* (Vol. 1, pp. 229–262). London: Wiley.

Landman, J., & Manis, M. (1983). Social cognition: Some historical and theoretical perspectives. In L. Berkowitz (Ed.), *Advances in experimental social psychology* (Vol. 16, pp. 49–123). Orlando: Academic Press.

LaPiere, R. T. (1934). Attitudes versus action. *Social Forces, 13,* 230–237.

LeBon, G. (1897). *The crowd: A study of the popular mind.* London: T. Fisher.

Levine, J. M., & Russo, E. M. (1987). Majority and minority influence. In C. Hendrick (Ed.), *Group processes* (pp. 13–54). Newbury Park: Sage.

Lingle, J. H., & Ostrom, T. M. (1981). Principles of memory and cognition in attitude formation. In R. E. Petty, T. M. Ostrom, & T. C. Brock (Eds.), *Cognitive responses in persuasion* (pp. 399–420). Hillsdale, NJ: Lawrence Erlbaum.

Logan, G. D. (1988). Toward an instance theory of automatization. *Psychological Review, 95,* 492–527.

Logan, G. D. (1989). Automaticity and cognitive control. In J. S. Uleman & J. A. Bargh (Eds.), *Unintended thought* (pp. 52–74). New York: Guilford.

Lord, C. G., Lepper, M. R., & Ross, L. (1979). Biased assimilation and attitude polarization: The effects of prior theories on subsequently considered evidence. *Journal of Personality and Social Psychology, 37,* 2098–2109.

Lord, C. G., Lepper, M. R., & Mackie, D. M. (1984). Attitude prototypes as determinants of attitude-behavior consistency. *Journal of Personality and Social Psychology, 46,* 1254–1266.

Maass, A., & Clark, R. D. (1983). Internalization versus compliance: Differential processes underlying minority influence and conformity. *European Journal of Social Psychology, 13,* 197–215.

Maass, A., & Clark, R. D. (1984). Hidden impact of minorities: Fifteen years of minority influence research. *Psychological Bulletin, 95,* 428–450.

Maass, A., West, S. G., & Cialdini, R. B. (1987). Minority influence and conversion. In C. Hendrick (Ed.), *Group processes* (pp. 55–79). Newbury Park: Sage.

McGuire, W. J. (1964). Inducing resistance to persuasion: Some contemporary approaches. In L. Berkowitz (Ed.), *Advances in experimental social psychology* (Vol. 1, pp. 191–229). San Diego, CA: Academic Press.

McGuire, W. J. (1968). Personality and attitude change: An information processing theory. In A. G. Greenwald, T. C. Brock, & T. M. Ostrom, (Eds.), *Psychological foundations of attitudes* (pp. 171–196). New York: Academic Press.

McGuire, W. J. (1969). The nature of attitudes and attitude change. In G. Lindzey & E. Aronson (Eds.), *The handbook of social psychology* (2nd ed) (Vol. 3, pp. 136–314). Reading, MA: Addison-Wesley.

McGuire, W. J. (1985). Attitudes and attitude change. In G. Lindsey & E. Aronson (Eds.), *The handbook of social psychology* (3rd ed.) (Vol. 2, pp. 233–246). New York: Random House.

Mackie, D. M. (1986). Social identification effects in group polarization. *Journal of Personality and Social Psychology, 50,* 720–728.

Mackie, D. M. (1987). Systematic and nonsystematic processing of majority and minority persuasive communications. *Journal of Personality and Social Psychology, 53,* 41–52.

Mackie, D. M., & Asuncion, A. G. (1990). On-line and memory-based processing of attitude change. *Journal of Personality and Social Psychology, 59,* 5–16.

Mackie, D. M., Worth, L. T., & Asuncion, A. G. (1990). Processing of persuasive in-group messages. *Journal of Personality and Social Psychology, 58,* 1–11.
Mackie, D. M., Gastardo-Conaco, M. C., & Skelly, J. J. (1992). Knowledge of the advocated position and the processing of in-group and out-group messages. *Personality and Social Psychology Bulletin, 18,* 145–151.
McLachlan, A. (1986). The effects of two forms of decision reappraisal on the perception of pertinent arguments. *British Journal of Social Psychology, 25,* 129–138.
Messick, D. M., & Mackie, D. M. (1989). Intergroup relations. *Annual Review of Psychology, 40,* 45–81.
Milgram, S. (1974). *Obedience to authority.* New York: Harper & Row.
Millar, M. G., & Tesser, A. (1986). Effects of affective and cognitive focus on the attitude-behavior relation. *Journal of Personality and Social Psychology, 51,* 270–276.
Millar, M. G., & Tesser, A. (1989). The effects of affective-cognitive consistency and thought on attitude-behavior relation. *Journal of Experimental Social Psychology, 25,* 189–202.
Moscovici, S. (1980). Toward a theory of conversion behavior. In L. Berkowitz (Ed.), *Advances in experimental social psychology* (Vol. 13, pp. 209–239). New York: Academic Press.
Moscovici, S., & Personnaz, B. (1980). Studies in social influence V: Minority influence and conversion behavior in a perceptual task. *Journal of Experimental Social Psychology, 10,* 270–282.
Moscovici, S., & Zavalloni, M. (1969). The group as a polarizer of attitudes. *Journal of Personality and Social Psychology, 12,* 125–135.
Nemeth, C. (1976). *A comparison between conformity and minority influence.* Paper presented to the International Congress of Psychology, Paris, France.
Nemeth, C. (1986). Differential contributions of majority and minority influence. *Psychological Review, 93,* 23–32.
Nemeth, C., Mayseless, O. Sherman, J., & Brown, Y. (1990). Exposure to dissent and recall of information. *Journal of Personality and Social Psychology, 58,* 429–437.
Newcomb, T. M. (1953). An approach to the study of communicative acts. *Psychological Review, 60,* 393–404.
Ostrom, T. M. (1981). Theoretical perspectives in the analysis of cognitive responses. In R. E. Petty, T. M. Ostrom, & T. C. Brock (Eds.), *Cognitive responses in persuasion* (pp. 283–290). Hillsdale, NJ: Erlbaum.
Peak, H. (1955). Attitude and motivation. In M. R. Jones (Ed.), *Nebraska symposium on motivation* (pp. 149–188). Lincoln: University of Nebraska Press.
Peak, H. (1958). Psychological structure and psychological activity. *Psychological Review, 65,* 325–347.
Personnaz, B. (1981). Researches in social influence; conversion in a perceptual task. Study with the spectrometer method. *European Journal of Social Psychology, 11,* 431–438.
Petty, R. E., & Cacioppo, J. T. (1977). Forewarning, cognitive responding, and resistance to persuasion. *Journal of Personality and Social Psychology, 35,* 645–655.
Petty, R. E., & Cacioppo, J. T. (1986a). The elaboration likelihood model of persuasion. In L. Berkowitz (Ed.), *Advances in experimental social psychology.* (Vol. 19, pp. 123–205). New York: Academic Press.
Petty, R. E., & Cacioppo, J. T. (1986b). *Communication and persuasion.* New York: Springer-Verlag.
Petty, R. E., Ostrom, T. M., & Brock, T. C. (Eds). (1981). *Cognitive responses in persuasion* Hillsdale, NJ: Erlbaum.
Pratkanis, A. R. (1989). The cognitive representation of attitudes. In A. R. Pratkanis, S. J. Breckler, & A. G. Greenwald (Eds.), *Attitude structure and function* (pp. 71–98). Hillsdale, NJ: Erlbaum.
Pratkanis, A. R., & Greenwald, A. G. (1989). A sociocognitive model of attitude structure and function. In L. Berkowitz (Ed.), *Advances in experimental social psychology* (Vol. 22, pp. 245–285). Orlando: Academic Press.

Pratkanis, A. R., Breckler, S. J., & Greenwald, A. G. (Eds.). (1989). *Attitude structure and function.* Hillsdale, NJ: Erlbaum.

Ratcliff, R., & McKoon, G. (1989). Memory models, text processing, and cue-dependent retrieval. In H. L. Roediger, & F. I. M. Craik (Eds.), *Varieties of memory and consciousness* (pp. 73–92). Hillsdale, NJ: Erlbaum.

Rokeach, M. (1956). Political and religious dogmatism: An alternative to the authoritarian personality. *Psychological Monographs, 70* (18, Whole No. 425).

Ronis, D. L., Yates, J. F., & Kirscht, J. P. (1989). Attitudes, decisions, and habits as determinants of repeated behavior. In A. R. Pratkanis, S. J. Breckler, & A. G. Greenwald (Eds.), *Attitude structure and function* (pp. 213–240). Hillsdale, NJ: Erlbaum.

Rosenberg, M., Hovland, C., McGuire, W., Abelson, R., & Brehm, J. (1960). *Attitude organization and change.* New Haven: Yale University Press.

Ross, L., Greene, D., & House, P. (1977). The "false consensus effect": an egocentric bias in social perception and attribution processes. *Journal of Experimental Social Psychology, 13,* 279–301.

Rumelhart, D. E., Smolensky, P., McClelland, J. L., & Hinton, G. E. (1986). Schemata and sequential thought processes in PDP models. In D. E. Rumelhart & J. L. McClelland (Eds.), *Parallel distributed processing: Explorations in the microstructure of cognition* (Vol. 2, pp. 7–57). Cambridge MA: Bradford.

Schneider, D. J. (1991). Social cognition. *Annual Review of Psychology, 42,* 527–562.

Schwarz, N., & Clore, G. L. (1983). Mood, misattribution, and judgments of well-being: Informative and directive functions of affective states. *Journal of Personality and Social Psychology, 45,* 513–523.

Shavitt, S. (1985). *Functional imperative theory of attitude formation and expression.* Unpublished doctoral dissertation. Ohio State University, Columbus, OH.

Shavitt, S. (1989). Operationalizing functional theories of attitude. In A. R. Pratkanis, S. J. Breckler, & A. G. Greenwald (Eds.), *Attitude structure and function* (pp. 311–338). Hillsdale, NJ: Erlbaum.

Sherif, M. (1936). *The psychology of social norms.* New York: Harper.

Sherif, M., & Cantril, H. (1945). The psychology of attitudes: I. *Psychological Review, 52,* 295–319.

Sherif, M., & Cantril, H. (1946). The psychology of attitudes: II. *Psychological Review, 53,* 1–24.

Sherif, M., & Sherif, C. W. (Eds.). (1967). *Attitude, ego-involvement, and change.* New York: Wiley.

Sherman, S. J. (1987). Cognitive processes in the formation, change, and expression of attitudes. In M. P. Zanna, J. M. Olson, & C. P. Herman (Eds.), *Social influence: The Ontario Symposium,* (Vol. 5, pp. 75–106). Hillsdale, NJ: Erlbaum.

Sherman, S. J., Chassin, L., Presson, C. C., & Agostinelli, G. (1984). The role of evaluation and similarity principles in the false consensus effect. *Journal of Personality and Social Psychology, 47,* 1244–1262.

Sherman, S. J., Judd, C. M., & Park, B. (1989). Social cognition. *Annual Review of Psychology, 40,* 281–326.

Sherman, S. J., Mackie, D. M., & Driscoll, D. M. (1990). Priming and the differential use of dimensions in evaluation. *Personality and Social Psychology Bulletin, 16,* 405–418.

Shiffrin, R. M., & Schneider, W. (1977). Controlled and automatic human information processing: II. Perceptual learning, automatic attending, and a general theory. *Psychological Review, 84,* 127–190.

Smith, M., Bruner, J., & White, R. (1956). *Opinions and personality.* New York: Wiley.

Snyder, M., & DeBono, K. G. (1987). A functional approach to attitudes and persuasion. In M. P. Zanna, J. M. Olson & C. P. Herman (Eds.), *Social influence: The Ontario Symposium* (Vol. 5, pp. 107–128). Hillsdale, NJ: Erlbaum.

Snyder, M., & DeBono, K. G. (1989). Understanding the functions of attitudes: Lessons from personality and social behavior. In A. R. Pratkanis, S. J. Breckler, & A. G. Greenwald (Eds.), *Attitude structure and function* (pp. 339–360). Hillsdale, NJ: Erlbaum.

Spielman, L. A., Pratto, F., & Bargh, J. A. (1988). Automatic affect: Are one's moods, attitudes, evaluations, and emotions out of control? *American Behavioral Scientist, 31,* 296–311.

Stasser, G., & Titus, W. (1987). Effects of information load and percentage of shared information on dissemination of unshared information during group discussion. *Journal of Personality and Social Psychology, 53,* 81–93.

Stoner, J. A. F. (1961). *A comparison of individual and group decisions including risk.* Unpublished thesis, Massachusetts Institute of Technology, MA.

Tannenbaum II, P. (1967). The congruity principle revisited: Studies in the reduction, induction, and generalization of persuasion. In L. Berkowitz (Ed.), *Advances in Experimental Psychology* (Vol. 3 pp. 271–320). New York, Academic Press.

Tesser, A., & Shaffer, D. R. (1990). Attitudes and attitude change. *Annual Review of Psychology, 41,* 479–523.

Thurstone, L. L., & Chave, E. J. (1929). *The measurement of attitude.* Chicago: University of Chicago Press.

Tourangeau, R., & Rasinski, K. A. (1988). Cognitive processes underlying context effects in attitude measurement. *Psychological Bulletine, 103,* 299–314.

Tourangeau, R., Rasinski, K. A., Bradburn, N., & D'Andrade, R. (1989). Belief accessibility and context effects in attitude measurement. *Journal of Experimental Social Psychology, 25,* 401–421.

Turner, J. C. (1985). Social categorization and the self-concept: A social cognitive theory of group behavior. *Advances in Group Processes, 2,* 77–121.

Turner, J. C. (1987). The analysis of social influence. In J. C. Turner, M. A. Hogg, P. J. Oakes, S. D. Reicher, & M. S. Wetherell (Eds.), *Rediscovering the social group: A self-categorization theory* (pp. 68–88). Oxford: Blackwell.

Turner, J. C. (1991). *Social influence.* Pacific Grove, CA: Brooks/Cole.

van der Pligt, J., & Eiser, J. R. (1984). Dimensional salience, judgment, and attitudes. In J. R. Eiser (Ed.), *Attitudinal judgment* (pp. 161–178). New York: Springer-Verlag.

Weber, S. J. (1972). *Opinion change as a function of the associative learning of content and source factors.* Unpublished doctoral dissertation, Northwestern University, Evanston, IL.

Wicker, A. W. (1969). Attitudes versus actions: The relationship of verbal and overt behavioral responses to attitude objects. *Journal of Social Issues, 25,* 41–78.

Wilder, D. A. (1977). Perception of groups, size of opposition, and social influence. *Journal of Experimental Social Psychology, 13,* 253–268.

Wilder, D. A. (1990). Some determinants of the persuasive power of ingroups and outgroups: Organization of information and attribution of independence. *Journal of Personality and Social Psychology, 59,* 1202–1213.

Wood, W. (1982). Retrieval of attitude-relevant information from memory: Effects on susceptibility to persuasion and on intrinsic motivation. *Journal of Personality and Social Psychology, 42,* 798–810.

Wood, W., Kallgren, C. A., & Preisler, R. M. (1985). Access to attitude-relevant information in memory. *Journal of Experimental Social Psychology, 21,* 73–85.

Wu, C., & Shaffer, D. R. (1987). Susceptibility to persuasive appeals as a function of source credibility and prior experience with the attitude object. *Journal of Personality and Social Psychology, 52,* 677–688.

Wyer, R. S., & Carlston, D. W. (1979). *Social cognition, inference, and attribution.* Hillsdale, NJ: Erlbaum.

Yi, Y. (1990). The indirect effects of advertisements designed to change product attribute beliefs. *Psychology and Marketing, 7,* 47–63.

Zajonc, R. B. (1968). Cognitive theories in social psychology. In G. Lindsey & E. Aronson (Eds.), *The handbook of social psychology* (Vol. 1, pp. 320–411). Reading, MA: Addison-Wesley.

Zajonc, R. B. (1980). Feeling and thinking: Preferences need no inferences. *American Psychologist, 35,* 151–175.

Zanna, M. P., & Rempel, J. K. (1988). Attitudes: a new look at an old concept. In D. Bar-Tal & A. Kruglanski (Eds.), *The social psychology of knowledge* (pp. 315–334). New York: Cambridge University Press.

Zanna, M. P., Kiesler, C. A., & Pilkonis, P. A. (1970). Positive and negative attitudinal affect established by classical conditioning. *Journal of Personality and Social Psychology, 14,* 321–328.

9

Social Cognition and the Study of Stereotyping

David L. Hamilton
Steven J. Stroessner
Denise M. Driscoll

> The human mind must think with the aid of categories . . . Once formed, categories are the basis for normal prejudgment. We cannot possibly avoid this process. Orderly living depends on it . . . Our experience in life tends to form itself into clusters (concepts, categories), and while we may call on the right cluster at the wrong time, or the wrong cluster at the right time, still the process in question dominates our entire mental life. A million events befall us every day. We cannot handle so many events. If we think of them at all, we type them. (Allport, 1954, p. 20)

> Modern life is hurried and multifarious. . . There is neither time nor opportunity for intimate acquaintance. Instead we notice a trait which marks a well known type, and fill in the rest of the picture by means of the stereotypes we carry about in our heads. . . The subtlest and most pervasive of all influences are those which create and maintain the repertory of stereotypes. We are told about the world before we see it. We imagine most things before we experience them. And those preconceptions . . . govern deeply the whole process of perception. They mark out certain objects as familiar or strange, emphasizing the difference, so that the slightly familiar is seen as very familiar, and the somewhat strange as sharply alien. . . They are aroused by small signs . . . Aroused, they flood fresh vision with older images, and project into the world what has resurrected in memory. (Lippmann, 1922, pp. 89–90)

These two quotations effectively summarize a couple of important principles that are central to current thinking about stereotypes. The first is a clear statement of the inevitability of categorization, the process on which all stereotyping is based. The second quotation describes the consequences of preexisting stereotypes for the process of social perception. Both of these topics have been the focus of a considerable amount of social cognition research in recent years. It is interesting, therefore, to note that the first quotation, on categorization, is from Gordon Allport's (1954) book *The Nature of Prejudice,* which was published 40 years ago; and that the second quotation, on how stereotypes influence social perception, is from Walter Lippmann's (1922) book *Public Opinion*, which was published more than 70 years ago.

Our purpose in dredging up these old quotes is simply to illustrate that, in the conceptualization of stereotypes, the cognitive emphasis has a long history. Still, the last 15–20 years of research on stereotyping from a social cognition perspective has had a qualitatively different flavor to it than the research literature that preceded it. What, then, is "new and different" about this more recent research? How has a social cognition perspective changed and advanced the way we think about, and do research on, stereotypes?

A social cognition analysis of stereotyping tries to understand the role of cognitive structures and processes in the perception of groups and group members. As such, it focuses on how an information processing system functions and how that system influences our perceptions of groups and group members. It emphasizes the role of information processing mechanisms as mediators between the information available in the stimulus world and the ultimate manifestations that we as social psychologists are interested in, such as perceptions of others and interpersonal behavior. The unique contribution that social cognition has made to research on stereotypes derives, we think, from this emphasis on the direct investigation of those cognitive mediators; for although the literature on stereotypes has always recognized a cognitive component, it is really only within the last 15 or so years that research has begun to inform us about how that cognitive component functions to influence group perceptions.

This chapter offers a perspective on the social cognition approach to stereotyping. We consider the place of the cognitive approach in the historical context of past work on stereotypes and stereotyping. We discuss the new theoretical and empirical developments of the last 15 or so years and how these developments have influenced the way researchers think about and investigate stereotypes and stereotyping. We conclude by speculating on some remaining issues and continuing quandaries that might benefit from applying this approach.

As a consequence of social cognition's impact, research on stereotypes today is quite different from research on stereotypes 20 years ago. To fully appreciate the nature and extent of these changes, we need to consider the historical context in which they took place.

STEREOTYPE THEORY AND RESEARCH: HISTORICAL CONTEXT

There is a lengthy history of both conceptual discussion of the nature of stereotypes and of empirical research investigating them. A thorough discussion of this history is well beyond the purview of this chapter, and a number of useful sources are available for the interested reader (Ashmore & Del Boca, 1981; Brigham, 1971; Cauthen, Robinson, & Krauss, 1971; Miller,

1982). Our brief overview is intended to provide some familiarity with the prevailing theory and research in this area until the mid-1970s, when social cognition became a major influence that changed the nature of this literature.

Conceptual Orientations

The term stereotype was introduced not by a behavioral scientist but by the journalist Walter Lippmann in his book, *Public Opinion* (Lippmann, 1922). As a commentator on current events, Lippmann was struck by the way different observers could "see" the same event in dramatically different ways, and he emphasized the role of preconceptions—or, to use his vividly descriptive phrase, "pictures in our heads"—in determining one's perceptions of people and events. When applied to group perceptions, these "pictures in our heads" are preconceptions that members of the group are all alike and not distinguishable from each other. To capture this idea, Lippmann borrowed the term "stereotype" from the printing industry, where it referred to a metal plate used in making duplicate pages of the same type. In doing so he gave a new, and lasting, meaning to the term.

In his highly insightful analysis, Lippmann offered a variety of ideas regarding the origins, functions, and consequences of stereotypes. As a commentator writing for a general audience, he was not concerned with the differences between or relationships among the various processes he identified. Rather, his purpose was to present a general characterization of stereotypes and to draw attention to their potentially detrimental effects on groups and group members. Thus, Lippmann's lasting contribution was the richness and diversity of his ideas, ideas which have provided the foundation for others to develop more systematic viewpoints.

Three main conceptual approaches to thinking about stereotypes have evolved, all of which have their roots in Lippmann's writing (see Ashmore & Del Boca, 1981; Hamilton & Sherman, 1994). From a *psychodynamic* perspective, stereotypes serve the motivational needs of the perceiver. Through the use of defense mechanisms, such as projection and displacement, negative attributes of the self or of one's in-group come to be perceived as characteristic of members of some out-group. And by perceiving out-groups in less favorable terms, one's in-group thereby becomes "better" than other groups. Moreover, to the extent that one's own self-esteem derives from the groups to which one belongs, then these mechanisms that enhance in-group evaluations also serve an important function for self-esteem maintenance as well. With its focus on intraindividual processes, it is not surprising that this approach has emphasized the role of personality functioning in stereotypes and prejudice. This emphasis is best illustrated in the research on the Authoritarian Personality (Adorno, Frenkel-Brunswik, Levinson, & Sanford, 1950), which was highly influential in the pre-social-cognition era.

From a *sociocultural* perspective, stereotypes are products of our social context and cultural heritage. This approach emphasizes the role of societal influences—family, peers, the media, cultural traditions—in both the formation and maintenance of stereotypes. Through social learning people acquire the intergroup beliefs and attitudes that prevail in their social environment, and through social reinforcement those belief systems are maintained.

From a *cognitive* perspective stereotypes are belief systems about the attributes characterizing various social groups. As indicated in the quote from Allport (1954), this approach emphasizes the role of categorization processes in both the initial formation of group concepts and in the subsequent perceptions of similarities within and differences between social categories. And as reflected in the quote from Lippmann (1922), these belief systems can "flood fresh vision with older images," biasing the way we perceive and interact with members of stereotyped groups.

Although the ideas defining each of these approaches have long been prevalent in writings about stereotypes, they have had only modest impact in guiding the nature of stereotype research. Historically, these conceptualizations—particularly the psychodynamic and sociocultural orientations—had noticeable influence on research investigating prejudice and intergroup relations (see Chapters 10 and 11, this volume), but less so on the study of stereotypes. As we shall see later in this chapter, social cognition changed this scenario by providing a theoretical framework that was highly effective in generating specific, testable research ideas.

Stereotype Research

One way to gauge the impact of social cognition on the nature of stereotype research is to note the dramatic change in the topics and issues that stereotype researchers investigate. To help make this point clearly, it is useful to consider an article published in 1971 by Brigham in which he reviewed the research literature on ethnic stereotypes. In a thorough and wide-ranging treatment, Brigham covered a variety of issues that had been predominant in the stereotype literature in the preceding decades. A brief summary of the topics Brigham discussed provides a useful insight into the problems and issues that captured the attention of stereotype researchers at that time.

Definitional Issues

One prominent characteristic of this early literature was a concern with defining what a stereotype is and with identifying its primary characteristics. However, there seemed to be only modest consensus among writers on these points, and hence Brigham devoted considerable space to discussing them. Two difficulties seemed to plague these efforts. First, a myriad of definitions was offered by various writers, reflecting different concerns and viewpoints. Some conceptions, for example, essentially equated stereotypes with myths, legend, and folklore, a view that seemingly captured the richness, breadth, and complexity of the concept. Others offered narrower, more focused conceptions, such as defining stereotypes as clusters of trait adjectives commonly associated with a social group. The latter attempts were intended to facilitate efforts to operationalize and measure stereotypes. The diversity in these definitions made it difficult for researchers to communicate with a shared understanding of what is and is not conveyed by the term stereotype.

In addition to these definitional problems, a second difficulty concerned attempts to identify the special characteristics or unique properties of stereotypes. For example, some argued that stereotypes are the result of a "faulty reasoning process." The implicit argument was that, because stereotypes characterize all group members as having the same attributes, they must necessarily be incorrect (at least for some individuals). Given that they are incorrect, they must be based on "faulty reasoning." Hence, the overgeneralizations reflected in stereotypic descriptions were viewed as due to a failure of normal cognitive functioning.

Though prevalent for many years, this view always faced some important drawbacks. The assertion that stereotypes are incorrect because they ascribe the same attributes to all group members is reasonable; stereotypes undermine the perception of within-group variability. However, this assertion of incorrectness, when applied to stereotypes as group-level characterizations, was more problematic. Validating the claim that stereotypes are incorrect in this sense requires some criterion of what accurate perceptions of a particular group would be. Such a criterion is not usually available, and hence the proposition could rarely be tested empirically. Similarly, the nature of the "faulty reasoning" presumed to underlie those judgments was never specified.

This characterization of stereotypes as inaccurate was balanced by researchers pursuing the accuracy component or "kernel of truth" in stereotypes. In this view, stereotypes of groups, although overgeneralized, are based on some small but "real" differences between groups. Again, the absence of any means of validly assessing the magnitude of the "real" difference limited the ability to evaluate the extent to which perceivers overgeneralized those differences.

Stereotypes were also characterized as being rigid, as reflected in their persistence over time and their resistance to change. This assumption of rigidity was particularly compatible with the psychodynamic perspective, in which the rigidity of stereotypes was viewed as deriving from a comparable characteristic in the stereotype holder. It is interesting to note that the rigidity of stereotypes was interpreted as evidence both for the accuracy of stereotypes (i.e., stereotyped group members have inherent and unchanging characteristics) and for their inaccuracy (i.e., perceivers are invariant in their response to stereotyped group members).

This focus on defining and characterizing stereotypes as correct or incorrect, as reasonable generalizations or as overgeneralizations based on faulty reasoning, and as reflecting inherent group differences or rigidly biased perceptions, encouraged methods for assessing whether there is agreement about the trait characteristics of various groups. The problem was to develop a way (1) to assess the content of the stereotype for particular groups, (2) to understand the rationale for assigning the content to a particular group, and (3) to track changes in the content of the stereotype for groups over time. For many years the empirical efforts to pursue these goals relied on a single methodology.

The Katz–Braly Method

Empirical research on stereotypes dates back to 1933 when Katz and Braly published their now-classic study of stereotypes held by college students. Their study became an important landmark for several reasons. First, at an early stage in the development of social psychology as a scientific discipline, they demonstrated that something as amorphous, and as socially significant, as racial and national stereotypes could be studied empirically. Second, they provided a method by which stereotypes could be measured with relative ease. Subjects were given a list of trait-descriptive adjectives and were asked to indicate which ones they felt described members of a particular group. Those attributes that were checked with highest frequency were considered to define the stereotype of that group. The procedure was straightforward, subjects had no difficulty completing the task, and because it took little time, one could assess the stereotypes of several groups within a relatively short time span (such as the experimental or classroom hour). Third, given its apparent usefulness, the Katz–Braly procedure (occasionally with minor modifications) became the standard methodology used in stereotype research for the next several decades. This point is documented not only by the fact that the Katz and Braly (1933) study itself was replicated literally (same materials, same university, etc.) on two subsequent occasions (Gilbert, 1951; Karlins, Coffman, & Walters, 1969), but also by the hundreds of other studies that have used the same basic procedure to study stereotypes (cf. Brigham, 1971; Cauthen et al., 1971; Ehrlich, 1973, for reviews).

Despite its wide usage, the Katz–Braly method had a number of problems that limited its usefulness (see Brigham, 1971). First, it could be used only for the purpose of assessing the content of stereotypes (Hamilton, 1976). Second, it restricted the content of stereotypes to trait language, and more specifically, to trait terms provided (on the checklist) by the researcher. Third, it was unclear what checking a trait on the list meant. Did it mean that the subject felt that *all* members of the group possess the trait? Or most? Or some? Or more members of this group than of other groups (cf. McCauley & Stitt, 1978)? Fourth, with this method subjects may be reporting, but not endorsing, the prevailing stereotype of a group. Fifth, subjects could easily distort their responses in a socially desirable manner (Sigall & Page, 1971).

Consensual Beliefs

One additional consequence that derives from the Katz–Braly method is that a stereotype consists only of traits that are consensually shared among the respondents; that is, the stereotype was usually defined as the 5–10 traits that had been checked by the largest percentage of a group of subjects. Consequently, in this method the stereotype only exists in, and cannot be defined apart from, the group of respondents. An important question concerns whether this agreement is an essential component of the definition of stereotypes. Some writers (e.g., Gardner, 1973; Vinacke, 1957) have explicitly advocated that this consensual property is an important element in the conceptualization (as well as the measurement) of stereotypes. More recently, others (e.g., Ashmore & Del Boca, 1981; Hamilton, 1979) have argued that stereotypes are belief systems that reside in the minds of individuals. The extent to which the same beliefs are shared in some subject population then becomes an empirical question. In this view, therefore, neither the definition nor the measurement of stereotypes should be constrained by the necessity of consensual agreement.

Properties of Stereotypes and Relations to Other Variables

In spite of these problems and limitations, the Katz–Braly method was the primary research tool for studying stereotypes for several decades. A great deal of knowledge was amassed about the content of various ethnic stereotypes, their properties, and their relationships with other variables. Here, we simply highlight some of the foci of that research (see Brigham, 1971, for a more thorough review).

One issue concerned the stability of stereotypes over time and their susceptibility to change. This tradition is most notably represented by the "Princeton trilogy" in which the original Katz and Braly (1933) study was subsequently replicated on two later occasions (Gilbert, 1951; Karlins et al., 1969). These and other studies documented a considerable degree of stability in major ethnic stereotypes over extended periods of time. The changes that did occur were seen as largely in response to major shifts in political, international, or economic conditions.

As noted earlier, there was considerable interest in the notion that a "kernel of truth" regarding intergroup differences underlies the diverging stereotypic conceptions of various groups (Campbell, 1967). These small but "real" differences are then overgeneralized in the group stereotypes. Attempts to empirically test this hypothesis were plagued, of course, by the lack of any adequate means of validly assessing the actual difference between groups on various attributes. Nevertheless, several approximations were attempted, usually comparing two or more assessments of the stereotype of the same group. For example, one might compare the stereotypes held by members of Group A and of Group B regarding what Group C is like. If there is considerable overlap in A's and B's stereotypes of C (particularly given extensive interaction with C), then there may be some valid basis for those perceptions of C. A second strategy consisted of comparing one group's stereotype of another group with that second group's perceptions of itself (i.e., its self-stereotype). Third, some efforts were made to compare both stereotypes and self-stereotypes of a group with independent measures of the same attributes assessed by personality questionnaires.

Although these analyses were often informative, none could provide solid evidence regarding stereotype validity. In the first strategy, agreement between two groups' stereotypes of a third group could reflect shared misconceptions. In the second strategy, agreement between stereotype and self-stereotype could be due to the minority's internalization of the majority's stereotype. The third strategy assumes validity of the personality questionnaire, itself a self-report measure.

Finally, there was some (though surprisingly little) research investigating the relationships of stereotypes with prejudicial attitudes and with behavior. A correlation between stereotypes and prejudice was generally assumed, and for some writers, stereotypes served to rationalize prejudicial attitudes. Similarly, it was assumed that one's stereotype of a group would influence one's behavior toward members of that group, although little evidence relevant to that relationship was available. In fact, Brigham (1971, p. 29) was forced to conclude that "discussion of the stereotype–behavior relationship will have to remain at a largely speculative level."

These were the issues that had dominated the stereotype literature ever since empirical research on the topic began with Katz and Braly's (1933) classic paper. Brigham's (1971) article provided an excellent review of this literature. It was both thorough and thoughtful, and it immediately became an authoritative and widely cited reference for anyone working in the area. In fact it still is.

THE SOCIAL COGNITION ANALYSIS: NEW DIRECTIONS

Brigham's review article was published in 1971, which means that it preceded by just a few years the advent of social cognition. Social cognition provided a new conceptual framework for thinking about stereotyping, and it generated research on a whole new set of questions (Hamilton, 1979, 1981). Within that framework a stereotype is a cognitive structure that can influence the way information about groups and group members is processed. Given this viewpoint, research has focused on issues pertaining to both the nature of that cognitive structure and the mechanisms by which that structure influences the processing of information about groups and group members.

Stereotypes As Cognitive Structures

In the extensive literature using the Katz–Braly technique, a stereotype consisted of the collection of trait attributes considered most typical of the social group in question. There was little if any discussion or analysis of a stereotype as a mental representation, of its structure, or its organization. Influenced by developments in cognitive psychology, more recent analyses of stereotypes have expanded this conception and have led to several different and more complex viewpoints regarding the nature of these structures. We can illustrate these changes by briefly highlighting two such developments.

One approach views stereotypes as prototypes within a hierarchical categorization system (Rosch, 1978). From this perspective perceivers develop mental representations not only of large social and ethnic groups (e.g., blacks), but also of subgroups within that broad classification (e.g., ghetto blacks, black athletes, black businessmen, etc.) that are characterized by distinct sets of attributes (Devine & Baker, 1991; see also Brewer, Dull, & Lui, 1981; Cantor & Mischel, 1979). Stereotyping can occur at any level within the hierarchy. Thus, when an individual group member is encountered, the features of that individual are "matched" to those of the prototypes or stereotypic conceptions of the various subcategories. These features are not limited to trait attributes and may include physical features, demographic characteristics, and a variety of other dispositionlike properties, such as attitudes, values, lifestyle, and the like (Andersen & Klatzky, 1987; Brewer, 1988; Cantor & Mischel, 1979). The person is then categorized as a member of the group to which there is greatest fit between individual and category feature sets. Thus, our mental representations of large social and ethnic groups can be much more complex than the conception implied in earlier stereotype research, and may include several distinct subtypes within that broader classification, each with its own stereotype (i.e., associated sets of features). In fact, some writers (e.g., Brewer et al., 1981) have argued that most stereotyping occurs at the level of these subtype categories, rather than at the superordinate level.

Ever since Katz and Braly's (1933) original efforts toward measuring the traits comprising various national and ethnic stereotypes, researchers have assumed that a stereotype is an abstract, generalized representation of the features and attributes most typical of the group's members. However, even that assumption is being challenged and scrutinized in some current work. Specifically, some researchers have recently argued that our conceptions of groups are less "abstract" then traditionally assumed, and that instead we rely heavily on our knowledge of specific group members and/or of particular experiences we have had with them (e.g., Linville, Fischer, & Salovey,

1989; Smith, 1990; Smith & Zárate, 1992). For example, some have argued that, without knowledge of individual group members stored as a part of the group concept, we would not be able to assess the degree of variability among members within a group. Yet perceivers are quite capable of detecting differences between groups in their variability (e.g., Park & Hastie, 1987). "Exemplar" theories emphasize the importance of these specific instances, retrieved from memory, in determining the perceiver's judgments of the group. In fact, in their "pure" form, these theories recognize little if any role of abstract, inference-based representations, arguing that knowledge is stored strictly in exemplar form and that generalized judgments are based solely on the set of exemplars that are retrieved from memory at the time these judgments are made (Smith & Zárate, 1992). Less extreme positions posit that conceptions of stereotypes need to include abstract, generalized characterizations of typical attributes as well as more specific, instance-based knowledge of group members, and that judgments of the group typically reflect the combined influence of both of these aspects of the group representation (see Hamilton & Sherman, 1994, for a more extended discussion of these viewpoints).

Contemporary conceptions of stereotypes, then, have advanced considerably beyond the notion of a cluster of traits that define a group stereotype. In fact, these newer conceptions raise a number of challenging questions regarding, for example, the nature of the "features" comprising stereotypes of groups; the structure of the group representation in memory; the way group-relevant information and experiences are organized as they are stored in memory; the retrieval and use of both generalized beliefs and specific knowledge about groups for various purposes, such as making judgments, reaching decisions, and guiding behavior; and how the nature of this cognitive structure might affect strategies of and prospects for stereotype change. These are issues that were considered only briefly, if at all, in the "old" stereotype literature, yet have moved to the forefront of current inquiry in the study of stereotypes.

Stereotypes and Information Processing

The analysis of stereotypes as cognitive structures is, as just noted, an important change in this research area. However, another shift seems even more fundamental to social cognition's impact on this literature. Specifically, this research has focused not simply on the nature of the cognitive structure itself but, even more so, on how that structure influences subsequent information processing, perception, and behavior. These are issues that the "old" approach to stereotypes, with its emphasis on measuring the content of stereotypes, was virtually incapable of addressing.

Stereotypes have been shown to influence information processing in a variety of ways. First, stereotypes affect what information is attended to and encoded. Activation of a stereotype directs attention such that perceivers are more likely to process and encode information that is stereotype consistent than information that is irrelevant to the stereotype (Bodenhausen, 1988; Cohen, 1981; Zadny & Gerard, 1974). Thus, one is more likely to remember that a bowling ball is present in a waitress's apartment than in a librarian's (Cohen, 1981). There is some evidence, however, that information that is inconsistent with a stereotype is more likely to be processed than consistent information (see Rojahn & Pettigrew, 1992; Stangor & McMillan, 1992). Because information that is inconsistent with a stereotype tends to be surprising, it draws attention as the perceiver attempts to account for the inconsistency (Clary & Tesser, 1983; Hastie, 1984; Sherman & Hamilton, in press). If, however, perceivers have limited capacity available to process (e.g., they must remember a multi-digit number while processing information), then they are less likely to engage in resolution of an inconsistency (Macrae, Milne, & Bodenhausen, 1994; Srull, 1981; Stangor & Duan, 1991). Under these conditions, then, subjects are as likely to recall both stereotype-consistent and -inconsistent information.

Second, stereotypes can influence how information is construed or interpreted (Darley & Gross, 1983; Duncan, 1976; Kunda & Sherman-Williams, 1993; Sagar & Schofield, 1980), especially when the information is ambiguous. For example, Sagar and Schofield (1980) presented subjects with several drawings depicting children performing a series of behaviors. The targets' behaviors were ambiguous in that they could be construed to represent either playful or threatening acts (e.g., one child is shown poking another child with the eraser end of his pencil). The target was portrayed as being either white or black. Subjects evaluated the behaviors as being more mean or threatening when performed by black children than when the same behaviors were performed by white children.

Even when behavior is unambiguous, stereotypes can change the standards against which an act is judged (Biernat, Manis, & Nelson, 1991). Activation of a stereotype evokes a set of expectancies about how the members of the group typically behave. For example, men are expected to be more assertive, on average, than are women. If a woman performs a behavior that is relatively assertive for a woman, yet would be considered unassertive for a man, then the behavior itself is likely to be seen as very assertive. Because people believe that men are more assertive than women, a woman's assertive acts are seen to be more discrepant from her group's standard, and therefore as more assertive than the same behaviors performed by a man.

Third, by influencing how information is processed, stereotypes also affect how people behave when interacting with members of other groups (Hamilton, Sherman, & Ruvolo, 1990; Snyder, Tanke, & Berscheid, 1977; Word, Zanna, & Cooper, 1974). When a person is categorized as a member of a group, a stereotype about the group is activated. The stereotype then serves both as a basis of expectancies about how that person is likely to behave and as a guide to how one should behave when interacting with that person.

These effects were demonstrated in research by Word et al. (1974) in which white subjects interviewed white or black confederates. When interviewing black confederates, white subjects conducted shorter interviews, made more speech errors, and made less eye contact. Because the confederates were all trained to act in a uniform fashion, the subjects' abrupt behavior toward the black confederates was likely due to the subjects' negative expectancies about blacks. Unfortunately, this stereotype-driven behavior can then influence the behavior of those with whom that person interacts. Word et al. (1974) showed that the abrupt manner demonstrated toward the black confederates in the first study can affect the quality of an interviewee's performance, regardless of the race of the interviewee. In a second study, confederates were trained to use one of two interviewing styles. They were trained to interview either in the manner exhibited by those interviewing blacks in the first study or in the manner of those who interviewed whites. Subjects who were interviewed in the former fashion were evaluated (by naive observers) more poorly than subjects in the latter condition. Studies such as these demonstrate that a perceiver's stereotype-based behavior can actually elicit behavior that confirms that stereotype, which would then serve to justify the maintenance of that stereotype.

Thus, research in the social cognition tradition has investigated how stereotypes affect the perceiver's selective attention to particular aspects of the information available; how they influence the interpretation of ambiguous information and the inferences one draws from it; how they affect the way that information becomes organized and represented in memory; and how they influence the retrieval of that information and its impact on judgments and behavior. None of these issues was addressed in the literature that Brigham had reviewed in 1971. Yet the number of articles published on these topics in the last 20 years is almost staggering (for reviews, see Hamilton, 1979, 1981; Hamilton & Sherman, 1994; Hamilton et al., 1990; Hamilton & Trolier, 1986; Jones, 1982; Stephan, 1985).

We can summarize these changes as a shift from the investigation of *content* to the investigation of *process*. To put it in other terms, there has been a change from research on *stereotypes*—their content and correlates—to research on *stereotyping*—the processes underlying intergroup perceptions. The important contributions that social cognition has made to research on stereotypes derive, we believe, from its emphasis on the direct investigation of cognitive mediators. For although the literature on stereotypes has always recognized a cognitive component, it is only within the last two decades that research has begun to inform us about how that cognitive component functions to influence intergroup perceptions and behavior. The consequence has been a dramatic change in the nature of our empirical research on stereotypes.

The changes instigated by the social cognition approach have not been limited, however, to the research issues investigated and the nature of experimentation in this literature. For these developments have been accompanied by equally fundamental shifts at the conceptual level, including some basic changes in how we think about stereotypes. Research from the cognitive approach has altered conceptions about how stereotypes are formed, how they are maintained, and, by extension, how they can be altered.

Assumptions About Stereotype Formation

Historically, intergroup perceptions were viewed as deriving from the existing relationships between groups. In fact, there is ample evidence that stereotypes of nations reflect the prevailing political and economic relations between countries and that changes in political alliances can result in dramatic shifts in stereotypic perceptions. For example, Americans' stereotypes of Germans and Japanese became more negative after the beginning of World War II (Dudycha, 1942; Seago, 1947) and improved soon after the end of the conflict (Gilbert, 1951). Competition between groups for scarce economic and political resources was also believed to underlie many negative stereotypes. One study, for instance, documented the case of a small American community where anti-German stereotypes emerged as German immigrants moved to the town and competed with residents for jobs (Dollard, 1938).

Experimental research also provided evidence that intergroup competition could promote negative stereotyping. In the classic field experiment by Sherif and his colleagues (Sherif, Harvey, White, Hood, & Sherif, 1961), 22 twelve-year-old boys were brought separately to a camp in two groups, each group originally being unaware of the existence of the other group. When the groups were brought together to engage in a series of competitive contests, name calling and derogation of the out-group quickly ensued. The formation of negative stereotypes about the out-group was accompanied by increased feelings of solidarity within the in-group, and the negative stereotypes of the out-group proved resistant to change.

These research findings, demonstrating the powerful impact of intergroup competition on evaluations of own and other groups, contributed to the predominant view that stereotypes and intergroup attitudes are based on the conflictual relationships between groups. More recent research, however, has shown that intergroup competition and conflict are not *essential* prerequisites for the development of negative stereotypes. This point has been demonstrated in several ways.

An important series of experiments initiated by Tajfel (see reviews in Brewer, 1979; Diehl, 1990; Tajfel, 1970, 1978) has shown that mere separation into in-groups and out-groups has powerful effects on intergroup perceptions. In this research, subjects were assigned membership in one of two groups, ostensibly based on performance on a trivial, seemingly unimportant task (e.g., whether subjects supposedly underestimated or overestimated the number of dots on a briefly presented card). Thus, there was no prior contact, conflict, or history of hostility between the groups. Nonetheless, these studies showed that mere division into groups—creating social categories in the mind of the subjects—can produce both evaluative differentiation and discriminatory behavior, benefiting the in-group and derogating the out-group, with consequent biases in perception, attribution, and memory. The categorization process itself, then, can lead to stereotyping and discrimination.

Other research has also shown that basic cognitive processes can underlie the formation of group stereotypes, even when no actual group differences exist. For example, as perceivers we tend to focus on information that is perceived to be unusual or infrequent. We notice a woman in a room full of men; we stare at a person with a physical handicap; we pay more attention to infrequent or unusual behaviors.

What are the implications of attending to unusual individuals? First, perceptions of distinctive individuals tend be exaggerated. In one series of studies (see Taylor, 1981), perceptions of individuals who were made salient by their social context were compared with perceptions of the same individuals in contexts where they were not distinctive. For example, in one study subjects listened to an audiotape of a group conversation while viewing photographs of the individuals who supposedly made each comment. The photographs either portrayed the group as being composed of three blacks and three whites or of five whites and one black. Because the conversation was identical in both conditions, there should have been no basis for perceiving the solo black any differently than when he was one of three blacks. However, the same individual was perceived to be more active, talkative, and influential, and was rated more extremely on personality characteristics, when he was the only black in a group of five whites. Thus, attending to individuals who are unusual in a context can lead to more extreme perceptions of that individual, which in turn may lead to biased perceptions of group differences.

Second, the predisposition to attend to unusual information can lead to group perceptions that are unjustified based on available information. Erroneous perceptions of group differences are especially likely to arise when the members of a numerically infrequent group perform infrequent behaviors (Hamilton & Gifford, 1976). For example, most whites in our culture have relatively little contact with blacks. Thus, for most whites, encounters with blacks would be infrequent and thus distinctive. In addition, certain behaviors (e.g., unfriendly behaviors) are also relatively infrequent. The results of a large number of studies indicate that the cooccurrence of two distinctive events is especially distinctive and can influence subsequent group perceptions. These cooccurrences of infrequent events are processed longer than other types of information (Stroessner, Hamilton, & Mackie, 1992), are more accessible in memory (Hamilton, Dugan, & Trolier, 1985; Johnson & Mullen, 1994), and bias group evaluations (see Hamilton & Sherman, 1989; Mullen & Johnson, 1990, for reviews). These effects emerge even though the proportion of undesirable behaviors for the infrequent group is equivalent to that for the majority group. Thus, this extra processing of cooccurring, infrequent information can lead to perception of an illusory correlation between group membership and behavioral desirability. These unjustified differential perceptions of majority and minority groups can provide the basis for the subsequent development of group stereotypes.

In sum, research generated by a social cognition perspective has shown that conflict and competition are not necessary prerequisites for the development of negative stereotypes. Basic cognitive processes by themselves can lead to biased perceptions of group differences. Categorization of others as members of in-groups and out-groups creates differential perceptions of the groups. Differential attention to unusual information can also lead to divergent perceptions of members of different groups, perceptions that are unwarranted based on the available information. These findings were of central importance. Stereotype formation rests on the perception of group differences, as these categorical distinctions must exist before different sets of beliefs (stereotypes) can become associated with them. By generating the initial perception of group differences, these cognitive mechanisms can constitute (or at least contribute to) the foundation for stereotype development.

These analyses produced an enhanced recognition of the important role of basic information processing mechanisms in the creation of group stereotypes. It was no longer assumed that stereotypes of different groups *necessarily* derived from aspects of their intergroup history, or even that they reflected the overgeneralization of some kernel of truth. Basic cognitive processes were shown to play a more central role than was previously presumed.

Assumptions about Stereotype Effects on Thought Processes

This recognition of the central role of information processing mechanisms in stereotype *formation* led to another important change in how contemporary researchers think about stereotyping, specifically, the nature of the thought processes involved in the *use* of stereotypes in intergroup perception. Traditionally, stereotyping was considered to be the product of thought processes that had been biased or distorted by motivational and affective factors. Stereotypes were often described as having three main characteristics —they are gross overgeneralizations, they have little basis in fact, and they are adhered to even in the face of contradictory evidence. Moreover, stereotypes seem to influence perception without conscious intent, thought, or awareness. Such apparent irrationality was assumed to have motivational roots.

The research of the last 20 years, however, indicates that apparent distortions in perception and seemingly irrational judgments do not *necessarily* reflect motivational influences. Rather, such judgments may derive from some rather common biases that are inherent in our normal information processing mechanisms. An earlier section (see Stereotypes and Information Processing) discussed evidence showing that stereotypes can bias the perceiver's attention to elements in the social situation, can influence the inferences, evaluations, and attributions the perceiver draws from that information, and can guide the perceiver's own behavior in social interaction contexts (see Hamilton & Sherman, 1994). Moreover, these processes tend to "reinforce" the stereotype that generated them: we tend to notice features and behaviors that fit with our stereotypic expectancies, and stereotype-based interpretations, inferences, and evaluations are, of course, consistent with that stereotype. This confirmatory trend achieves its ultimate influence in the self-fulfilling prophecy, in which the stereotype holder induces, from an out-group member, behavior that confirms stereotypic expectancies. Through these processes stereotypes can create their own supporting evidence, making them resistant to change.

Our intuitive experience that stereotypes impinge on our perceptions and judgments without intent or awareness seems to imply some unconscious, motivational roots of stereotyping, as noted by many previous authors, including Lippmann (1922) and Allport (1954). Until recently, however, researchers lacked adequate empirical tools to investigate these ideas. Now, conceptual developments and methodological advances in cognitive psychology have provided a basis for reinterpretation of this question. In social cognitive terms, the issue concerns automaticity, and recent research has investigated whether both social categorization and the use of stereotypes are automatic processes (see Bargh, 1989; Brewer, 1988; Devine, 1989; Fiske, 1989; Fiske & Neuberg, 1990).

Some studies have measured the speed with which various category judgments are made (Stroesnner, 1992; Zárate & Smith, 1990). Subjects were shown a number of stimulus person photos and asked to identify the race or gender of each one. The results suggest that categorizations denoting membership in a nonnormative category may be made automatically. For example, judgments of a black male's race are made quickly, and judgments of his gender are made slowly, compared to judgments of white males. These findings provide preliminary evidence suggesting that some kinds of categorization may occur automatically as the stimulus person is perceived. Other studies have presented category-relevant information outside the perceiver's conscious awareness and then determined its effect on subsequent judgments. Some evidence (e.g., Devine, 1989; Macrae et al., 1994) indicates that an activated stereotype, even when activated outside of awareness, can influence how subsequent information is processed. These lines of research are still in an early stage of development. Nevertheless, they do demonstrate that questions of "unconscious" influences of stereotypes can be conceptualized and investigated within a cognitive processing framework.

The cognitive processes that generate the findings discussed in this section are mechanisms that typically facilitate our adjustment to a complex social stimulus environment. These mechanisms may, however, lead us to make oversimplified and even grossly erroneous judgments (cf. Dawes, 1976; Hamilton, 1976). In other words, our cognitive processes can by themselves result in group perceptions that are overgeneralizations, that have little basis in fact, and that are highly resistant to change, and these effects can occur without conscious intent or awareness—the same patterns of "evidence" from which motivational forces were inferred. Moreover, rather than simply assuming that these perceptual manifestations reflect a particular underlying process, research from a social cognition perspective has been successful at pinpointing, and documenting with evidence, the specific cognitive mechanisms that produced the obtained results.

The consequence of this research has been a considerable change in the way we *think about* stereotyping. Perceptions, judgments, and decisions that are seemingly unjustified, given the information available, are no longer routinely viewed as irrational or as by-products of motivational forces. They may simply reflect biases in our normal cognitive functioning.

Stereotype Research in the Context of Social Psychology

There is a final consequence of the social cognition research on stereotypes that we believe is also important. Despite its long history, the study of stereotypes has traditionally been a somewhat isolated topic within social psychology. Textbooks often have a separate chapter on stereotypes and prejudice. And until recently there was little overlap between the conceptual and research questions being debated in the stereotype literature on one hand and the more basic literature on social perception on the other. For example, at the time Brigham (1971) reviewed the state of the stereotype literature, other social perception researchers were concerned with a quite different set of issues, such as the nature of information integration rules in impression formation, the structure of implicit personality theories, and the bases of internal and external attributions. These topics seemingly had little bearing on the kinds of questions that were prominent in the stereotype literature (which we summarized earlier). Hence, research on these two subparts of social perception (perception of persons, perception of groups) had virtually no interface.

This situation has changed considerably in recent years, as the social cognition approach to stereotyping has essentially brought this subject matter into the mainstream of experimental social psychology. Because stereotypes are viewed as cognitive structures, like other cognitive structures, they are assumed to influence information processing in ways that reflect some rather general principles. As a consequence, contemporary research on stereotyping and on social perception more generally share considerable overlap, both of them investigating a variety of questions concerning the relationships among structure, process, representation, and judgment. In fact, investigators' hypotheses about these relationships can be, and often are, tested in experiments on stereotypes, or on impressions, or on the self—which become largely interchangeable research contexts. The consequence is that stereotyping is no longer viewed as a separate, "special interest" topic in social psychology.

In sum, social cognition has changed the way we think about stereotypes and stereotyping, it has changed the kind of questions studied in our research, and it has brought this subject matter into the mainstream of experimental social psychology.

EXTENDING THE SOCIAL COGNITION ANALYSIS

These changes in the stereotype literature brought about by social cognition have clearly had a substantial impact. Yet we think it is important that these developments be viewed in a larger perspective as well. In particular, it would be unwise to lose sight of what we now talk about as the "old" literature on stereotypes. The issues raised and debated in that literature—the issues that Brigham (1971) discussed in his review article—are no less important now than they were then. Can a social cognition analysis be applied to some of the issues that historically were important topics in this literature? Are there new directions in which this approach might be extended, broadening its domain of relevance? In this section we speculate briefly on these possibilities and highlight some new extensions.

Stereotype Measurement

As we noted earlier, for many years research on stereotypes focused on assessing the content of various national and ethnic stereotypes. What does the social cognition literature have to say about procedures for measuring stereotypes?

There has been surprisingly little research on this question. In fact, the emphasis in recent years on questions of process can be viewed, in part, as a reaction against the overriding concern with measuring the content of stereotypes that characterized earlier periods. The consequence is that the procedures typically used to measure stereotypes today do not differ substantially from those that have always been used, namely, subjects make ratings of a group on a series of trait rating scales. These techniques have been criticized because of their susceptibility to biases due to social desirability and self-presentation concerns. Does a social cognition analysis suggest anything new?

A stereotype consists of the beliefs that are associated with a particular social group. The problem then is to determine the content of those beliefs that are most strongly associated with a perceiver's concept of that group. Cognitive research has provided some techniques for investigating the strength of association between a concept and various features. These methodologies—such as the lexical decision task and priming paradigms—involve measuring subjects' reaction times in response to questions regarding pairs of stimulus items, such as a group concept and a trait attribute. The rationale in these paradigms is that the more closely associated two stimulus items are in memory, the faster will be the subject's response. These techniques have the potential advantage of assessing stereotype content, while avoiding the transparency and other inadequacies of self-report measures (see Dovidio, Evans, & Tyler, 1986; Gaertner & McLaughlin, 1983). They are not as quick and easy as questionnaire measures, but in this age of computers their use seems quite feasible for many purposes, even on a relatively large scale. There are interesting possibilities here that need to be explored.

The Content of Stereotypes

A related question concerns the determinants of the specific content of a group stereotype. Stereotypes are often overgeneralizations based on small but real differences between groups. However, groups differ in many ways. Some of the attributes that differentiate one group from other groups will become stereotypic of the group, whereas other such attributes will not. What determines which differences between groups will become central to the content of the stereotype? This is an important question, but it is one that has been relatively neglected by social cognitive research.

The reason for this neglect is clear. The social cognition approach brought about a shift in emphasis from content to process. Given the focus on process, it is assumed that all stereotypes, as cognitive structures, function in the same way and have similar effects on information processing. Consequently, to identify how stereotypes affect information processing, the specific content of the stereotypes used in any given study usually has been of only secondary concern. So in the recent literature, one can find studies of stereotyping not only about significant stereotyped groups, like blacks and women, but also about fraternity members, librarians, and even Groups A and B.

Despite this relative neglect, research has provided some important preliminary evidence concerning the bases of stereotype content. First, it has been suggested that observing members of different groups in different roles can influence the actual content of stereotypes (Eagly & Steffen, 1984). A perceiver may see a disproportionate number of a group's members filling a certain role in a society. The content of the group's stereotype might then derive largely from the requirements of the role that group members typically fill.

For example, one of the authors of this chapter spent a year as a high-school exchange student in the Republic of South Africa. Groups of supervised black prisoners were often seen in local parks and on municipal property performing gardening and maintenance tasks. White prisoners, on the other hand, were not required to perform these tasks in public. What might be the implication of seeing only black prisoners fill these roles? First, one might conclude that blacks are more likely to engage in criminal behavior than whites. Whereas relatively few white prisoners were ever seen in public, black convicts were regularly on display in the community. Second, one might conclude that blacks are particularly adept at tasks such as gardening and maintenance, given that they are seen performing these tasks every day. Thus, the white South Africans' stereotype that blacks are criminally prone and capable primarily of certain types of labor may arise from seeing them on a daily basis in these roles.

The content of a stereotype, then, may be based on the unequal distribution of members of different groups in different social roles. This effect has been interpreted as reflecting perceivers' failure to perform an "intuitive analysis of covariance" (Schaller & O'Brien, 1992). In other words, perceivers view an unequal distribution of group members into social roles and make the inference that a group's members are particularly suited to the role that they fill. They fail to correct for the fact that social role acts as a confounding "third variable," and hence the stereotype appears to be completely justified based on the available information.

Second, there is some evidence that the attributes that best differentiate groups are likely to be the basis of stereotypes (Ford & Stangor, 1992; McCauley & Stitt, 1978). According to this approach, when perceivers encounter members of a group, they ascertain the central tendency and the variability of group members on various attribute dimensions. Members of a group will on average possess a number of different attributes (e.g., they typically watch television, hold full-time jobs, are politically active). Not all of these attributes, however, will likely be the basis for the stereotype of the group. The attributes on which the group is most differentiated from other groups (e.g., they are politically active) are likely to form the content of the stereotype of that group.

This research is reminiscent of the earlier notion that stereotypes reflect a "kernel of truth" regarding actual intergroup differences (Campbell, 1967). Stereotype content may be based on attributes that, in fact, do distinguish members of one group from members of another group. However, the preceding analysis begins to address why only a subset of the traits that characterize group members become central to the stereotype of the group, and suggests that small but significant differences may become overgeneralized; that is, members of a particular group may be quite similar to members of other groups in many respects. The stereotype of that group, however, will reflect the subset of attributes that best differentiates members of the group from other groups. In one sense, then, stereotypes may to some degree capture actual group differences. However, to the extent that the stereotype discourages recognition of the ways that group members are similar to others (i.e., nonmembers), the stereotype promotes a misrepresentation of what group members are actually like.

These issues have not been adequately addressed in past research. It seems to us that these issues might be fertile ground for future research and that the knowledge base provided by a social cognition analysis may be useful in approaching them.

Bases of Categorization

The cognitive approach to stereotyping has emphasized the role of categorization in stereotyping. As we noted earlier, categorization is both ubiquitous and highly functional; without it, we would have difficulty functioning in a world that inundates us with countless pieces of information.

One lingering question concerns what specific information people use in categorizing others. Any person can be categorized in a multitude of ways, based on any observable feature or combination of features. We might notice a person's skin color, facial or vocal characteristics, clothing style, or hair style, or we may observe the types of behaviors that the person performs. Any of this information could provide the basis for categorizing the individual as a member of a certain social group. However, theorists have long argued that we are not likely to categorize others on the basis of all available information (Allport, 1954; Bruner, 1957). Rather, it is likely that "there exists a near infinitude of ways of grouping events in terms of discriminable properties, and we avail ourselves of only a few of these" (Bruner, Goodnow, & Austin, 1956, p. 7).

What determines which categorizations we make? One approach has been to identify a subset of categories, often called "primitive categories" (Bruner, 1957), that are consistently used when perceivers encounter others. Consistent with this notion, two recent models of impression formation (Brewer, 1988; Fiske & Neuberg, 1990) argue that perceivers categorize individuals on certain dimensions so frequently and consistently that categorization occurs "unconsciously and without intention" (Brewer, 1988, p. 6). Gender, race, and age are most commonly cited as "primitive" categories that are routinely and automatically used in perceiving others.

The question remains, however, why these and not other potential categorizations are used so frequently that they become automatized. Why, for instance, are perceivers more likely to automatically categorize others as members of racial groups than to categorize them as members of groups who wear different styles of clothing? Both pieces of information are readily observable, yet it is more likely that we will categorize by race than by clothing style (Brewer, 1988; Fiske & Neuberg, 1990).

One possible answer to this question is offered by Rothbart and Taylor (1992), who propose that categories differ in the degree to which they are perceived to be based on deep, underlying, structural differences such as innate potential or biology. According to these authors, categories that are believed to reflect basic underlying commonalities among group members are assumed to be unalterable. More importantly, these categories are also believed to reflect differences on a variety of other attributes even when, in reality, the category provides little diagnostic information. Therefore, Rothbart and Taylor argue, perceivers are more likely to associate group membership and possession of personality traits when the group is based on biological rather than cultural factors. Features that imply biological differences (such as the features assumed basic to primitive categorization) may have a "special status" and are especially potent. In summary, categories that are believed to be based on biology are likely to be frequently activated and therefore are likely to be used automatically. Rothbart and Taylor's (1992) analysis provides an interesting perspective on why some categories, such as those that are assumed to reflect underlying structural differences, are more likely to be consistently used rather than other potentially informative classifications.

However, not all biologically based categorizations are likely to be made when perceivers encounter others (Smith & Zárate, 1992; Stroessner, 1992; Zárate & Smith, 1990). Even though information regarding, for instance, race, sex, and age is simultaneously available, these three categorizations are not equally likely to be used. Some recent evidence suggests that information that denotes membership in an unusual category receives special processing (Stroessner, 1992; Zárate & Smith, 1990). Within a culture, particular category memberships may be perceived as "normal" or as "default values" (Smith & Zárate, 1992, p. 15). In American culture, for example, being white may be perceived as more "normal" than being black, due to the relative infrequency of blacks in the general population, the historical dominance of whites in our culture, and the prominence of whites in the mass media. For similar reasons (except for numerical infrequency), being female also may be perceived as less "normal" than being male.

Information that denotes membership in a group that differs from the "white male norm" is likely to be salient and receive extra attention, and hence will likely be the basis for categorizing a person. Thus, black males, who differ from the perceived norm in terms of their race but not in terms of their sex, are more likely to be categorized as black than as males, even though both categorizations would be equally appropriate. Black females, who differ from the perceived norm in terms of both their race and their gender, appear to be categorized on both dimensions (Stroessner, 1992).

Thus, there has long been an interest in identifying the bases of categorization. Although an individual can be categorized as a member of an almost limitless number of groups, it is unlikely that perceivers do so. In this section we have summarized some recent conceptual ideas regarding factors that influence the categories likely to be used in intergroup perception. Some of these "new" ideas relate directly to the "old" notion of primitive categories and suggest new ways of thinking about that concept. Still, we lack an adequate framework for understanding the bases of social categorization, an issue that promises to be a focus of continuing research and theoretical debate.

Cognitive and Affective Determinants

One common complaint about the social cognition approach is that, by focusing on cognitive processes, it excludes consideration of other factors that are important for understanding stereotyping. In particular, it is argued that this approach neglects the important role of affective and motivational factors in intergroup perceptions, as well as the interactions of these variables with the cognitive underpinnings on which this literature has focused.

It is true that a lot of the research inspired by the cognitive approach has focused exclusively on cognitive variables, and as an attempt to understand how the *cognitive component* of stereotyping functions, such a strategy seems quite legitimate. However, the approach is not necessarily *limited* to such an exclusive focus. In fact, recently there has been a marked renewal of interest in the role of affective variables, and this new research on the interface of affect and cognition demonstrates the utility of the cognitive approach for understanding the impact of other, noncognitive factors as well (see Mackie & Hamilton, 1993). That is, stereotyping involves biased perception of groups based on the information one processes about those groups or group members. Any independent variable that affects group perceptions probably does so through its impact on the way that information is processed. As a result of the recent emphasis on cognitive processing, we now have available a number of experimental paradigms and methodological tools that can be used to determine exactly how, say, some motivational goal or mood state affects the perceiver's use of the available information. For example, does that motivation or mood state affect the perceiver's attention to selected aspects of the information available? Does it influence how thoroughly that information is processed, the inferences that are drawn, how the information is represented in and retrieved from memory? Does it influence the extent to which judgments are based on the information at hand as opposed to relying on preexisting stereotypic beliefs about the group? These questions are now more amenable to empirical analysis than they were in previous times.

One line of recent research has examined the influence of one's current mood state on how group-relevant information is processed and used by the perceiver. Some studies, for example, have shown that induced affective states can undermine information processing biases that underlie the formation of distinctiveness-based illusory correlations, thereby diminishing the likelihood of unwarranted perceptions of differences between groups (Stroessner et al., 1992). Other studies have shown that mood states (Stroessner & Mackie, 1992, 1993) and anxiety (Wilder, 1993; Wilder & Shapiro, 1989) can reduce the perceiver's sensitivity to differences among members of a group, contributing to the perception of homogeneity among group members. In these ways affect can influence the likelihood that stereotypes will be formed as information about group members is acquired. Other research has shown that the perceiver's arousal (Kim & Baron, 1988) and mood states (Bodenhausen, 1993; Forgas & Moylan, 1991; Mackie et al., 1989) can increase the perceiver's use of preexisting stereotypes in judgments of groups. Thus, the perceiver's current affective state can influence stereotyping in a variety of ways.

Affect can also be generated in the intergroup context itself; that is, whereas stereotype research has typically focused on the attributes inferred about members of specific social and ethnic groups, recent research has shown that these stereotypes have affective components as well, such that perceivers experience important affective reactions to members of various out-groups (Dijker, 1987; Jackson & Sullivan, 1989; Vanman & Miller, 1993). These affective responses can be quite predictive of intergroup attitudes (Esses, Haddock, & Zanna, 1993; Stangor, Sullivan, & Ford, 1991; Stephan & Stephan, 1993). Moreover, the nature of the interpersonal relationship between group members can have affective concomitants that influence the course and outcome of the intergroup interactions (Fiske & Ruscher, 1993; Stephan & Stephan, 1985; Wilder, 1993).

These findings illustrate the variety of ways that affective variables can have effects on perceptions on groups and group members. Most of this research has explicitly examined the interplay of affective and cognitive variables in intergroup contexts, and in doing so it documents the benefits to be gained from an extension of the social cognition approach to studying the role of affect in stereotyping.

Stereotype Change

Finally, there is the question of how we can change stereotypes. This question is as important today as it was before the social cognition approach came along. Despite several recent efforts to pinpoint the factors underlying stereotype change (see Hamilton & Sherman, 1994, for a review), there still are no good answers. In fact, in the last two decades we have learned a lot more about how stereotypes are maintained than about how they can be changed. That is, stereotypes tend to bias information processing in ways that maintain and preserve the existing belief system. People tend to seek and remember information that confirms their stereotypes, and hence at the level of the perceiver's subjective experience, those stereotypes are verified. Thus the use of a stereotype serves to reinforce its apparent usefulness. The clear implication is that changing stereotypes will not be easy.

However, by identifying processes and mechanisms that contribute to stereotyping, the cognitive approach has thereby identified possible targets for efforts aimed at changing stereotypes. That is, if a particular cognitive mechanism is involved in the use of stereotypes, then changing that mechanism somehow ought to reduce the extent to which stereotyping occurs. For example, if categorization in social perception is inevitable, one might try to change the kinds of categories that are used, or to make perceivers cognizant of multiple possible categorizations. If stimulus salience influences perception, then there may be instances in which the salience of some cue can be reduced, or the salience of other cues can be increased. If some groups are novel or distinctive because of their infrequency in the perceiver's experience, then one might try to diminish this distinctiveness through greater exposure to these groups. At this point these are little more than speculations, but the strategy in each case is the same: if a cognitive mechanism is involved in stereotyping, find a way to alter it or to undermine its influence, and the extent of stereotyping should decrease. Little research in the stereotype literature fits this prescription. We believe this strategy would be a worthwhile extension of the social cognition analysis of stereotyping.

A CONCLUDING PERSPECTIVE

In summary, it is clear that social cognition has changed the nature of stereotype research. We can anticipate that this approach will continue to evolve and to open up new lines of inquiry. In addition, we believe that this perspective offers new possibilities for reexamining some of the longstanding, yet still unresolved, issues in the stereotype literature.

Yet, research on stereotypes will not continue to have the singularly cognitive focus that has characterized the last two decades. New issues will arise, and other conceptual analyses will be proposed. As we have indicated, some new directions can already be detected. As the study of stereotypes continues to develop and to change, what will be the enduring legacy of the social cognition approach? What will be social cognition's lasting impact on this literature?

There are a number of ways one could address these questions. One could cite the innovative conceptual breakthroughs generated by adopting this information processing perspective. One could enumerate the many important empirical discoveries fostered by this approach. Either of these responses would provide impressive documentation of social cognition's contribution to this literature (cf. Hamilton & Sherman, 1994). In our view, however, these answers would miss the heart of the matter, for social cognition's influence extends well beyond any specific theoretical positions or empirical findings.

We believe that the enduring legacy of the social cognition approach is that it has focused our attention on issues of processing. Regardless of what future direction the field takes, issues regarding how information is processed and how underlying mechanisms function will be central to the analysis. If one examines how affect, emotion, and motivation influence stereotyping, for example, the analysis will be enriched by specifically investigating how these variables influence attention, encoding, retrieval, or any other mechanism, as group-relevant information is processed. If one takes a sociocultural view, issues of how the culture's beliefs and values become internalized can now be addressed and studied in terms more precise than those utilized earlier. An intrapsychic approach will be able to analyze and investigate more specifically how threats to the ego influence one's attention to various pieces of information or the inferences and elaborations made from it. Although conceptual orientations and terminology may change, the advances of future research will benefit from the emphasis on analyzing underlying processes, which has been central to the social cognition approach.

ACKNOWLEDGMENTS

Preparation of this chapter was supported by NIMH Grant MH 40058. The authors are grateful to Patricia G. Devine, Diane M. Mackie, and Thomas M. Ostrom for their comments on a preliminary version of this chapter.

REFERENCES

Adorno, T. W., Frenkel-Brunswik, E., Levinson, D. J., & Sanford, R. N. (1950). *The authoritarian personality.* New York: Harper.

Allport, G. W. (1954). *The nature of prejudice.* Reading, MA: Addison-Wesley.

Andersen, S. M., & Klatzky, R. L. (1987). Traits and social stereotypes: Levels of categorization in person perception. *Journal of Personality and Social Psychology, 53,* 235–246.

Ashmore, R. D., & Del Boca, F. K. (1981). Conceptual approaches to stereotypes and stereotyping. In D. L. Hamilton (Ed.), *Cognitive processes in stereotyping and intergroup behavior* (pp. 1–35). Hillsdale, NJ: Erlbaum.

Bargh, J. A. (1989). Conditional automaticity: Varieties of automatic influence in social perception and cognition. In J. S. Uleman & J. A. Bargh (Eds.), *Unintended thought* (pp. 3–51). New York: Guilford.

Biernat, M., Manis, M., & Nelson, T. F. (1991). Stereotypes and standards of judgment. *Journal of Personality and Social Psychology, 60,* 485–499.

Bodenhausen, G. V. (1988). Stereotypic biases in social decision making and memory: Testing process models of stereotype use. *Journal of Personality and Social Psychology, 55,* 726–737.

Bodenhausen, G. V. (1993). Emotion, arousal, and stereotypic judgments: A heuristic model of affect and stereotyping. In D. M. Mackie & D. L. Hamilton (Eds.), *Affect, cognition, and stereotyping: Interactive processes in group perception* (pp. 13–37). San Diego, CA: Academic Press.

Brewer, M. B. (1979). In-group bias in the minimal intergroup situation: A cognitive-motivational analysis. *Psychological Bulletin, 86,* 307–324.

Brewer, M. B. (1988). A dual process model of impression formation. In T. K. Srull & R. S. Wyer, Jr. (Eds.), *Advances in social cognition* (Vol. 1, pp. 1–36). Hillsdale, NJ: Erlbaum.

Brewer, M. B., Dull, V., & Lui, L. (1981). Perceptions of the elderly: Stereotypes and prototypes. *Journal of Personality and Social Psychology, 41,* 656–670.

Brigham, J. C. (1971). Ethnic stereotypes. *Psychological Bulletin, 76,* 15–33.

Bruner, J. S. (1957). On perceptual readiness. *Psychological Review, 64,* 123–152.

Bruner, J. S., Goodnow, J. J., & Austin, G. A. (1956). *A study of thinking.* New York: Wiley.

Campbell, D. T. (1967). Stereotypes and the perception of group differences. *American Psychologist, 22,* 817–829.

Cantor, N., & Mischel, W. (1979). Prototypes in person perception. In L. Berkowitz (Ed.), *Advances in experimental social psychology* (Vol. 12, pp. 3–52). New York: Academic Press.

Cauthen, N. R., Robinson, I. E., & Krauss, H. H. (1971). Stereotypes: A review of the literature 1926–1968. *The Journal of Social Psychology, 84,* 103–125.

Clary, E. G., & Tesser, A. (1983). Reactions to unexpected events: The naive scientist and interpretive activity. *Personality and Social Psychology Bulletin, 9,* 609–620.

Cohen, C. E. (1981). Person categories and social perception: Testing some boundaries of the processing effects of prior knowledge. *Journal of Personality and Social Psychology, 40,* 441–452.

Darley, J. M., & Gross, P. H. (1983). A hypothesis-confirming bias in labeling effects. *Journal of Personality and Social Psychology, 44,* 20–33.

Dawes, R. M. (1976). Shallow psychology. In J. S. Carroll & J. W. Payne (Eds.), *Cognition and social behavior* (pp. 3–11). Hillsdale, NJ: Erlbaum.

Devine, P. G. (1989). Stereotypes and prejudice: Their automatic and controlled components. *Journal of Personality and Social Psychology, 56,* 5–18.

Devine, P. G., & Baker, S. M. (1991). Measurement of racial stereotype subtyping. *Personality and Social Psychology Bulletin, 17,* 44–50.

Diehl, M. (1990). The minimal group paradigm: Theoretical explanations and empirical findings. In W. Stroebe & M. Hewstone (Eds.), *European Review of Social Psychology* (Vol. 1, pp. 263–292). Chichester, England: Wiley.

Dijker, A. G. M. (1987). Emotional reactions to ethnic minorities. *European Journal of Social Psychology, 17,* 305–326.

Dollard, J. (1938). Hostility and fear in social life. *Social Forces, 17,* 15–26.

Dovidio, J. F., Evans, N., & Tyler, R. B. (1986). Racial stereotypes: The contents of their cognitive representations. *Journal of Experimental Social Psychology, 22,* 22–37.

Dudycha, G. J. (1942). The attitude of college students toward war and the Germans before and during the second world war. *Journal of Social Psychology, 15,* 317–324.

Duncan, B. L. (1976). Differential social perception and attribution of intergroup violence: Testing the lower limits of stereotyping of blacks. *Journal of Personality and Social Psychology, 34,* 590–598.

Eagly, A. H., & Steffen, V. J. (1984). Gender stereotypes stem from the distribution of women and men into social roles. *Journal of Personality and Social Psychology, 46,* 735–754.

Ehrlich, H. J. (1973). *The social psychology of prejudice.* New York: Wiley.

Esses, V. M., Haddock, G., & Zanna, M. P. (1993). Values, stereotypes, and emotions as determinants of intergroup attitudes. In D. M. Mackie & D. L. Hamilton (Eds.), *Affect, cognition, and stereotyping: Interactive processes in group perception* (pp. 137–166). San Diego, CA: Academic Press.

Fiske, S. T. (1989). Examining the role of intent: Toward understanding it's role in stereotyping and prejudice. In J. S. Uleman & J. A. Bargh (Eds.), *Unintended thought* (pp. 253–283). New York: Guilford.

Fiske, S. T., & Neuberg, S. L. (1990). A continuum of impression formation, from category-based to individuating processes: Influences of information and motivation on attention and interpretation. In M. P. Zanna (Ed.), *Advances in experimental social psychology* (Vol. 23, pp. 1–74). New York: Academic Press.

Fiske, S. T., & Ruscher, J. B. (1993). Negative interdependence and prejudice: Whence the affect? In D. M. Mackie & D. L. Hamilton (Eds.), *Affect, cognition, and stereotyping: Interactive processes in group perception* (pp. 239–268). San Diego, CA: Academic Press.

Ford, T. E., & Stangor, C. (1992). The role of diagnosticity in stereotype formation: Perceiving group means and variances. *Journal of Personality and Social Psychology, 63,* 356–367.

Forgas, J. P., & Moylan, S. J. (1991). Affective biases in stereotype judgments. *Cognition and Emotion, 5,* 379–395.

Gaertner, S. L., & McLaughlin, J. P. (1983). Racial stereotypes: Associations and ascriptions of positive and negative characteristics. *Social Psychology Quarterly, 46,* 23–30.

Gardner, R. C. (1973). Ethnic stereotypes: The traditional approach, a new look. *The Canadian Psychologist, 14,* 133–148.

Gilbert, G. M. (1951). Stereotype persistence and change among college students. *Journal of Abnormal and Social Psychology, 46,* 245–254.

Hamilton, D. L. (1976). Cognitive biases in the perception of social groups. In J. S. Carroll & J. W. Payne (Eds.), *Cognition and social behavior* (pp. 81–93). Hillsdale, NJ: Erlbaum.

Hamilton, D. L. (1979). A cognitive-attributional analysis of stereotyping. In L. Berkowitz (Ed.), *Advances in experimental social psychology* (Vol. 12, pp. 53–84). New York: Academic Press.

Hamilton, D. L. (Ed.). (1981). *Cognitive processes in stereotyping and intergroup behavior.* Hillsdale, NJ: Erlbaum.

Hamilton, D. L., & Gifford, R. K. (1976). Illusory correlation in interpersonal perception: A cognitive basis of stereotypic judgments. *Journal of Experimental Social Psychology, 12,* 392–407.

Hamilton, D. L., & Sherman, J. W. (1994). Stereotypes. In R. S. Wyer, Jr., & T. K. Srull (Eds.), *Handbook of social cognition* (2nd ed.). Hillsdale, NJ: Erlbaum.

Hamilton, D. L., & Sherman, S. J. (1989). Illusory correlations: Implications for stereotype theory and research. In D. Bar-Tal, C. F. Graumann, A. W. Kruglanski, & W. Stroebe (Eds.), *Stereotypes and prejudice: Changing conceptions* (pp. 59–82). New York: Springer-Verlag.

Hamilton, D. L., & Trolier, T. K. (1986). Stereotypes and stereotyping: An overview of the cognitive approach. In J. F. Dovidio & S. L. Gaertner (Eds.), *Prejudice, discrimination, and racism* (pp. 127–163). Orlando FL: Academic Press.

Hamilton, D. L., Dugan, P. M., & Trolier, T. K. (1985). The formation of stereotypic beliefs: Further evidence for distinctiveness-based illusory correlations. *Journal of Personality and Social Psychology, 48,* 5–17.

Hamilton, D. L., Sherman, S. J., & Ruvolo, C. M. (1990). Stereotype-based expectancies: Effects on information processing and social behavior. *Journal of Social Issues, 46(2),* 35–60.

Hastie, R. (1984). Causes and effects of causal attribution. *Journal of Personality and Social Psychology, 46,* 44–56.

Jackson, L. A., & Sullivan, L. A. (1989). Cognition and affect in evaluations of stereotyped group members. *The Journal of Social Psychology, 129,* 659–672.

Johnson, C., & Mullen, B. (1994). Evidence for the accessibility of paired distinctiveness in distinctiveness-based illusory correlation in stereotyping. *Personality and Social Psychology Bulletin, 20,* 65–70.

Jones, R. A. (1982). Perceiving other people: Stereotyping as a process of social cognition. In A. G. Miller (Ed.), *In the eye of the beholder: Contemporary issues in stereotyping* (pp. 41–91). New York: Praeger.

Karlins, M., Coffman, T. L., & Walters, G. (1969). On the fading of social stereotypes: Studies in three generations of college students. *Journal of Personality and Social Psychology, 13,* 1–16.

Katz, D., & Braly, K. (1933). Racial stereotypes in one hundred college students. *Journal of Abnormal and Social Psychology, 28,* 280–290.

Kim, H-S., & Baron, R. S. (1988). Exercise and the illusory correlation: Does arousal heighten stereotypic processing? *Journal of Experimental Social Psychology, 24,* 366–380.

Kunda, Z., & Sherman-Williams, B. (1993). Stereotypes and the construal of individuating information. *Personality and Social Psychology Bulletin, 19,* 90–99.

Linville, P. W., Fischer, G. W., & Salovey, P. (1989). Perceived distributions of the characteristics of in-group and out-group members: Empirical evidence and a computer simulation. *Journal of Personality and Social Psychology, 57,* 165–188.

Lippman, W. (1922). *Public Opinion.* New York: MacMillan.

McCauley, C., & Stitt, C. L. (1978). An individual and quantitative measure of stereotypes. *Journal of Personality and Social Psychology, 39,* 929–940.

Mackie, D. M., & Hamilton, D. L. (1993). *Affect, cognition, and stereotyping: Interactive processes in group perception.* San Diego, CA: Academic Press.

Mackie, D. M., Hamilton, D. L., Schroth, H. A., Carlisle, C. J., Gersho, B. F., Meneses, L. M., Nedler, B. F., & Reichel, L. D. (1989). The effects of induced mood on illusory correlations. *Journal of Experimental Social Psychology, 25,* 524–544.

Macrae, C. N., Milne, A. B., & Bodenhausen, G. V. (1994). Stereotypes as energy-saving devices: A peek inside the cognitive toolbox. *Journal of Personality and Social Psychology, 66,* 37–47.

Miller, A. G. (1982). Historical and contemporary perspectives on stereotyping. In A. G. Miller (Ed.), *In the eye of the beholder: Contemporary issues in stereotypes.* New York: Praeger.

Mullen, B., & Johnson, C. (1990). Distinctiveness-based illusory correlations and stereotyping: A meta-analytic integration. *British Journal of Social Psychology, 29,* 11–28.

Park, B., & Hastie, R. (1987). Perception of variability in category development: Instance-versus abstraction-based stereotypes. *Journal of Personality and Social Psychology, 53,* 621–635.

Rojahn, K., & Pettigrew, T. F. (1992). Memory for schema-relevant information: A meta-analytic resolution. *British Journal of Social Psychology, 31,* 81–110.

Rosch, E. H. (1978). Principles of categorization. In E. Rosch & B. B. Lloyd (Eds.), *Cognition and categorization.* Hillsdale, NJ: Erlbaum.

Rothbart, M., & Taylor, M. (1992). Category labels and social reality: Do we view social categories as natural kinds? In G. R. Semin & K. Fiedler (Eds.), *Language, interactions, and social cognition* (pp. 11–36). London: Sage.

Sagar, H. A., & Schofield, J. W. (1980). Racial and behavioral cues in black and white children's perceptions of ambiguously aggressive acts. *Journal of Personality and Social Psychology, 39,* 590–598.

Schaller, M., and O'Brien, M. (1992). "Intuitive analysis of covariance" and group stereotype formation. *Personality and Social Psychology Bulletin, 18,* 776–785.

Seago, D. W. (1947). Before Pearl Harbor and after. *Journal of Psychology, 23,* 55–63.

Sherif, M., Harvey, O. J., White, B. J., Hood, W. R., & Sherif, C. W. (1961). *Intergroup conflict and cooperation: The Robbers' Cave experiment.* Norman, OK: University of Oklahoma Press.

Sherman, J. W., & Hamilton, D. L. (in press). On the formation of interitem links in person memory. *Journal of Experimental Social Psychology.*

Sigall, H., & Page, R. (1971). Current stereotypes: A little fading, a little faking. *Journal of Personality and Social Psychology, 18,* 247–255.

Smith, E. R. (1990). Content and process specificity in the effects of prior experiences. In T. K. Srull, & R. S. Wyer, Jr. (Eds.), *Advances in social cognition* (Vol. 3, pp. 1–59). Hillsdale, NJ: Erlbaum.

Smith, E. R., & Zárate, M. A. (1992). Exemplar-based model of social judgment. *Psychological Review, 99,* 3–21.

Snyder, M., Tanke, E. D., & Berscheid, E. (1977). Social perception and interpersonal behavior: On the self-fulfilling nature of social stereotypes. *Journal of Personality and Social Psychology, 35,* 656–666.

Srull, T. K. (1981). Person memory: Some tests of associative storage and retrieval models. *Journal of Experimental Psychology: Human Learning and Memory, 7,* 440–462.

Stangor, C., & Duan, C. (1991). Effects of multiple task demands upon memory for information about social groups. *Journal of Experimental Social Psychology, 27,* 357–378.

Stangor, C., & McMillan, D. (1992). Memory for expectancy-congruent and expectancy-incongruent information: A review of the social and social developmental literatures. *Psychological Bulletin, 111,* 42–61.

Stangor, C., Sullivan, L. A., & Ford, T. E. (1991). Affective and cognitive determinants of prejudice. *Social Cognition, 9,* 359–380.

Stephan, W. G. (1985). Intergroup relations. In G. Lindzey & E. Aronson (Eds.), *Handbook of social psychology* (3rd ed.) (Vol. 2). New York: Random House.

Stephan, W. G., & Stephan, C. W. (1985). Intergroup anxiety. *Journal of Social Issues, 41(3),* 157–175.

Stephan, W. G., & Stephan, C. W. (1993). Cognition and affect in stereotyping: Parallel interactive networks. In D. M. Mackie & D. L. Hamilton (Eds.), *Affect, cognition, and stereotyping: Interactive processes in group perception* (pp. 111–136). San Diego, CA: Academic Press.

Stroessner, S. J. (1992). *Target-based determinants of social categorization: Extension of the "white male norm" hypothesis.* Unpublished Doctoral dissertation, University of California, Santa Barbara.

Stroessner, S. J., & Mackie, D. M. (1992). The impact of induced affect on the perception of variability in social groups. *Personality and Social Psychology Bulletin, 18,* 546–554.

Stroessner, S. J., & Mackie, D. M. (1993). Affect and perceived group variability: Implications for stereotyping and prejudice. In D. M. Mackie & D. L. Hamilton (Eds.), *Affect, cognition, and stereotyping: Interactive processes in group perception* (pp. 63–86). San Diego, CA: Academic Press.

Stroessner, S. J., Hamilton, D. L., & Mackie, D. M. (1992). Affect and stereotyping: The effect of induced mood on distinctiveness-based illusory correlations. *Journal of Personality and Social Psychology, 62,* 564–576.

Tajfel, H. (1970). Experiments in intergroup discrimination. *Scientific American, 223(5),* 96–102.

Tajfel, H. (1978). *Differentiation between social groups: Studies in the social psychology of intergroup relations.* London: Academic Press.

Taylor, S. E. (1981). A categorization approach to stereotyping. In D. L. Hamilton (Ed.), *Cognitive processes in stereotyping and intergroup behavior* (pp. 88–114). Hillsdale, NJ: Erlbaum.

Vanman, E. J., & Miller, N. (1993). Applications of emotion theory and research to stereotyping and intergroup relations. In D. M. Mackie & D. L. Hamilton (Eds.), *Affect, cognition, and stereotyping: Interactive processes in group perception* (pp. 213–238). San Diego, CA: Academic Press.

Vinacke, W. E. (1957). Stereotypes as social concepts. *Journal of Social Psychology, 46,* 229–243.

Wilder, D. A. (1993). The role of anxiety in facilitating stereotypic judgment of outgroup behavior. In D. M. Mackie & D. L. Hamilton (Eds.), *Affect, cognition, and stereotyping: Interactive processes in group perception* (pp. 87–109). San Diego, CA: Academic Press.

Wilder, D. A., & Shapiro, P. (1989). Role of competition-induced anxiety in limiting the beneficial impact of positive behavior by an out-group member. *Journal of Personality and Social Psychology, 56,* 60–69.

Word, C. O., Zanna, M. P., & Cooper, J. (1974). The nonverbal mediation of self-fulfilling prophecies in interracial interaction. *Journal of Experimental Social Psychology, 10,* 109–120.

Zadny, J., & Gerard, H. B. (1974). Attributed intentions and informational selectivity. *Journal of Experimental Social Psychology, 10,* 34–52.

Zárate, M. A., & Smith, E. R. (1990). Person categorization and stereotyping. *Social Cognition, 8,* 161–185.

10

Prejudice and Prejudice Reduction: Classic Challenges, Contemporary Approaches

Margo J. Monteith
Julia R. Zuwerink
Patricia G. Devine

Over the years, many psychologists, sociologists, anthropologists, and historians have attempted to specify the factors that contribute to the development of negative intergroup attitudes, often with the underlying goal of understanding how such attitudes might be changed. Interest in these issues, however, has not been limited to intellectual exercises of social scientists. Indeed, intergroup prejudice has been a concern of politicians, legislators, educators, and lay persons.

In this chapter we focus on social psychological research on prejudice. As reviews of the literature reveal, specifying the origins of prejudice has proved to be a vexing problem, and efforts to reduce prejudice have met with only mixed success (see Duckitt, 1992a,b; Harding, Kutner, Proshansky, & Chein, 1954; Katz, 1976; Stephan, 1985). The prominent trends in the history of social psychological research on prejudice include the measurement of ethnic attitudes and prejudice during the 1920s and 1930s, the study of attitude change during the 1950s, and investigations of discrimination (following the "social problems approach") during the 1950s through the 1960s. Throughout these decades, major efforts were made to propose various individual- and societal-level theories concerning the origins of prejudice, and investigators attempted to identify strategies for reducing prejudice. Around the 1960s, cognitive approaches to understanding prejudice emerged and grew (see Ashmore & Del Boca, 1981; Billig, 1985) until, at present, much of the work in the area of prejudice draws heavily upon social cognition analyses.

Our goal in this chapter is to explore the contributions of social cognition to understanding issues related to prejudice. As evidenced in the chapters comprising this volume, social cognition has given social psychologists studying a variety of phenomena new ways to address classic theoretical and empirical controversies. Furthermore, application of the social cognition approach has allowed researchers in many areas to ask questions of a fundamentally different quality than was possible previously. This conceptual shift is most commonly characterized as representing a change from content-oriented to process-oriented research. The emphasis on process has arisen because social cognition provides the tools for examining the cognitive mediators of social behavior. In so doing, the social cognition approach has provided a broader understanding of the phenomena of interest to social psychologists.

In defining the scope of this chapter, we chose to focus on theoretical accounts of the origins of prejudice and how such work has been related to understanding and promoting the prejudice reduction process. The work that we examine derives from individual-level (as opposed to societal-level) theories of prejudice because most contemporary social psychological theories focus on individual-level processes involved in prejudice, and because change strategies often focus on the individual. Our central thesis is that attempts to understand how cognitive processes contribute to or underlie prejudice have provided the insight necessary for identifying promising strategies for reducing prejudice.

CLASSIC THEORIES AND CHANGE STRATEGIES: AN OVERVIEW

The main issue addressed in older theories of prejudice concerned the etiology of highly prejudiced attitudes, thoughts, and behaviors. For example, according to one classic approach, social learning, part of a child's learning experiences involves differentiating between various social groups and acquiring positive or negative evaluations of the groups. The child's parents, peers, schools, and the mass media all can serve as influential agents in the development of prejudiced attitudes, thoughts, and behaviors (Allport, 1954; Ashmore, 1970; Ashmore & Del Boca, 1976; Katz, 1976; Pettigrew, 1958; Proshansky, 1966). Such prejudiced responses need not be transmitted through explicit teachings. They might be more or less subtly reinforced by socializing agents, children may imitate others' prejudiced attitudes, or prejudiced attitudes may be learned by association. The data supporting the social learning perspective are striking (Ashmore, 1970; Katz, 1976). For example, Goodman (1952) found that children at ages 3 to

4 already possess racial awareness, and 25% of 4-year-olds expressed strong racial attitudes.

The impact of social learning on the development of prejudiced attitudes figures importantly in some contemporary theories of prejudice (e.g., Devine, 1989). An interesting implication of the perspective concerns possible strategies for reducing prejudice. Specifically, one might reason that prejudiced attitudes acquired through social learning can be changed by learning new, more positive attitudes. However, social cognitive analyses of this problem suggest that the cliche "easier said than done" is quite apropos; that is, as discussed in greater detail later, changing prejudiced attitudes does not necessarily serve to eliminate people's prejudiced responses (Devine, 1989; Dovidio & Gaertner, 1986).

A second classic approach to understanding the origins of prejudice relies on analyses of personality processes. The most widely cited and influential personality explanation for prejudice is Adorno and his colleagues' work on the authoritarian personality (Adorno, Frenkel-Brunswik, Levinson, & Sanford, 1950). According to this view, prejudice is rooted in psychopathology. Specifically, harsh parental child-rearing practices produce individuals with personality characteristics that make them especially prone to developing and maintaining prejudiced attitudes. The authoritarian personality is characterized by, for example, an obdurate obedience to conventional and conservative values, a strong tendency to make categorical (e.g., "us" vs. "them") distinctions, and feelings of generalized hostility. Adorno et al.'s original findings, as well as more recent investigations (Altemeyer, 1981; Weigel & Howes, 1985), revealed that authoritarianism does predict prejudice toward a variety of target groups.

Several other personality-focused explanations, stimulated by Freudian psychoanalytic theory, maintain that intrapsychic factors or personality conflicts give rise to prejudice (see Ashmore & Del Boca, 1976; Harding et al., 1954). For example, prejudiced people supposedly project their negative tendencies onto out-group members in order to protect themselves from anxiety-arousing id or ego impulses, which sets the stage for degradation of out-groups. Alternatively, the displacement explanation (or scapegoat theory) of prejudice maintains that prejudiced people repress their everyday frustrations, thus building up aggression that subsequently is displaced onto out-groups.

Although Adorno's work on the authoritarian personality and more psychodynamic orientations have had a pervasive impact on thinking about prejudice, they have not escaped criticism (see Altemeyer, 1981). Foremost among the concerns is the lack of explanatory power of the theories; that is, they appear to explain prejudiced attitudes among only a fairly small proportion of the population of highly prejudiced persons. Other criticisms have focused on methodological concerns, such as response bias in the measurement of authoritarianism. Despite these criticisms, the goal of this perspective—to explain how and why individuals develop highly prejudiced attitudes, thoughts, and behaviors—is still an important one. However, it receives relatively little attention in contemporary work on prejudice (but see Altemeyer, 1981, 1988).

In contrast to the emphasis on individuals with deeply entrenched and highly prejudiced attitudes, other classic work has focused on the intrapersonal psychological processes contributing to prejudicial biases among *all* people. According to this perspective, the tendency to categorize and stereotype people arises from the need to simplify one's understanding of the complex social environment (see Hamilton, 1981a; and Chapters 9 and 11, this volume for reviews of the relevant literature). Thus, to the extent that prejudiced feelings, thoughts, and behaviors follow from such categorization and stereotyping tendencies, prejudice is thought to result from *normal* cognitive processes. The seminal contributions to this cognitive perspective were made by Allport (1954) and Tajfel (1969), although similar ideas were expressed as early as 1922 by Lippman. Such work constitutes the historical precursors to modern analyses of prejudice using the social cognition approach.

One might imagine that the various psychological processes underlying prejudice that classic theorists identified would provide fruitful ground for generating prejudice reduction techniques. However, the tactics for promoting change that emerged during these early years were mostly atheoretical in nature. This fact is demonstrated well in the major reviews of the prejudice literature: researchers organized their coverage of change around "the various change-producing experiences that have been investigated rather than around the various psychological processes that were presumably at work" (Harding et al., 1954, p. 1046; see also Stephan, 1985). As a consequence of this nearly complete divorce between theories and change strategies, prejudice reduction techniques seemed to have a "hit-or-miss" quality about them; the processes responsible for the techniques' successes and failures often were—and remain—unknown.

For example, propaganda in the form of oral presentations, written materials, and movies has met with variable success in changing prejudiced attitudes (see Harding et al., 1954; Stephan, 1985; Williams, 1947). Likewise, the notion that specific school courses and, more generally, college education will have liberalizing effects on students' intergroup attitudes has failed to find support in as many studies as it has gained support (see Harding et al., 1954; Stephan, 1985). Identifying the reasons for the variable success of these change strategies is occasionally difficult because of inherent differences between the studies or because of methodological shortcomings of particular studies. However, the greatest impediment to understanding why the techniques worked only some of the time is the failure to identify theoretically relevant processes that either facilitated or hindered attitude change.

The same problem is found in prejudice reduction approaches that are based on therapeutic and group interaction techniques (see Stephan, 1985). For example, client-centered counseling, sensitivity training, therapeutic techniques, and systematic desensitization have proved somewhat successful in reducing prejudiced attitudes. However, the atheoretical context of this research leaves us unsure about what types of people at which stages of prejudice reduction are most likely to benefit from the techniques (Stephan, 1985). And the potential risks of inappropriately applying the techniques are great. For example, Myers and Bishop (1970) found that discussion groups actually increased prejudice among people holding highly prejudiced attitudes.

Other more rigorously investigated change strategies also have suffered from a "hit-or-miss" quality, as is the case in the literature on the effects of intergroup contact on reducing prejudice (summarized in Chapter 11, this volume; see also Amir, 1969, 1976; Cook, 1985; Harding et al., 1954; Stephan, 1985; Williams, 1977). Although intergroup contact proves to be a moderately successful tactic, several "favorable" conditions must first be met. Some of these conditions include pleasant interaction that involves cooperation, the pursuit of common or superordinate goals, intimacy, equal status, and the support of an outside authority figure. Although this list is representative, it is not exhaustive. As Stephan concluded, "The complexity of this literature makes it difficult to draw firm conclusions about what aspects of cooperative intergroup contact promote favorable relations" (1985, p. 643; see also Gaertner & Dovidio, 1986). In other words, we still do not have a good understanding of the processes involved in prejudice reduction via intergroup contact.

A final classic strategy for changing highly prejudiced attitudes is Rokeach's (1973) confrontation technique. An influential impetus for Rokeach's work was Gunner Myrdal's (1944) characterization of the American Dilemma. According to Myrdal, many white Americans, who are committed to the general egalitarian tenants of the "American Creed," but who simultaneously have specific prejudiced tendencies, experience an internal moral conflict. Rokeach reasoned that self-dissatisfaction should arise when people are encouraged to realize that their egalitarian self-conception is inconsistent with their prejudiced values, attitudes, and/or behaviors. This self-dissatisfaction should then motivate individuals to change the prejudiced aspects of their belief system and behaviors to be more in line with their egalitarian self-image.

Several experiments in which college instructors encouraged their students to recognize prejudice-related inconsistencies provided supported for Rokeach's analysis (see Rokeach, 1973). For example, some subjects initially ascribed little personal importance to the values "equality" and "freedom." However, these subjects viewed equality and freedom as very important after they were confronted with the inconsistency between their low rankings of the values and their views of themselves as fair, tolerant, democratic, and the like. This value change was eventually followed by attitude change, such that subjects revised their anti-Black attitudes to be consistent with their nonprejudiced values. Moreover, several behavioral measures also provided evidence for positive change as a consequence of the confrontation technique. In addition to these encouraging findings, Rokeach's program of research is impressive because it underscores the theoretical processes involved in changing prejudiced attitudes. In this respect, the work is unique among the classic prejudice reduction techniques.

Summary Remarks

Two key summary points can be made in connection with our (representative but nonexhaustive) consideration of classic issues in the study of prejudice. First, it is generally true that both theories of prejudice and suggested strategies for reducing it were concerned with fairly high prejudiced feelings, thoughts, and behaviors. An exception is the early cognitive analyses of prejudice, which emphasized the idea that people naturally develop biases toward out-group members (e.g., more favorable evaluation of in-group than out-group members; see Chapter 11, this volume). Although unquestionably negative, these biases are different from the extreme intolerance and bigotry of highly prejudiced persons. Second, even though several theoretical explanations have been advanced concerning the origins of prejudice, there has been a paucity of research that uses these theories in order to identify the processes involved in the reduction of prejudice. Without regard to process, classic prejudice reduction strategies seem to have a "hit-or-miss" quality to them. An exception is Rokeach's (1973) innovative work, which did not build on the classic theories of prejudice but, nonetheless, posited specific processes that underlie the modification of prejudiced attitudes.

CONTEMPORARY ANALYSES OF PREJUDICE

Contemporary analyses of prejudice differ substantially from the majority of the older work in terms of the forms of prejudice investigated. Rather than focusing on fairly blatant and extreme intolerance and bigotry, many researchers today focus on people who hold markedly less prejudiced attitudes, but continue to manifest subtle or covert response biases. The coexistence of nonprejudiced attitudes and prejudiced responses creates internal conflict within individuals (see Allport, 1954; Myrdal, 1944; Rokeach, 1973). In our opinion, contemporary work also differs from the older literature in that its theories are more precise and, therefore, better able to specify the processes involved in the reduction of prejudice. These characteristics equip current theories with considerable potential for understanding what strategies should successfully promote prejudice reduction.

However, we would argue that the change in focus from blatant to more subtle forms of prejudice is less related to the advent of the social cognition approach than it is to historical and cultural changes. The focus and the kinds of questions asked by social scientists are often shaped by changes in the social climate, and this observation is most certainly true in the history of social psychological research on prejudice (Duckitt, 1992b). For example, researchers became considerably more concerned with the evils of prejudice following World War II than they had been prior to the war. Further, after the Civil Rights legislation of the 1960s and the advent of the women's movement, expressing prejudiced attitudes and engaging in prejudiced behaviors became less socially acceptable. These historical events served to transform America's cultural framework, and changes in many individuals' attitudes followed suit (Dovidio & Gaertner, 1986). For example, whites' current attitudes toward Blacks are substantially less negative than they have been in the past (Schuman, Steeh, & Bobo, 1985).

Despite the decline of old-fashioned prejudiced *attitudes,* prejudiced tendencies apparently have evolved into a modern form in which subtle, prejudiced *responses* persist (see Crosby, Bromley, & Saxe, 1980; Devine, 1989; Gaertner & Dovidio, 1986; McConahay, 1986). Current prejudice theorists are interested in understanding why these subtle, prejudiced responses persist, what implications they have for individuals' psychological states, and how such responses might be eliminated.

Although the advent of social cognition is not, in our opinion, the primary catalyst for the change of interests among prejudice theorists (i.e., from blatant to more subtle forms of prejudice), it certainly has facilitated the change. Social cognition analyses unquestionably have afforded a great deal of theoretical precision with regard to the processes involved in the formation and expression of subtle forms of prejudice. With such precision, it becomes possible to draw from the theoretical work in order to propose strategies for reducing modern forms of prejudice. We turn now to an examination of the contemporary work on prejudice, with two central questions in mind: (1) What processes give rise to various modern forms of prejudice? and (2) What implications does this have for promoting change?

Sources of Modern Forms of Prejudice

A premise of many of the contemporary models of prejudice is that the persistence of prejudiced responses, coupled with more egalitarian and less prejudiced attitudes, creates a self-threatening state of conflict within many individuals (Devine, Monteith, Zuwerink, & Elliot, 1991; Gaertner & Dovidio, 1986; Katz, Wackenhut, & Hass, 1986). Before turning to these models, it is important to note that the implications of this conflict were spelled out by Allport (1954) many years ago in his writings on "inner conflict" (see also Myrdal, 1944). Allport suggested that the conflict can be handled in a number of ways. Prejudiced tendencies can be repressed, thus protecting the self from inner conflict and feelings of compunction (i.e., guilt and self-criticism). Defensive rationalizations might be used that support one's prejudiced attitudes, thereby eliminating the conflict. Or, compromise solutions may be adopted in which the individual alternates between nonprejudiced and prejudiced expressions. Finally, Allport argued that some people will view repression, rationalization, and compromising as inadequate solutions. These people instead attempt to achieve a "true resolution" of their conflict by gradually eliminating their prejudiced tendencies.

Although Allport's work foreshadows the basic concerns and theoretical frameworks of contemporary researchers in the area of prejudice, he provided little more than anecdotal evidence to support his ideas. For example, no empirical evidence of the various processes that produce inner conflict was provided. Although subsequent, related research efforts attempted to demonstrate that compunction was experienced when low-prejudiced individuals engaged in prejudiced responses (Campbell, 1961; Friedrichs, 1959; Westie, 1965), the results were clouded by methodological shortcomings (see Devine et al., 1991). Finally, no empirical evidence documented the various strategies that people might use to reduce their inner conflict.

Nevertheless, the primary aim of various contemporary theories of prejudice has been to identify and empirically investigate these issues involving individual-level conflict and ambivalence. This work is much more specific about the processes giving rise to inner conflict and about the implications of these processes for reducing the conflict. Furthermore, a number of contemporary theories have direct implications for understanding how the occurrence of prejudiced responses can be reduced.

The contemporary theories that we summarize here utilize the social cognition approach in order to address these issues.[1] According to Sherman, Judd, and Park (1989), a defining characteristic of the social cognition approach is that it emphasizes the type of social information that is stored in memory. Moreover, Sherman et al. note that this approach underscores the impact of stored information on the judgments and choices that people make, the behaviors in which people engage, and the way in which they process information. Consideration of such issues in the context of studying prejudice has been extremely enlightening. Specifically, the conflict that characterizes modern forms of prejudice is often rooted in the conflicting types of

[1]Because of our focus on frameworks that use the social cognition approach, certain theories are not discussed herein. Most notably, we do not discuss the theory of symbolic racism (e.g., Kinder & Sears, 1981) and the theory of modern racism (e.g., McConahay, 1986).

social information that are represented in memory. Further, the type of conflict experienced helps to explain the persistence of prejudiced responses among people who profess to be low in prejudice.

Conflicting Value and Attitude Structures

One framework for understanding contemporary forms of prejudice underscores the importance of considering the values and attitudes that people possess about certain stereotyped groups. Specifically, according to Irwin Katz and his colleagues' theory of ambivalence-induced behavior amplification (e.g., Katz, 1981; Katz et al., 1986; Katz & Hass, 1988), many white Americans simultaneously hold two sets of conflicting values. One of these core value orientations is egalitarianism, which supports democratic and humanitarian principles. The other is individualism, which is grounded in principles associated with the Protestant ethic, such as personal freedom, self-reliance, devotion to work, and achievement. According to Katz, each of these value orientations encourages the development of other memory-based representations, which take the form of more specific attitudes. That is, egalitarian values give rise to genuine pro-Black sentiments, including sympathy for and favorable stereotypes about the target group. The simultaneous endorsement of individualism, however, gives rise to anti-Black sentiments, based on attributions of negative patterns among Blacks (e.g., high crime, drug addiction, unemployment) to personal weaknesses rather than to situational factors. Overall then, such "attitude duality" creates ambivalence.

Katz and Hass (1988, Study 1) developed four scales with the aim of examining whether the proposed value–attitude structures do indeed coexist in connection with Blacks. The Pro-Black and Anti-Black scales tapped into individuals' attitudes toward Blacks, whereas the Protestant Ethic (PE) and Humanitarianism-Egalitarianism (HE) scales tapped into their more general value orientations. Correlations between the Pro-Black and HE scales and between the Anti-Black and PE scales were significant in several northern samples (although they were not significant for the southern samples). Furthermore, the crossover correlations between the different attitude–value scales were generally low in the northern samples, suggesting that the pro-Black–HE and the anti-Black–PE structures were independent of one another.

Katz and Hass (1988, Study 2) also demonstrated the associative link in memory between the PE value orientation and the anti-Black attitude structure, as well as the link between the HE value orientation and the pro-Black attitude structure. This was accomplished by using a priming task, a methodology that is highly characteristic of the social cognition approach. Priming a given value orientation raised subjects' scores on the theoretically related attitude measure. Likewise, priming a given attitude resulted in higher scores on the corresponding value orientation scale. Thus, the value–

attitude structures do appear to be linked in memory. Further evidence of the independence of these structures also was obtained, as the priming tasks did not raise scores on the theoretically *un*related value or attitude structure.

The simultaneous existence of largely independent negative and positive cognitive structures has implications for peoples' responses toward the target group. Specifically, Katz and his colleagues maintain that ambivalent attitudes give rise to psychological discomfort and behavioral instability (Hass, Katz, Rizzo, Bailey, & Moore, 1992; Katz, 1981; Katz et al., 1986). Responses are either positive or negative, depending on which component of the ambivalent attitude is activated in a given situation. Furthermore, either a positive or negative response would threaten the ambivalent person's self-esteem because the response would discredit the opposite component of the ambivalent disposition. In order to reduce this threat, either the positive or negative response is amplified (Katz, Glass, & Cohen, 1973; Katz, Glass, Lucido, & Farber, 1979); that is, "the ambivalent subject's extreme evaluations of the Black are viewed theoretically as an attempt to disavow the contradicted attitude and thereby restore positive self-regard" (Katz et al., 1986, p. 54).

In sum, Katz and his colleagues' work suggests that two core value orientations commonly held by Americans are associatively linked in memory with attitude structures, one being pro-Black and the other anti-Black. Such ambivalence helps to explain the persistence of prejudiced responses among people who sometimes appear to be low in prejudice. Despite the existence of genuine pro-Black sentiments, situations that activate the unfavorable attitude structure will give rise to negative responses. Further, considering motivational factors (i.e., efforts to protect one's self-esteem) as well as cognitive factors helps to explain the amplification of behaviors (although the link between amplification and self-esteem has not yet been empirically explored).

Conflict between Egalitarian Values and Prejudiced Beliefs and Feelings

A second framework for understanding modern forms of prejudice is Gaertner and Dovidio's (1986) theory of aversive racism. According to Gaertner and Dovidio, most Americans are highly committed to egalitarian values. Therefore, they desire to maintain an image of the self as fair, just, and nonprejudiced, which causes them to report nonprejudiced, nondiscriminatory attitudes. Such attitudes are not to be confused with genuinely positive attitudes toward stereotyped groups. Instead, they reflect peoples' attempt to respond consistently with their egalitarian self-image.

Gaertner and Dovidio (1986) characterize aversive racists as people who possess egalitarian tendencies but, at the same time, also have negative feelings and beliefs toward the members of the racial group. The development of these negative tendencies is viewed as highly commonplace owing to a variety of contributing factors. America's historically racist culture certainly contributes to the development and persistence of negative stereotypes and prejudiced tendencies. Gaertner and Dovidio especially emphasize how easily and frequently biases toward out-groups or members of stereotyped groups develop because of certain cognitive information processing biases (see Dovidio, Gaertner, Anastasio, & Sanitioso, 1992; Hamilton, 1981a; Hamilton & Trolier, 1986). These biases are thought to stem from basic social categorization processes, which serve to distinguish groups that include the self from those that do not. Once the in-group and the out-group are defined, differential treatment is likely. For example, the in-group is evaluated more favorably and is treated more positively than the out-group (see Chapter 11, this volume, for greater detail).

Gaertner and Dovidio (1986) maintain that aversive racists will alternate between positive and negative behaviors toward members of the racial group. The type of response generated is thought to depend on the normative structure in a given situation and the potential for generating a nonracial justification for a prejudiced response. If the situation clearly calls for a nonprejudiced response or if a justification or rationalization for engaging in a prejudiced response cannot be generated, the response will be positive. When normative prescriptions are weaker or more ambiguous, or when a justification is handy, aversive racists' negative tendencies will be manifested. Their biased responses go unacknowledged by the self, however, so that their egalitarian self-image will not be threatened. Thus, although aversive racists' prejudiced feelings and beliefs are in conflict with their egalitarian values, the conflict supposedly is not consciously recognized.

Based on the aversive racism framework, prejudiced tendencies among people who often appear to be nonprejudiced can be explained in terms of coexisting egalitarian values and prejudiced feelings and beliefs. Because people are motivated to protect their egalitarian self-image, they will respond based on their egalitarian values in a limited set of circumstances, most notably when the situation clearly calls for a nonprejudiced response. However, in many other more ambiguous situations responses will be subtly biased, largely because of normal cognitive processes that presumably operate spontaneously.

Conflict between Stereotype-Based Responses and Personal Beliefs

A final model that explains the persistence of prejudiced responses among people who espouse nonprejudiced attitudes is the dissociation model developed by Devine (1989). Devine argued that to understand the nature of contemporary forms of prejudice one must distinguish between two types of stored information: (1) stereotypes and (2) personal beliefs (or attitudes) about group members. In the dissociation model, a stereotype is defined as *knowledge* of the attributes that are stereotypically associated with a particular group. Prejudiced personal beliefs are defined as the endorsement or acceptance of the content of a negative cultural stereotype. However, being knowledgeable about the stereotype does not necessarily entail endorsement of the stereotype, so that the content of the stereotype would not be a part of the low-prejudiced individual's personal beliefs about the target group.

Conceptualizing stereotypes and beliefs as distinct cognitive structures differs from the long-standing tradition of essentially equating the two; that is, a stereotype is often defined as "a set of beliefs about the personal attributes of a group of people" (Stroebe & Insko, 1989, p. 5; see also Ashmore & Del Boca, 1981; Brigham, 1971). Yet Devine argued that the distinction is important because the activation of stereotypes and personal beliefs is governed by different cognitive processes: automatic and controlled processes, respectively (Posner & Snyder, 1975; Shiffrin & Schnieder, 1977; Schnieder & Shiffrin, 1977).

One implication of this analysis is that the two cognitive structures should provide the basis for responses under different circumstances. To understand this suggestion, it is important to understand the distinction between automatic and controlled processes. Automatic processes involve the unintentional (spontaneous) activation of previously developed associations in memory that have been established through a history of repeated activation. Thus, these processes can be initiated by the presence of relevant environmental cues without requiring conscious attention, and they are difficult to bypass (Neely, 1977; Shiffrin & Dumais, 1981). In contrast, controlled processes involve the intentional activation of information stored in memory. They are more flexible than automatic processes, but they can be initiated only with active attention and not under conditions in which one's cognitive capacity is limited; that is, automatically activated responses can be inhibited by controlled processes only if there is enough time and cognitive capacity for a conscious expectancy to develop and to inhibit the more spontaneous, automatic response (Neely, 1977).

Because stereotypes typically have a long socialization history and have been frequently activated, Devine argued that they can be automatically activated, providing a "default" basis for responding in the presence of members of the stereotyped group or their symbolic equivalent. As demonstrated empirically (Devine, 1989, Study 2; Klinger & Beal, 1992), low- and high-prejudiced people (i.e., those who renounce prejudice vs. those who do not, respectively) are equally susceptible to the automatic activation and use of stereotypes because they are equally knowledgeable about the cultural stereotype (Devine, 1989, Study 1; Brigham, 1972; Katz, 1976). In contrast to stereotypes, personal beliefs about a target group are often developed after the initial, early learning of the stereotype (see Allport, 1954; Katz, 1976; Proshansky, 1966). As a result, they are less accessible cognitive structures than stereotypes and rely on controlled processing for their activation. The important implication of this analysis is that the default response, even among low-prejudiced people, is stereotype-based (see Higgins & King,

1981; Klinger & Beal, 1992; Kruglanski & Freund, 1983; Jamieson & Zanna, 1989; Sherman & Gorkin, 1980). As a consequence, even low-prejudiced people can only inhibit stereotype-based responses if they have the time and the cognitive capacity to initiate controlled processes so as to bring their personal beliefs to mind.

Based on this analysis, many low-prejudiced people appear to be prone to a conflict between their nonprejudiced beliefs and their actual prejudiced responses that arise due to automatic stereotype activation. Moreover, many people appear to be aware of this conflict. That is, they recognize and are willing to admit that in a variety of situations their responses are more prejudiced than their personal beliefs indicate is appropriate (Devine et al., 1991; Monteith, Devine, & Zuwerink, 1993; Pressly & Devine, 1992; Zuwerink, Monteith, Devine, & Cook, 1993). The goal, then, becomes learning how to inhibit and replace well-learned, stereotype-based responses with belief-based responses, which likely takes considerable attention and time (see Devine & Monteith, 1993). This analysis suggests that subtle, contemporary forms of prejudice exist because many low-prejudiced people have not progressed far enough in the prejudice reduction process in order to be efficient and effective at generating nonprejudiced responses that are consistent with their nonprejudiced beliefs.

Summary Remarks

We believe that the theories summarized above are complementary rather than competing. Although each framework specifies different cognitive mechanisms as giving rise to the conflict apparent in contemporary forms of prejudice, different mechanisms may operate for different people. For example, Devine et al. (1991) suggested that Katz and his colleagues' (1986) model of ambivalence may explain the conflict experienced by people who have not developed a firm commitment to nonprejudiced beliefs. Consistent with this suggestion, Devine et al. found that the higher subjects scored on a measure of prejudice toward homosexuals, the more likely they were to report that their personal beliefs about male homosexuals contained both egalitarian and discriminatory tendencies. Subjects with lower prejudice scores showed no such ambivalence. Their nonprejudiced beliefs were well internalized (i.e., linked to the self-concept and defined as important), and subjects were highly committed to responding consistently with their beliefs. Thus, the occurrence of prejudiced responses might be best explained for some people in terms of value–attitude ambivalence, but for others in terms of the effect of spontaneous stereotype activation on their responses.

Likewise, the aversive racism theory may provide the best explanation for prejudiced responses among people who have not adopted genuinely positive attitudes that are independent of their egalitarian ideals and who protect their self-image by rationalizing or justifying their prejudiced responses. Our findings, however, have not been consistent with this reasoning. The majority of our subjects in several samples recognized that they sometimes engaged in prejudiced responses (Devine et al., 1991; Monteith et al., 1993; Pressly & Devine, 1992; Zuwerink et al., 1993). Nevertheless, it is possible that even those who recognize prejudiced responses in certain situations (such as the responses targeted in our laboratory research) generate rationalizations under different conditions or for other responses.

REDUCING CONTEMPORARY FORMS OF PREJUDICE

The identification of the cognitive structures and mechanisms that underlie contemporary forms of prejudice has important implications for potential change strategies. By increasing our understanding of what exactly needs to change, contemporary models of prejudice better equip us to approach the prejudice reduction process. Thus, because contemporary forms of prejudice apparently exist for a variety of reasons that presumably differ across people and possibly across situations, change strategies must be carefully devised to target the type of conflict that underlies a given prejudiced response. Further, the success of various change strategies is likely to depend on whether the nature of the conflict has been appropriately identified. In fact, it is possible that some of the classic change strategies proved largely ineffective because they were not targeted at the appropriate individuals.

Katz and Hass (1988) suggested that educational techniques, in which the egalitarian outlook is stressed and linked directly to minority rights, may be effective for reducing prejudiced responses among people with ambivalent attitudes. Yet a potential problem with this approach is that strengthening the favorable value and belief structures may not affect the negative structures because of the independence of these structures. Further, Katz and Hass suggest that anti-Black sentiments may persist because the negative attitudes are so firmly grounded in values associated with the Protestant ethic. One way to undermine this relation between negative attitudes and PE values, suggested by these authors, is to communicate the idea that adherence to PE values is laudable only when equal opportunity and incentives are possible for everyone.

Gaertner and Dovidio (1986; Dovidio & Gaertner, 1991) offer a couple of ways in which aversive racism can be reduced. First, increasing peoples' awareness of their subtle, prejudiced responses should motivate change because of the inconsistency between such responses and the aversive racists' strong egalitarian values. Along a similar line, we believe that educating aversive racists about the types of justifications and rationalizations people generate for their prejudiced responses would prove useful. If people generate rationalizations without being aware that they are doing so, achieving change would require both becoming conscious of the problem and initiating more careful, controlled processing in the future. Second, Gaertner and

Dovidio point out that change may take place as a function of societal reforms. Just as the Civil Rights legislation and other public policies and programs were critical in altering racism from the overt to the covert forms, future legislation that confronts modern forms of racism may prove effective in bringing about further change (Blanchard, Lilly, & Vaughn, 1991).

Although the speculations about how prejudice reduction might be encouraged among people with ambivalent attitudes and among aversive racists are few in number, and the suggested strategies have not been empirically investigated, the potential for future research that identifies useful prejudice reduction strategies is great. In our work, we have addressed how people who are firmly committed to their low-prejudiced beliefs but remain prone to the automatic activation of stereotypes can eliminate their prejudiced responses. The central challenge for such individuals appears to involve bringing their personal beliefs to mind so that these beliefs can provide a basis for responding before automatically activated stereotypes are used in the response-generation process.

A straightforward strategy for eliminating prejudiced responses that result from spontaneous stereotype activation might involve increasing the frequency of activation of low-prejudiced persons' attitudes or beliefs, with the aim of making the attitudes at least as accessible as the stereotypes. The more accessible attitudes are, the more likely they should be to guide behavior (Fazio, 1986), and this should especially be the case if other cognitive structures (i.e., stereotypes) are not encouraging rival responses. Along these lines, we recently found that people who have extremely low-prejudiced attitudes do have more accessible personal standards than those higher in prejudice (Zuwerink & Devine, 1993). Still, the implications of such findings for behavior have yet to be investigated, and it is important to do so.

Nevertheless, because stereotypes often are highly accessible and easily used (Devine, 1989; Klinger & Beal, 1992), simply increasing the ease with which one's personal beliefs come to mind may not be entirely effective in eliminating stereotype-based responses. Thus, the elimination of prejudiced responses among low-prejudiced individuals may require more than implementing tactics aimed directly at making low-prejudiced attitudes more accessible. Prejudice reduction may instead require the initiation of processes that enable individuals to control or to *inhibit* the prejudiced responses that stem from spontaneous stereotype activation. In other words, the initiation of careful, controlled processing when stereotype-based responses are possible should enable individuals to inhibit prejudiced responses and then to generate responses that are consistent with their low-prejudiced attitudes.

It is important to note that when low-prejudiced individuals engage in prejudiced responses, they experience *discrepancies* between their actual responses and their low-prejudiced beliefs. Insight into the processes that may facilitate the elimination of prejudice-related discrepancies may be gained by examining research relevant to the motivational, learning, and self-regulatory consequences of discrepant responses. To this end, Monteith (1993) drew from this literature in developing a model relevant to the process of acquiring the ability to control prejudiced responses and to replace them with attitude-consistent responses.

Based on previous research (Devine, 1989), the model posits that prejudice-related discrepancies arise when stereotypes are spontaneously activated and used so that a prejudiced response occurs. Further, when low-prejudiced individuals become aware that they have engaged in a prejudiced response, several consequences follow. First, negative self-directed affect should increase (Devine et al., 1991; Monteith et al., 1993; Pressly & Devine, 1992; Zuwerink et al., 1993; see also Allport, 1954; Myrdal, 1944; Rokeach, 1973). Theoretically, engaging in a prejudiced response that conflicts with low-prejudiced beliefs represents a personally significant discrepancy that is arousing and quite disconcerting to low-prejudiced persons, threatening an important part of their self-image and giving rise to guilt-related feelings. The experience of such affect should then serve as a punishment (Gray, 1982; Fowles, 1980) and motivate discrepancy reduction (Aronson, 1968; Bandura, 1986; Bandura & Jourden, 1991; Duval, Duval, & Mulilis, 1992; Duval & Wicklund, 1972; Festinger, 1957; Rokeach, 1973).

According to the model, a second consequence of becoming aware of a prejudice-related discrepant response is that self-focused attention is heightened. This, in turn, instigates attempts to regulate or to control subsequent responses that are relevant to the discrepancy (Pyszczynski & Greenberg, 1986, 1987). Third, environmental stimuli that are relevant to the discrepancy are given special attention, and, fourth, exploratory-investigative behavior is initiated to search for cues associated with the discrepant response. The third and fourth consequences work in concert so that cues present when the discrepancy occurred can be noted. For example, one might take note of the situation in which the discrepancy occurred or think about what prompted the prejudiced response. Consequently, associations between the cues present when the discrepancy occurred, the discrepant response, and the punishment (i.e., guilty feelings) are built. Such associations serve to establish cues for punishment (see Figure 1; Gray, 1982; Fowles, 1980).

According to the model, these discrepancy-associated consequences serve the adaptive function of increasing the likelihood that future prejudiced responses will be inhibited (see boxed portion of Figure 1). Specifically, when the stereotype is spontaneously activated on subsequent occasions and the cues for punishment that were previously established are present, a "warning signal" of sorts is set off. Consequently, the response-generation process is slowed and executed more carefully (Gray, 1982). Low-prejudiced beliefs can therefore be brought to mind so that the prejudiced response can be inhibited and a low-prejudiced response can be generated. In this way, control can be achieved over prejudiced responses.

Research investigating a number of aspects of this model of the self-

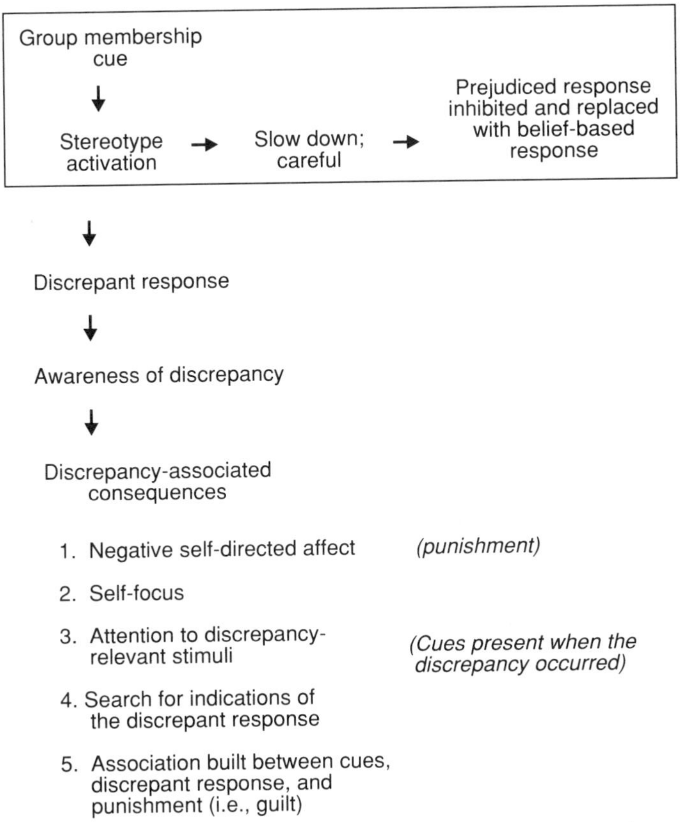

FIGURE 1.

A model of the self-regulation of prejudiced responses.

regulation of prejudiced responses produced results that were consistent with the model (Monteith, 1993). For example, low-prejudiced subjects who believed they had engaged in prejudiced responses experienced guilt, showed heightened self-focus, and appeared to engage in behaviors that are theoretically related to the activities necessary for the establishment of cues for punishment. Most importantly, when low-prejudiced individuals believed they had engaged in a prejudiced response, they were less likely to generate prejudiced responses in a subsequent task. This finding supports the idea that the processes activated as a consequence of engaging in prejudice-related discrepant responses facilitate the future inhibition of prejudiced responses. Thus, it is possible that low-prejudiced individuals can reach their goal of eliminating prejudiced responses, provided they are willing to devote effort, attention, and time to their goal. However, considerably more research is needed that investigates the self-regulation of prejudiced responses.

If future results are consistent with the notion that individuals can learn to inhibit prejudiced responses arising from spontaneous stereotype activation, it will be important to investigate the long-term implications of the practiced self-regulation of prejudiced responses (see Monteith, 1993). Note that, according to the model shown in Figure 1, the stereotype continues to be activated in the presence of group membership cues even after the ability to inhibit prejudiced responses and replace them with belief-based responses has been acquired. This is because the consequences of prejudice-related discrepancies may not necessarily decrease the accessibility of the stereotype; it may continue to come to mind in the presence of group membership cues. The implication is that prejudiced responses may continue to be generated due to stereotype activation when individuals lack the time or cognitive ability (e.g., when drinking at a crowded party) either to process cues for punishment in the environment or to bring their low-prejudiced beliefs to mind.

Nevertheless, there are two reasons for suspecting that the processes involved in learning to inhibit prejudiced responses may also decrease the likelihood of stereotype activation. First, the cues for punishment that are established based on the association between prejudice-related discrepant responses and the punishment (i.e., guilt) might also become associated with stereotype activation. For example, if a person says "typical for a woman" when observing a crying woman and the person believes that such a response is inappropriate, guilt should be experienced. Cues for punishment that develop due to this sequence of events may not only be associated with saying "typical for a woman" but also with the activation of the stereotype that women are emotional. If this is the case, stereotype activation itself should be inhibited in the future. Second, low-prejudiced beliefs should be activated and used more frequently as individuals become more adept at self-regulating their prejudiced responses, whereas stereotype use should become less frequent. The low-prejudiced beliefs, therefore, may become relatively more accessible than the stereotypes.

CONCLUSIONS

Compared to more classic approaches to understanding prejudice and prejudice reduction, the contemporary approaches that we have reviewed take a more theory-driven approach. As highlighted in the previous section, an important goal of contemporary researchers has been to understand theoretically how prejudiced responses can be eliminated by changing the cognitive structures that come to mind and are used to guide peoples' responses to members of stereotyped groups. In contrast to this theory-driven, process approach, classic approaches to prejudice reduction looked for global prejudice reduction strategies that might work for all people at all levels of prejudice. But this search took place in a hit-or-miss way, outside of a guiding theoretical framework. From our contemporary vantage point, it is not surprising, then, that these global prejudice reduction strategies were less than completely successful.

In addition to providing a useful conceptual framework, the social cognition approach has provided important new methodological approaches to the study of prejudice. These new methods have allowed investigators to empirically investigate some of Allport's (1954) early theorizing about how different individuals deal with the conflict between prejudiced responses and more egalitarian attitudes. Allport suggested that some individuals may deal with this conflict by rationalizing it away—a strategy consistent with Gaertner and Dovidio's analysis of aversive racism. A second suggestion was that individuals may alternate between prejudiced and nonprejudiced responses —a strategy reflected in Katz and colleagues' ambivalence model. Finally, work by Devine, Monteith, and their colleagues has provided confirmatory evidence for Allport's suggestion that some people explicitly acknowledge the conflict between their nonprejudiced attitudes and prejudiced responses, that this conflict gives rise to feelings of guilt, and that this guilt can motivate attempts to eliminate prejudiced responses.

Note that the starting point and focus for these contemporary models is primarily on individual-level conflict between more egalitarian and less prejudiced attitudes and persistent prejudiced responses. This emphasis on more or less low-prejudiced individuals represents a shift in focus from the classic concern with understanding extremely high-prejudiced people. Despite this shift, it would be a mistake to assume that extremely high-prejudiced people no longer exist. Hochschild and Herk (1989), for example, have noted that a hard core of real racists still exist in our society; for example, as many as 15% of white adults still agree that "blacks are inferior to white people." Thus, a fundamental challenge remains to discover ways of changing "hard-core" prejudiced beliefs. Whereas social cognition has helped us gain insight into the nature of the cognitive structures that need to be changed and into what must be done to facilitate the process of change, it seems less effective in helping us understand how to *initiate* belief change. Perhaps a bridge between classic and contemporary concerns can be built via a revival of Rokeach's self-confrontation technique for the production of genuine belief change. According to Rokeach (1973), realizing the inconsistency between one's self-conception as fair, tolerant, and democratic and one's prejudiced attitudes should give rise to self-dissatisfaction. This dissatisfaction, in turn, should motivate a change in the prejudiced attitude to be more consistent with one's self-defining egalitarian values. Once such genuine attitude change has been initiated by the individual, the knowledge gleaned from research employing the social cognition approach can offer insight into the process of working out the implications of such belief change for everyday thought and interaction.

One caveat to the application of Rokeach's technique, however, is that it may not work with equal effectiveness for all individuals. One key individual difference, for example, may be the specific function served by the prejudiced attitude (see Monteith et al., 1993, for a more detailed discussion). Rokeach's method may be especially effective for reducing prejudiced attitudes that serve an instrumental function. Because such attitudes are not self-defining but, rather, are based on the costs and benefits that may be derived from the attitude object (Abelson & Prentice, 1989), the conflict between the attitude and one's self-concept as fair minded and egalitarian should favor revision of the specific prejudiced attitude.

In contrast, attitudes that serve a symbolic function (Abelson & Prentice, 1989) are used as a means of expressing and/or protecting one's self-identity. They are, by definition, self-defining. Thus, for people whose negative attitudes serve a symbolic function, Rokeach's method results in bringing two important aspects of one's self-concept into conflict. Resolving such an inconsistency requires changing at least one aspect of the self-concept. Because people generally resist such change, Rokeach's method may prove less effective in this case. Rather than resolving the inconsistency by changing the prejudiced attitude, people may seek alternative ways to cope with the conflict (e.g., repress it or rationalize it away).

In conclusion, we believe that the social cognition approach has provided a framework for understanding the importance of attending to individual differences in the expression and reduction of prejudice (e.g., people may be at different stages in the prejudice reduction process). The challenge now is to continue research that fleshes out these key individual differences and explores the implications of such differences for prejudice reduction. Although we believe that cognitive analyses have contributed greatly to our understanding of the process of prejudice reduction, we do not believe that this approach alone will enable us to solve the problem of intergroup prejudice. Other affective, motivational, and learning processes appear to play a central role in mediating the cognitive change necessary for the elimination of prejudiced responses (Devine & Monteith, 1993; Hamilton, 1981b; Monteith, 1993; Rokeach, 1973). Thus, as we further our understanding of how all of these processes work together to affect behavior, we may be able to develop truly effective strategies for producing long-lasting change.

REFERENCES

Abelson, R. P., & Prentice, D. A. (1989). Beliefs as possessions: A functional perspective. In A. R. Pratkanis, S. J. Breckler, & A. G. Greenwald (Eds.), *Attitude structure and function* (pp. 361–381). Hillsdale, NJ: Erlbaum.

Adorno, T. W., Frenkel-Brunswik, E., Levinson, D. J., & Sanford, R. N. (1950). *The authoritarian personality.* New York: Harper.

Allport, G. W. (1954). *The nature of prejudice.* Reading, MA: Addison-Wesley.

Altemeyer, B. (1981). *Right-wing authoritarianism.* Winnipeg: University of Manitoba Press.

Altemeyer, B. (1988). *Enemies of freedom: Understanding right-wing authoritarianism.* San Francisco: Jossey-Bass.

Amir, Y. (1969). The contact hypothesis in ethnic relations. *Psychological Bulletin, 71,* 319–342.

Amir, Y. (1976). The role of intergroup contact in changes of prejudice and ethnic relations. In P. A. Katz (Ed.), *Towards the elimination of racism* (pp. 245–308). New York: Pergamon.

Aronson, E. (1968). The theory of cognitive dissonance: A current perspective. In L. Berkowitz (Ed.), *Advances in experimental social psychology* (Vol. 4, pp. 1–34). New York: Academic Press.

Ashmore, R. D. (1970). The problem of intergroup prejudice. In B. E. Collins (Ed.), *Social psychology* (pp. 245–296). Reading, MA: Addison-Wesley.

Ashmore, R. D., & Del Boca, F. K. (1976). Psychological approaches to understanding intergroup conflict. In P. Katz (Ed.), *Towards the elimination of racism* (pp. 73–123). New York: Pergamon.

Ashmore, R. D., & Del Boca, F. K. (1981). Conceptual approaches to stereotypes and stereotyping. In D. L. Hamilton (Ed.), *Cognitive processes in stereotyping and intergroup behavior* (pp. 1–35). Hillsdale, NJ: Erlbaum.

Bandura, A. (1986). *Social foundations of thought and action: A social cognitive theory.* Englewood Cliffs, NJ: Prentice-Hall.

Bandura, A., & Jourden, F. (1991). Self-regulatory mechanisms governing the impact of social comparison on complex decision making. *Journal of Personality and Social Psychology, 60,* 941–951.

Billig, M. (1985). Prejudice, categorization, and particularization: From a perceptual to a rhetorical approach. *European Journal of Social Psychology, 15,* 79–103.

Blanchard, F. A., Lilly, T., & Vaughn, L. A. (1991). Reducing the expression of racial prejudice. *Psychological Science, 2,* 101–105.

Brigham, J. C. (1971). Ethnic stereotypes. *Psychological Bulletin, 76,* 15–38.

Brigham, J. C. (1972). Racial stereotypes: Measurement variables and stereotype–attitude relationship. *Journal of Applied Social Psychology, 2,* 63–76.

Campbell, E. Q. (1961). Moral discomfort and racial segregation—an examination of the Myrdal hypothesis. *Social Forces, 39,* 228–234.

Cook, F. W. (1985). Experimenting on social issues: The case of school desegregation. *American Psychologist, 40,* 452–460.

Crosby, F., Bromley, S., & Saxe, L. (1980). Recent unobtrusive studies of black and white discrimination and prejudice: A literature review. *Psychological Bulletin, 87,* 546–563.

Devine, P. G. (1989). Stereotypes and prejudice: Their automatic and controlled components. *Journal of Personality and Social Psychology, 56,* 5–18.

Devine, P. G., & Monteith, M. J. (1993). The role of discrepancy associated affect in prejudice reduction. In D. M. Mackie & D. L. Hamilton (Eds.), *Affect, cognition, and stereotyping: Interactive processes in intergroup perception* (pp. 317–344). Orlando, FL: Academic Press.

Devine, P. G., Monteith, M. J., Zuwerink, J. R., & Elliot, A. J. (1991). Prejudice with and without compunction. *Journal of Personality and Social Psychology, 60,* 817–830.

Dovidio, J. F., & Gaertner, S. L. (1986). Prejudice, discrimination, and racism: Historical trends and contemporary approaches. In J. F. Dovidio & S. L. Gaertner (Eds.), *Prejudice, discrimination, and racism* (pp. 1–34). New York: Academic Press.

Dovidio, J. F., & Gaertner, S. L. (1991). Changes in the expression of racial prejudice. In H. Knopke, J. Norrell, & R. Rogers (Eds.), *Opening doors: An appraisal of race relations in contemporary America* (pp. 201–241). Tuscaloosa: University of Alabama Press.

Dovidio, J. F., Gaertner, S. L., Anastasio, R. A., & Sanitioso, R. (1992). Cognitive and motivational bases of bias: Implications of aversive racism for attitudes toward hispanics. In S. B. Knouse, P. Rosenfeld, and A. L. Culbertson (Eds.), *Hispanics in the workplace* (pp. 75–106). Newbury Park: Sage.

Duckitt, J. (1992a). Psychology and prejudice: A historical analysis and integrative framework. *American Psychologist, 47,* 1182–1193.

Duckitt, J. (1992b). *The social psychology of prejudice.* New York: Praeger.

Duval, S., & Wicklund, R. A. (1972). *A theory of objective self-awareness.* New York: Academic Press.

Duval, T. S., Duval, V. H., & Mulilis, J. (1992). Effects of self-focus, discrepancy between self and standard, and outcome expectancy favorability on the tendency to match self to standard or to withdraw. *Journal of Personality and Social Psychology, 62,* 340–348.

Fazio, R. H. (1986). How do attitudes guide behavior? In R. M. Sorrentino & E. T. Higgins (Eds.), *Handbook of motivation and cognition* (pp. 204–243). New York: Guilford.

Festinger, L. (1957). *A theory of cognitive dissonance.* Stanford, CA: Stanford University Press.

Fowles, D. C. (1980). The three-arousal model: Implications of Gray's two factor learning theory for heart rate, electrodermal activity, and psychopathy. *Psychophysiology, 17,* 87–104.

Friedrichs, R. W. (1959). Christians and residential exclusion: An empirical study of a Northern dilemma. *Journal of Social Issues, 15,* 14–23.

Gaertner, S. L., & Dovidio, J. F. (1986). The aversive form of racism. In J. F. Dovidio & S. L. Gaertner (Eds.), *Prejudice, discrimination, and racism* (pp. 61–89). New York: Academic Press.

Goodman, M. E. (1952). *Race awareness in young children.* Reading, MA: Addison-Wesley.

Gray, J. A. (1982). *The neuropsychology of anxiety: An enquiry into the functions of the septo-hippocampal system.* New York: Oxford University Press.

Hamilton, D. L. (Ed.). (1981a). *Cognitive processes in stereotyping and intergroup behavior.* Hillsdale, NJ: Erlbaum.

Hamilton, D. L. (1981b). Stereotyping and intergroup behavior: Some thoughts on the cognitive approach. In D. L. Hamilton (Ed.), *Cognitive processes in stereotyping and intergroup behavior* (pp. 333–353). Hillsdale, NJ: Erlbaum.

Hamilton, D. L., & Trolier, T. K. (1986). Stereotypes and stereotyping: An overview of the cognitive approach. In J. Dovidio & S. L. Gaertner (Eds.), *Prejudice, discrimination, and racism* (pp. 127–163). New York: Academic Press.

Harding, J., Kutner, B., Proshansky, H., & Chein, I. (1954). Prejudice and ethnic relations. In G. Lindzey (Ed.), *The handbook of social psychology.* (Vol. 2, pp. 1021–1061). Cambridge, MA: Addison-Wesley.

Hass, R. G., Katz, I., Rizzo, N., Bailey, J., & Moore, L. (1992). When racial ambivalence evokes negative affect, using a disguised measure of mood. *Personality and Social Psychology Bulletin, 18,* 786–797.

Higgins, E. T., & King, G. (1981). Accessibility of social constructs: Information-processing consequences of individual and contextual variability. In N. Cantor & J. F. Kihlstrom (Eds.), *Personality and social interaction* (pp. 69–121). Hillsdale, NJ: Erlbaum.

Hochschild, J. L., & Herk, M. (1989). "Yes but . . .": Principles and caveats in American racial attitudes. In J. Chapman (Ed.), *NOMOS: Majorities and minorities: Political and philosophical perspectives* (pp. 308–335). New York: New York University Press.

Jamieson, D. W., & Zanna, M. P. (1989). Need for structure in attitude formation and expression. In A. R. Pratkanis, S. J. Breckler, & A. G. Greenwald (Eds.), *Attitude structure and function* (pp. 383–406). Hillsdale, NJ: Erlbaum.

Katz, I. (1981). *Stigma: A social psychological analysis.* Hillsdale, NJ: Erlbaum.

Katz, I., & Hass, R. G. (1988). Racial ambivalence and American value conflict: Correlational and priming studies of dual cognitive structures. *Journal of Personality and Social Psychology, 55,* 893–905.

Katz, I., Glass, D. C., & Cohen, S. (1973). Ambivalence, guilt, and the scapegoating of minority group victims. *Journal of Experimental Social Psychology, 9,* 423–436.

Katz, I., Glass, D. C., Lucido, D. J., & Farber, J. (1979). Harm-doing and victim's racial or orthopedic stigma as determinants of helping behavior. *Journal of Personality, 47,* 430–434.

Katz, I., Wackenhut, J., & Hass, R. G. (1986). Racial ambivalence, value duality, and behavior. In J. F. Dovidio & S. L. Gaertner (Eds.), *Prejudice, discrimination, and racism* (pp. 35–60). New York: Academic Press.

Katz, P. A. (1976). The acquisition of racial attitudes in children. In P. A. Katz (Ed.), *Towards the elimination of racism* (pp. 125–154). New York: Pergamon Press.

Kinder, D. R., & Sears, D. O. (1981). Prejudice and politics: Symbolic racism versus threats to the good life. *Journal of Personality and Social Psychology, 40,* 414–431.

Klinger, M., & Beal, P. (1992). Conscious and unconscious effects of stereotype activation. Paper presented at the 64th annual meeting of the Midwestern Psychological Association, Chicago, May.

Kruglanski, A. W., & Freund, T. (1983). The freezing and unfreezing of lay inferences: Effects on impressional primacy, ethnic stereotyping and numerical anchoring. *Journal of Experimental Social Psychology, 19,* 448–468.

Lippman, W. (1922). *Public opinion.* New York: Harcourt & Brace.

McConahay, J. G. (1986). Modern racism, ambivalence, and the modern racism scale. In. J. F. Dovidio & S. L. Gaertner (Eds.), *Prejudice, discrimination, and racism* (pp. 91–125). New York: Academic Press.

Monteith, M. J. (1993). Self-regulation of prejudiced responses: Implications for progress in prejudice-reduction efforts. *Journal of Personality and Social Psychology, 65,* 469–485.

Monteith, M. J., Devine, P. G., & Zuwerink, J. R. (1993). Self-directed vs. other-directed affect as a consequence of prejudice-related discrepancies. *Journal of Personality and Social Psychology, 64,* 198–210.

Myers, D. G., & Bishop, G. D. (1970). Discussion effects on racial attitudes. *Science, 169,* 778–789.

Myrdal, G. (1944). *An American dilemma.* New York: Harper & Row.

Neely, J. H. (1977). Semantic priming and retrieval from lexical memory: Roles of inhibitionless spreading activation and limited-capacity attention. *Journal of Experimental Psychology, 106,* 226–254.

Pettigrew, T. F. (1958). Personality and sociocultural factors in intergroup attitudes: A cross-national comparison. *Journal of Conflict Resolution, 2,* 29–42.

Posner, M. I., & Snyder, C. R. R. (1975). Attention and cognitive control. In R. L. Solso (Ed.), *Information processing and cognition: The Loyola Symposium* (pp. 55–85). Hillsdale, NJ: Erlbaum.

Pressly, S. L., & Devine, P. G. (1992). Gender, prejudice and affect. Paper presented at the 64th annual meeting of the Midwestern Psychological Association, Chicago, May.

Proshansky, H. M. (1966). The development of intergroup attitudes. In L. Hoffman & M. L. Hoffman (Eds.), *Review of child development research.* (Vol. 2, pp. 311–371). New York: Sage.

Pyszczynski, T., & Greenberg, J. (1986). Persistent high self-focus after failure and low self-focus after success: The depressive self-focusing style. *Journal of Personality and Social Psychology, 50,* 1039–1044.

Pyszczynski, T., & Greenberg, J. (1987). Self-regulatory perseveration and the depressive self-focusing style: A self-awareness theory of reactive depression. *Psychological Bulletin, 102,* 122–138.

Rokeach, M. (1973). *The nature of human values.* New York: Free Press.

Schneider, W., & Shiffrin, R. M. (1977). Controlled and automatic human information processing: I. Detection, search and attention. *Psychological Review, 84,* 1–66.

Schuman, H., Steeh, C., & Bobo, L. (1985). *Racial attitudes in America: Trends and interpretations.* Cambridge, MA: Harvard University Press.

Sherman, S. J., & Gorkin, L. (1980). Attitude bolstering when behavior is inconsistent with central attitudes. *Journal of Experimental Social Psychology, 16,* 388–403.

Sherman, S. J., Judd, C. M., & Park, B. (1989). Social cognition. *Annual review of psychology, 40,* 281–326.

Shiffrin, R. M., & Dumais, S. T. (1981). The development of automatism. In J. R. Anderson (Ed.), *Cognitive skills and their acquisition* (pp. 111–140). Hillsdale, NJ: Erlbaum.

Shiffrin, R. M., & Schneider, W. (1977). Controlled and automatic human information processing: II. Perceptual learning, automatic attending, and a general theory. *Psychological Review, 84,* 127–190.

Stephan, W. G. (1985). Intergroup relations. In G. Lindzey & E. Aronson (Eds.), *The handbook of social psychology* (3rd ed.) (Vol. 2, pp. 559–658). Hillsdale, NJ: Erlbaum.

Stroebe, W., & Insko, C. A. (1989). Stereotype, prejudice, and discrimination: Changing conceptions in theory and research. In D. Bar-Tal, C. F. Graumann, A. W. Kruglanski, & W. Stroebe (Eds.), *Stereotyping and prejudice: Changing conceptions* (pp. 3–34). Berlin: Springer.

Tajfel, H. (1969). Cognitive aspects of prejudice. *Journal of Social Issues, 25,* 79–97.

Weigel, R. H., & Howes, P. W. (1985). Conceptions of racial prejudice: Symbolic racism reconsidered. *Journal of Social Issues, 41,* 117–138.

Westie, F. R. (1965). The American dilemma: An empirical test. *American Sociological Review, 30,* 527–538.

Williams, Jr., R. M. (1947). The reduction of intergroup tensions: A survey of research on problems of ethnic, racial, and religious group relations. New York: Social Science Research Council, Bulletin 57.

Williams, Jr., R. M. (1977). *Mutual accommodation: Ethnic conflict and cooperation.* Minneapolis: University of Minnesota Press.

Zuwerink, J. R., & Devine, P. G. (1993). Prejudice, internalization, and the accessibility of personal standards. Paper presented at the 65th annual meeting of the Midwestern Psychological Association, Chicago, May.

Zuwerink, J. R., Monteith, M. J., Devine, P. G., & Cook, D. (1993). Prejudice toward Blacks: With and without compunction? Unpublished manuscript, University of Wisconsin, Madison.

11

Cognitive Processes and Intergroup Relations: A Historical Perspective

Myron Rothbart
Scott Lewis

INTRODUCTION

The goal of this chapter is to identify and assess the contribution of the cognitive perspective to the study of intergroup relations. To fully appreciate the impact of this perspective, we offer a highly selective and largely historical view of the continuities and changes in theories of intergroup relations. We begin with a detailed discussion of a critical review published shortly after the end of World War II to provide some perspective on the field prior to the recent cognitive influences. Modern cognitive theories and techniques have had a major influence on contemporary research, yet it is also clear that a number of these important ideas were anticipated by others, most notably by Lippmann and Allport. Following a discussion of their work, we examine the contributions of Sherif, and Levine and Campbell, and then consider more modern contributions to intergroup relations. Our goal is to emphasize the continuities with the past, as well as the divergences, and to assess the value and limits of the cognitive perspective.

THE COGNITIVE REVOLUTION AND SOCIAL PSYCHOLOGY

Psychology's cognitive revolution beginning in the late 1950s and 1960s represented a significant departure from earlier behaviorist and functionalist traditions. Although the change may have been more of degree than kind, the focus shifted away from defining the relationship between stimulus and response, and toward a systematic exploration of the nature of mental representations. Posner and Shulman (1979) identify Bartlett's *Thinking* (1958) and Bruner, Goodnow, and Austin's *A Study of Thinking* (1956) as "[freeing] many researchers from the belief that the higher mental processes were not amenable to experimental investigation." Given this shift in perspective, there was a renewed interest in mental processes, and particularly in those mechanisms that allowed a processing system of limited capacity to deal with large amounts of information (e.g., Broadbent, 1958; Miller, 1956).

The impact of the cognitive revolution may have been less on social psychology than on psychology as a whole, because social psychology had never abandoned an interest in mental processes. Although a behaviorist influence was evident in a number of areas of social psychology, a continued strong focus on the content and organization of social attitudes, opinions, and beliefs throughout the 1930s, 1940s, and 1950s indicates that an interest in the nature of social thought persisted throughout the behaviorist period. Although the effect of the cognitive revolution on social psychology did not alter the already strong interest in mental processes, it did shift the focus away from affective processes toward cognitive processes. In the area of opinions and beliefs, the concept of attitude, as an affective proclivity, had been considered causally paramount. In the area of belief systems, theories of cognitive consistency had been proposed, but could as easily have been labeled theories of "affective consistency," since they were based on grouping by affective similarity. In the area of intergroup relations, the emphasis on scapegoating, with its psychodynamic origins, also had placed affective processes at the center of theories of prejudice and intergroup hostility.

The effect of the cognitive revolution in the area of intergroup relations was twofold. First, it shifted the inquiry away from affective processes and, consistent with the dominant theme of a limited capacity system coping with a surfeit of information, focused instead on those mental processes that allow us to simplify our images of the social world. Second, the same important methodological advances that enabled cognitive psychologists to systematically study covert mental processes allowed social psychologists to explore the effects of memory, attention, and categorization on social judgment and social perception. The goal of this chapter is to examine these contributions in its historical context. To appreciate the state of intergroup relations prior to the strong influences of cognitive psychology, it is useful to consider an influential critique published at midcentury.

ZAWADSKI'S CRITIQUE

In an article written shortly after the end of World War II, titled "Limitations of the Scapegoat Theory of Prejudice," Zawadski (1948) identified two extant theories to account for intergroup hostility. The first, the Well-Earned

Reputation Theory, located the source of hostility toward a group in the truly objectionable characteristics possessed by that group. The second, the Scapegoat Theory, located the cause of hostility in the perceiver, through the following causal chain: (1) frustration leads to aggression, (2) this aggression is displaced away from the frustrating source and toward a powerless minority group, and (3) the hostility is then rationalized by ascribing "plausible" negative attributes to the minority group. Zawadski characterized the first theory as a pure "stimulus" theory and the second as a pure "drive" theory. Since most social scientists, including Zawadski, rejected the well-earned reputation theory, the second or Scapegoat theory remained the most popular explanation for hostility directed against minorities.

Zawadski then identified problems with the Scapegoat Theory as the "single and sovereign" explanation for the origins of intergroup hostility. He argued, with caveats, that a reasonable theory of intergroup hostility must take into account *both* the internal dynamics of the perceiver, and the nature of the stimulus group; he labeled this dual approach a "convergence theory." Zawadski approached the issue of a group's "real" character with caution, if not apprehension. To suggest, as the world was learning of the Nazi death camps, that a despised minority may have characteristics that warrant opprobrium, appeared to be more of an example of, rather than an explanation for, intergroup hostility. Zawadski's argument was not naive, however, and deserves further examination.

Zawadski disliked the Scapegoat Theory for a number of reasons, not the least of which was its implications for ameliorating intergroup relations. A variant of the frustration-aggression theory, the Scapegoat Theory implied that hostility was inevitable, because frustration of impulses and goals was inevitable. The Well-Earned Reputation Theory would be preferable due to its ameliorating potential, *assuming* that people could adopt an enlightened view of the nature of group characteristics. In particular, it was important that people perceive a group's negative attributes as (1) learned rather than innate, (2) a product of social conditions and therefore malleable, and (3) often a reaction to prejudice and discrimination. Zawadski's last point is of particular significance, because it suggests that an observer's pejorative view of a group may itself perpetuate the group's undesired characteristics.

For historic as well as intellectual reasons, Zawadski's arguments are interesting, particularly if we realize that his article preceded the soon-to-be-published work on the Authoritarian Personality (Adorno, Frenkel-Brunswick, Levinson, & Sanford, 1950), which itself was a variation on the scapegoat model. In retrospect, there are a number of problems with Zawadski's analysis. First, in his view, the causes of intergroup perception reside in only two domains, the motivational/affective needs of the observer, and the observer's evaluative response to the group's "actual" characteristics. Both influences are affective in character, and do not consider the possibility that other powerful perceptual and conceptual processes may be implicated. Second, there are at least two questionable underlying assumptions regarding the "real" characteristics of the stimulus group: that there is invariance in encoding group characteristics, and that given a negative evaluation of a trait, hostility to the group is a *warranted* response.

The problem with the first assumption is the problem of the stimulus error (e.g., Rothbart & Birrell, 1977), in that it assumes only one response is demanded by a given stimulus. Allport clarified this issue when he asked why ambition was a trait admired in Abraham Lincoln but despised in the Jews. The second assumption concerns the prescriptive issue of what response is "warranted" by the presence of an undesirable trait. Again the link between stimulus and response is not invariant, and an undesirable characteristic can be responded to with sympathy or disdain, as Zawadski himself recognized. To the extent that Zawadski admonished us to consider the nature of the stimulus group in accounting for intergroup perception, his argument is unassailable. His error, in our view, was in assuming invariance in the representation of group characteristics, and in assuming that affective responses alone dominate intergroup perception and intergroup relations.

It is important to note two additional ideas mentioned only in passing by Zawadski. The first is an implicit recognition of the importance of cognitive/perceptual processes and notes that the naive perception of group characteristics ". . . seems to follow some as yet unknown laws of perception. It is possible that experiments on perception of group characteristics in physical objects may throw some light on the peculiarities of social perception" (1948, p. 136). The second is a qualification of his "convergence theory" as an account of the *origins* of prejudice, acknowledging the incompleteness of his theory for understanding the *maintenance* of intergroup hostility. Maintenance, he argued, could be understood in terms of the economic, social, and other material gains that accrue to the majority group as a result of dominance over the minority.

Zawadski's article represents an important benchmark against which other views can be compared. From a contemporary perspective, we are struck by both the simplicity of the models being contrasted, and the minimal role they accord to cognitive processes. The prevailing explanations for intergroup hostility reside either in the perceiver's internal mechanisms for drive reduction (the pure "drive" theory), or in the target group's actual, offensive qualities (the pure "stimulus" theory). Although Zawadski increased the complexity of explanation by doubling the number of factors from one to two, he acknowledged only parenthetically two additional classes of explanation: the "unknown laws of perception" that influence our thinking about group characteristics, and "realistic" factors that allow the dominant group to gain from the disadvantaged position of the minority group.

Before considering the developments following Zawadski's analysis, we first examine Walter Lippmann's ideas about mental representation, published shortly after World War I. In our view, Lippmann's *Public Opinion*, Allport's *Nature of Prejudice*, Sherif's *The Robbers' Cave Experiment*, and Levine and Campbell's *Ethnocentrism* constitute four landmark contributions in the area of intergroup relations. It should become clear that a number of important ideas regarding cognitive processes appeared substantially before the mid-1970s, although the bulk of research has been undertaken since that time.

LIPPMANN'S *PUBLIC OPINION*

In 1922, Walter Lippmann, a journalist with a strong interest in psychology, published his analysis of the relations between public images and social policy. His analysis of stereotypes dealt with intergroup relations more by implication than direct analysis, yet the dominant impact of World War I is apparent in much of his thinking. Lippmann used the example of Plato's cave to argue that, just as Plato's observers could only know the shadows on the cave wall and not the external reality casting those shadows, contemporary observers know only their constructed or "pseudo" environment, not the environment itself. The problem is that different groups construct different pseudoenvironments:

> [We have] . . . to account for such facts as two nations attacking one another, each convinced that it is acting in self-defense; or two classes at war, each certain that it speaks for the common interest. They live, we are likely to say, in different worlds. More accurately, they live in the same world, but they think and feel in different ones. (p. 20)

Thus, social perception is vital for understanding conflict, and an understanding of stereotypes is vital for understanding social perception. Lippmann's view of the process of stereotyping is remarkably contemporary, and quite consistent with the simplification function (exaggeration of intercategory boundaries) later outlined by Tajfel (1969), Taylor (1981), and Levine and Campbell (1972). Although Lippmann's view of stereotypes has been described as emphasizing the stereotype's ". . . largely incorrect contents and . . . products of a faulty reasoning process" (Brigham, 1971), we believe this does not fully do justice to Lippmann's view. There is little question that Lippmann viewed stereotypes as oversimplifications, as frequently inaccurate, and resistant to change, but it is not clear that these shortcomings describe a faulty reasoning process:[1]

> For the real environment is altogether too big, too complex, and too fleeting for direct acquaintance. We are not equipped to deal with so much subtlety, so much

[1]It is not clear how one decides whether a process is faulty or not. One criterion is whether the system is capable of inaccuracy. A system that is never allowed inaccuracy may be unwieldy given demands of time and space, and therefore highly maladaptive, whereas a system that is generally accurate with some error, but swift and efficient, may be highly adaptive.

> variety, so many permutations and combinations. And although we have to act in that environment, we have to reconstruct it on a simpler model before we can manage with it. To traverse the world men must have maps of the world. Their persistent difficulty is to secure maps on which their own need, or someone else's need, has not sketched in the coast of Bohemia. (Lippmann, 1922, p. 16)

The idea of having to act on a complex world with a cognitive/perceptual system of limited capacity anticipates Simon's (1981) concept of "satisficing," and stresses the idea that simplification is necessary and desirable if we are to map a finite set of actions onto a near-infinitely complex world. The idea of a map that is "good enough" to enable us to traverse the environment is compelling. A map one yard square taking us from Eugene, Oregon to San Francisco, California cannot capture the intricacies of the environment over a distance of 500 miles. However, as long as it includes information relevant to getting on and off the freeway at the appropriate locations, it is functional. The fact that the map does not literally represent the environment is highly desirable, because the overwhelming detail would hamper our progress. The idea of a "good enough" representation is important, because it inextricably links the observer's goals with the fidelity of the stereotype.

Lippmann's metaphor of social representation as an internal map of the external world is helpful for a number of reasons. Maps are by definition simplifications stripped of unneeded details. Stereotypes are also summaries that fail to accurately describe differences among category members. Second, some parts of the map may show more detail than others, reflecting the needs and goals of the traveler, just as some aspects of the stereotype may be more relevant to some observers than to others. We suggest that in the intergroup context, the most relevant attributes of the out-group will be those that threaten the security or values of the in-group, leading to greater articulation of unfavorable than favorable attributes of the outgroup.[2]

We view Lippmann's metaphor of the stereotyping process as quite consistent with the view that was to be articulated almost half a century later regarding the simplifying nature of the information processing system. It is a view that is in marked contrast to the drive versus stimulus distinction advanced by Zawadski.

The discussion of Lippmann's work allows us to outline our major substantive theme in this chapter. We view the central contribution of the cognitive perspective to be an elaboration of Lippmann's argument that the complex social reality of the external world must be simplified in order to be mapped readily into belief, decision, and action. In our view, the term simplification will refer to psychological processes that have the effect of reduc-

[2]Campbell (1967) has argued that those attributes of a group most different from one's own are most likely to be encoded in the stereotype. This prediction, generated from a Hullian model, is based on the perceptual principle of distinctiveness. To the extent that a group views its own characteristics as favorable, it would be an out-group's most unfavorable characteristics that would be noted, leading to the same prediction as above.

ing both the complexity of information and the complexity of the mental structures that represent that information. The principles outlined by Lippmann clearly serve the function of reducing the complexity of the stimulus. But the functions of categorization, later outlined by Allport, Campbell, and Tajfel also serve the function of simplification by focusing on the features common to a class of objects rather than on the attributes that differentiate those objects. Smith (1989) has noted the tremendous economy that results from categorization: instead of having to learn separately that cats, dogs, lions, and tigers bear live young and regulate their own body temperature, we learn merely that they are mammals, and thus share the attributes of other mammals. Research on the nature and function of categorization, and the meaning of category boundaries has been a major contribution of the cognitive approach to intergroup relations, some of which will be reviewed later in this chapter.

ALLPORT'S *THE NATURE OF PREJUDICE*

One of the best early treatments of categorization appears in Allport's *The Nature of Prejudice* (1954). Allport's encyclopedic treatment of the causes of prejudice is far too extensive to be summarized adequately in this chapter. It is a brilliant overview of social and psychological factors implicated in intergroup hostility. Given the dearth of empirical research then available and the scarcity of work on cognitive processes, the book is amazing in its prescience. Zawadski's two factors are included, but their importance fades amidst a discussion that includes cognitive, linguistic, psychodynamic, and sociocultural determinants of intergroup hostility. The book is meant to be discursive, and is more concerned with an exegesis of relevant concepts than in comparing different theories, or in reducing the overwhelming array of ideas to a few contrasting theories.

One of the most novel aspects of Allport's work is its strong emphasis on cognitive processes. This probably would not be surprising for anyone familiar with his earlier collaboration on the psychology of rumor (Allport & Postman, 1947), which attempted to understand systematic changes in the description of a visual image as it was transmitted from person to person. One of the central concepts was *assimilation,* whereby new information is incorporated into existing knowledge about social categories. One of their stimulus sets used a multiracial scene on a New York subway, containing line drawings of whites (male and female), a black man, two Asians, and an Orthodox Jew, in which the well-dressed black man appears to be having an argument with a white worker, with the white man holding a straight razor. Allport and Postman observed that across five transmissions, with only the first individual having access to the original drawing, the razor changed hands from the white to the black for approximately 50% of the groups studied. Allport and Postman interpreted these findings as assimilation to (stereotypic) expectations. More generally, the process of assimilation, in which new information is structured by existing beliefs, can be thought of as a powerful simplifying mechanism.

This assimilation theme is continued in *The Nature of Prejudice*, under the heading of the "Normality of Pre-judgment," in which generalization is expected to occur on the basis of past experience. Perhaps the most noteworthy aspect of Allport's book was his concern with the nature of social categories, an emphasis that ran counter to two powerful contemporary trends. The first was the behaviorist's aversion to mental processes, and the second was the hegemony accorded the Scapegoat Theory, whose origins lay in the psychoanalytic notions of frustration-aggression and displacement. Allport argued that categories themselves differ on a number of attributes, including their susceptibility to modification by disconfirming evidence. A tendency to view individuals in simple, either/or categories was thought to be related to ". . . a belief in essence" in which, for example, every Jew or every black possesses some essential quality that renders the person similar to all other Jews and blacks and different from others who are not in those categories. The principle of psychological essentialism has recently achieved a renaissance (Medin, 1989; Medin & Ortony, 1989), and may be related to an implicit mutual exclusivity among some social categories (Rothbart & Taylor, 1992). Allport's ideas about categorization, including assimilation and generalization, must be considered among the most important antecedents to the later work on social cognition.

SHERIF'S *THE ROBBERS' CAVE EXPERIMENT*

While Allport tended to focus on the individual's "mental state" to understand the causes of prejudice, Sherif attempted to shift the focus to intergroup rather than intrapersonal processes. Sherif's recently reissued classic experiments on intergroup relations (Sherif, Harvey, White, Hood, & Sherif, 1988, originally published in 1961) differs in a number of ways from Allport's work. Notably, Sherif et al. explicate their own theoretical position, contrasting with other views of intergroup conflict. In the authors' words:

> . . . the conception of the present study differs markedly from existing theories that posit one factor or a few factors as sole or primary determinants of the course of intergroup relations. . .
>
> The functional relatedness of various factors leads us to the cardinal psychological principle of our whole plan of study: *in the study of intra- and intergroup relations, the relative contribution of given external stimulus factors and internal factors pertaining to participating individuals (hunger, sex, status desire, complexes, etc.) have to be analyzed within the framework of the ongoing interaction process among the members in question.* (p. 28)

Sherif et al. offers a "taxonomy" of the causes of intergroup hostility, listing five causes (not including their own): (1) inherent differences in superiority, (2) inherent differences among nations in aggressivity, (3) aggressive instincts, (4) frustrations (individually experienced), and (5) aggressivity of national leaders. His own sixth explanation, described below, may be labeled an "intergroup relations" model. The first cause is equivalent to Zawadski's Well-Earned Reputation principle, and is, along with the idea of "aggressive instincts," dismissed as implausible. Differences among nations, or among leaders of nations, in their hostility toward others (numbers 2 and 5, respectively) are listed as possible causes, as is *individually experienced* frustration (number 4).

All of these factors are considered subservient to the "functional relations between groups," central to the rationale for the Robbers' Cave experiment. Sherif's model is more complex than is generally believed. The elaborate taxonomy derived by Levine and Campbell (1972) originally considered it to be a "realistic conflict model," but later (Campbell, 1988, p. xix) argued for reclassification as a more social/organizational model. Sherif et al.'s argument is twofold: (1) every group establishes its own norms, beliefs, values, and intragroup structure (pattern of relations among group members); as a result, any two interacting groups will have different norms, beliefs, and values, and (2) the quality of intergroup relations will be determined by the functional relations between the groups. When the relations are defined by negative interdependence (e.g., competition), hostility will increase, and when they are defined by positive interdependence (e.g., cooperation), hostility will be diminished. Other factors, such as individually experienced frustration, or individual aggressiveness, will operate through the existing functional relations.

There are some ambiguities in Sherif's position in our view, and they can be illustrated by considering the procedures and results of the Robbers' Cave study. During the process of in-group formation, 24 eleven-year-old boys enrolled in a summer camp were assigned, in a quasi-random fashion, to one of two groups, and each group was taken to a different section of Robbers' Cave State Park. Each group named itself in accordance with their location (Eagles and Rattlers). Each group was initially unaware, but gradually became aware, of the other's presence. During the initial stage of the study each group developed somewhat different interests and activities, depending primarily on the physical location of each camp (e.g., how close it was to the water and to good swimming holes), and on the characteristics of each group's informal leaders. Evidence of antagonism of one group toward the other was seen shortly after the two groups became aware of each other's existence, even before actual contact.

When the groups came into contact, antagonism was exacerbated, and when competitive relations between the groups were contrived by the staff, antagonism increased with each subsequent interaction. Relations between groups were defined by a tournament, consisting of competitions based on baseball, tug-of-war, tent pitching, cabin inspections, skits, and a treasure hunt. The group with the highest cumulative score received a trophy, and each member of the winning group received a knife and a medal.

Since the goal of this research was to demonstrate the effects of cooperation as well as competition, the last phase of the research was to introduce cooperative interaction via the introduction of superordinate goals. It should be mentioned parenthetically that prior to the introduction of superordinate goals, the researchers assessed the effects of contact, without accompanying competition or cooperation, and found no diminution of hostility as a function of contact (in the context of otherwise competitive interaction), a conclusion that has recently been further supported by Hewstone and Brown (1986).

Interdependent cooperative situations with superordinate goals included fixing a tank that supplied water to the camp, pooling money to rent a desired movie, using the tug-of-war rope to pull a truck to get it started (converting a previously competitive activity to one that was cooperative), meal preparation, tent pitching, and traveling together in a single truck. Interestingly, not all of these activities involve a high level of cooperative interdependence. Nevertheless, as is well known, these activities had an important effect in reducing hostility between the groups.

The ingredients of the Robbers' Cave study are complex and include at least the following components: (1) real differences in values and talents between the two groups, (2) competition at a number of levels, (3) frustration, as a result of direct competition, by which each group blocks the goals of the other, (4) a competitive and cooperative orientation sanctioned implicitly, if not explicitly, by the adult authority figures, and (5) the salience of membership in one of two mutually exclusive dichotomous social categories (a factor whose importance would not be established for another decade). Given the highly multidimensional aspect of the critical experimental manipulations, it is not clear to what extent functional relations between groups were or were not the key ingredients to conflict and accord.

Although there is ambiguity in determining the subset of factors critical for generating conflict and accord in the Robbers' Cave experiment, the importance of this work cannot be overstated. At one level, the research emphasized the ubiquitous nature of intergroup conflict, a perspective to be reinforced by Tajfel's (1970) later work on the minimal group paradigm. When thinking about naturally occurring, historically based intergroup conflict, whether it is in the Mid-East, Northern Ireland, or the United States, there is a powerful bias toward *particularization;* that is, there is a tendency to analyze the conflict in terms of particular historical circumstances, or of the specific differences in goals, behaviors, or values of the conflicting groups. Sherif's experiment was also the first to create ahistorical intergroup conflict, in which there is virtually random assignment to category. Although there were differences between the groups, the differences themselves were produced by arbitrary assignment rather than "fundamental" incompatibilities. This experiment demonstrated that historical enmity and profound group differences were not essential to the establishment of hostile, even occasionally violent, conflict.

The ingredient deemed essential to intergroup hostility was that of intergroup competition, and it is worth exploring the nature of the competition used in the Sherif experiments. The two groups competed in a number of athletic contests, labeled as a tournament, and could win a trophy, jackknives, and emblems if victorious. Recall that Campbell originally classified these experiments as instances of "realistic conflict," but later changed his mind. Perhaps the reason for the change relates to the ambiguity of the term "realistic." In real-world conflict, where two groups compete over resources vital to existence, the meaning is clear; but is competition for trophies and emblems "realistic" in character? The problem, of course, is that the resources over which groups compete vary in importance, from resources necessary for survival (food, shelter, etc.) to those that convey only social dominance (winning a tournament). If we accept the Sherif experiment as demonstrating the power of unimportant social competition, then this research may anticipate some of the processes underlying the implicit social competition of the minimal group paradigm (Tajfel, 1970).

LEVINE AND CAMPBELL'S *ETHNOCENTRISM*

We turn now to the major systematic effort to compare and contrast different theories of intergroup conflict: Levine and Campbell's *Ethnocentrism* (1972). Adopting Sumner's (1906) concept of ethnocentrism "one's own group [as] the center of everything, and all others are rated and scaled with reference to it. . . ," as the primary phenomenon of intergroup perception, Levine and Campbell provide a comprehensive analysis of societal and sociopsychological theories of conflict regarding the predicted magnitude of ethnocentric belief and behavior. We focus on a subset of Levine and Campbell's types of explanations.

Realistic Group Conflict Theory

"[Realistic Group Conflict] theory assumes that group conflicts are rational in the sense that groups do have incompatible goals and are in competition for limited resources" (Levine & Campbell, 1972, p. 29). They note that realistic conflict theories were originally contrasted with psychological theories that emphasized "irrational" processes (e.g., displacement or projection) as the cause of intergroup hostility. Sherif et al. had regarded competition as one way of defining the functional relations between groups, and thus amalgamated a psychological approach with realistic conflict theory. It is worth noting that functional relations between groups was not even considered as a possibility in Zawadski's article.

Frustration-Aggression-Displacement Theory

Most, but not all, versions of the Scapegoat Theory involve the frustration-aggression-displacement principle (as outlined by Zawadski). The frustration-aggression principle was based on Freud's first theory of aggression, and was deemed a powerful explanation for a variety of social behaviors (cf. Dollard, Doob, Miller, Mowrer, & Sears, 1939). To the extent that displaced aggression is part of the explanation for the Authoritarian Personality (Adorno et al., 1950), this explanation generated the largest single body of research on prejudice and intergroup hostility.

Other Psychoanalytic Theories

Levine and Campbell make an important contribution by noting that the psychoanalytic contribution is not limited to the frustration-aggression hypothesis.

Group Narcissism

In Freud's *Group Psychology and the Analysis of the Ego,* Freud analyzes the psychic bond that attracts individuals to the group leader and, secondarily, to the group and its members. By identifying with a powerful or glorious group leader and with the group, individuals are able to enhance their own sense of worth. Although the language of psychoanalysis uses the term narcissism to describe this process, it is not difficult to see conceptual similarity between "group narcissism" and more contemporary work on people's preference to associate themselves with valued groups (Cialdini et al., 1976), and the now-popular social identity theory (Tajfel & Turner, 1986). To quote from Freud:

> Every time two families become connected by a marriage, each of them thinks itself superior to or of better birth than the other. Of two neighboring towns each is the other's most jealous rival; every little canton looks down upon the others with contempt. Closely related races keep one another at arm's length; the South German cannot endure the North German, the Englishman casts every kind of aspersion upon the Scot, the Spaniard despises the Portuguese. We are no longer astonished that greater differences should lead to an almost insuperable repugnance, such as the Gallic people feel for the German, the Aryan for the Semite, and the white races for the colored. (1959/1926, p. 33)

Freud described this kind of thought as "the narcissism of small differences," indicating that meaninglessly small differences may be exaggerated for the purpose of invidious comparison.[3] In our view, Freud's quote is somewhat ambiguous, however, in that it implies that (1) trivial differences can become the basis for intense hostility, and (2) larger "real" differences generate even greater hostility. If the lack of differences do not deter us from disparaging the out-group, as implied by the narcissism of small differences, why then assume that "real" differences invariably lead to hostility? It strikes us that Freud does not take his own psychological determinism far enough. If the lack of differences can generate profound distinctions, is it not also possible that "real" differences can be construed as inconsequential? In short, whether a dimension becomes the basis for hostility cannot be predicted from the "reality" of the similarity or difference, but from the social and psychological meaning of that dimension.

Projection

In projection, impulses or fantasies unacceptable to the perceiver are projected onto an out-group. This concept is actually closer to the biblical use of the "scapegoat" concept than is the frustration–aggression–displacement model. The Bible (Leviticus, 16:20–22) describes a process whereby hands are placed on the head of a live goat, transgressions and sins of Israelites are transferred to the goat, and the goat is sent into the wilderness. Frazer's (1919) *The Golden Bough* has an extensive discussion of scapegoating among preliterate peoples, and notes the common practice of transferring a physical or psychic malady onto another object.

Deutsch (1990), in a most interesting analysis, suggests a link between the concept of "splitting" in object relations theory, and the tendency to view human groups as either good or bad. The infant/child's need to split the caregiver into the good mother, as distinct from the bad mother, and the corresponding tendency to split the self into the good-me and the bad-me, find expression in the adult's need to identify enemies in the world to serve as the focus for negative affect. The object relations model sees the origins of intergroup conflict not in the displacement of aggressive impulses, but as an external projection of the self's need to keep the good-self distinct from the bad-self.

Authoritarianism

The single largest body of research on prejudice emanates from work on the Authoritarian Personality (Adorno et al., 1950), derived largely from

[3]We note that Thorsten Veblen's *Theory of the Leisure Class* (Veblen, 1902) considered "the need for invidious comparison" to be a basic human need. Veblen, an economist attempting to understand the low social value associated with meaningful work, and the high social value placed on meaningless (conspicuous) consumption, based his theory on the premise that people, individually or collectively, are highly motivated to view themselves as superior to others. These ideas have been developed more recently by Messick (Messick & Thorngate, 1967) in his work on maximizing difference in group settings, in Turner's work on esteem and social identity (Turner, 1982), and in the function of downward comparison (Wills, 1981).

psychoanalytic theory. It focuses on individual differences, predicting that guilt over ambivalent attitudes toward parents is resolved by idealizing authority figures and directing hostile feelings away from parents and toward out-groups. Although the mechanism for out-group hostility lies in guilt over ambivalence, its consequences are manifested through effects on cognitive processes, with sharp category boundaries preferred over graded continua. Interestingly, later work on category boundaries stresses the importance of category accentuation processes, but without invoking psychosexual conflict (e.g., Krueger, 1992).

Perception of Out-group Attributes

In this section, Levine and Campbell deal with a number of issues that anticipate later work in the social cognition area. The first is the attributional principle whereby observers misattribute behaviors emanating from social roles to "inherent" dispositions. Behaviors evoked by roles, or by victimizing discrimination are erroneously thought to be enduring qualities of the group. The importance of this idea is immediately apparent, because it acknowledges the "reality" of the behaviors that underlie the attribution, but notes the erroneous causal locus of that attribution.

Another perceptual principle acknowledging the contribution of the stimulus group is the work on in-group–out-group perception. Basing their argument in part on Peabody's (1968) important distinction between the descriptive domain (e.g., that "Group X tends to not spend much money"), while differing in the evaluation of that domain (e.g., a group is described as "thrifty" by in-group members, but as "stingy" by out-group members). This can be viewed as a variant of the "kernel of truth" perspective, inasmuch as the real characteristics of the stimulus group structure the domain of attribution, but the observer's perspective structures the evaluation of that domain. It should be noted that it is exactly this line of argument that creates problems for the well-earned reputation theory. What is the reality of Group X? Thriftiness? Stinginess? To the extent that the differences between these two attributions lie in evaluation rather than description, it is not a question that can be settled empirically.

In the domain of category boundaries, Levine and Campbell argue that group differences will be perceptually exaggerated:

> Such effects correspond to pervasive cognitive processes, noted in perception research as the enhancement of contrast through homogenization of differences within gestalt boundaries and the exaggeration of differences across boundaries. (p. 169)

This quote accurately summarizes the predictions of an earlier paper by Tajfel and Wilkes (1963), and a later paper by Taylor, Fiske, Etcoff, and Ruderman (1978). Campbell (1956), in a neglected article entitled "Enhancement of Contrast as Composite Habit," derived predictions from learning theory regarding stimulus generalization that predicted exaggeration of differences across category boundaries, and confirmed these predictions experimentally. One can only speculate that if the phrase "category accentuation" had been substituted for the original "composite habit," this article may have been more readily incorporated into the social cognition literature.

Research and theory on the enhancement of category boundaries raises interesting questions about the accuracy of intergroup perception. Issues of accuracy in social perception are complex, but have tended to focus on interpersonal, in contrast to intergroup, accuracy. Clarke and Campbell (1955) found that white judges perceived larger differences between the test scores of whites and blacks than were warranted by the actual scores. Dawes, Singer, and Lemons (1972) found that Doves and Hawks during the Vietnam War overestimated the extremity of the attitudes held by the "other" side in the conflict. Judd, Ryan, and Park (1991) compared judgments about University of Colorado engineering and business majors, with the self-ratings of a random sample of each of those groups. Using self-ratings as the benchmark of "reality" they found that (1) perceived differences were greater than actual differences, and (2) estimated variability was more accurately judged by in-group than by out-group members (with out-group members perceiving more homogeneity).

Outside of the domain of social perception, Krueger, Rothbart, and Sriram (1989) presented subjects with an abstract category learning task, in which two intermixed sets of three-digit numbers were presented. Different font styles defined category membership, and the two sets of numbers described two adjacent but nonoverlapping frequency distributions. The subjects' task was to periodically estimate the mean or average of each of the two sets of numbers. This is a demanding task, but subjects were remarkably accurate. Midway through the experiment, the numbers presented for one of the two categories started to "move" the central tendency of that distribution. The question was, to what extent would the subjects incorporate the new values into their perception of central tendency? Krueger et al. predicted, and found, that new information was more likely to be incorporated into estimates of central tendency when the new information accentuated category differences (i.e., when the changing category moved away from the adjacent category) rather than blurred category differences (i.e., when the changing category moved toward the adjacent category). Given that there was no meaning attached to the numbers, they took their findings as evidence for a pervasive tendency to prefer information that simplifies category relations, in this case by maintaining clear boundaries between categories. Earlier, Dawes (1964, 1966) argued that subjects show systematic errors in their memory for set relations. He found that subjects were more likely to misremember overlapping sets as either nonoverlapping or inclusive, whereas the latter two types of sets were rarely remembered as overlapping. These findings were consistent with Krueger et al.'s arguments favoring simplification of category relations.

Lewis (1990) conducted a category learning experiment, and compared subjects' judgments about the central tendency of two categories with the actual central tendency. He presented subjects with two types of faces on a CRT, where the faces differed on an important feature (e.g., width of nose). When he then asked subjects to recreate the actual facial features on the computer screen, he found that subjects systematically overestimated the differences between the two sets of faces on the critical features, and judged the central tendencies to be more extreme than the central tendency of the actual exemplars. This study has some interesting implications for our later discussion of category-exemplar dynamics in stereotype change, but for now we wish to argue that all of the above studies point in the direction of a category accentuation process that simplifies category relations, as predicted by Allport, Tajfel, and Campbell.

Cognitive Congruity Theories

One of the most powerful explanations for hostility against out-groups is that out-groups possess attitudes, beliefs, and values different from our own, and because of that dissimilarity, they are less admired. The assumption is that real differences in attitudinal similarity exist, and that attraction is a function of similarity to one's self or one's group (Rokeach, 1960; Rokeach & Mezei, 1966). This was one of the possible explanations for some of the findings in the Robbers' Cave experiment.

There are two points to be made regarding this view. First, is this a variant of realistic conflict theory? To us, the answer is both yes and no. That is, to the extent that the values between two groups are antithetical to the well-being of either group, this view is synonymous with realistic conflict theory. For example, to the extent that the Nazis' values preclude the survival of the Jews, or that white South African values deny political or economic power to black South Africans, the value similarity and realistic conflict views become indistinguishable. To the extent that the bases of value differences concern trivial issues, for example, preference for vanilla versus chocolate ice cream, then we are no longer in the domain of realistic conflict.

Second, to the extent that hostility is based on trivial value differences (e.g., preference for flavor of ice cream), does the value similarity approach make sense at all? That is, is the concept of a trivial value an oxymoron? Do not values have to be of importance to be applicable to intergroup hostility? To the extent that significant hostility emanates from trivial differences, we seem to be back in the domain of Freud's "narcissism of small differences," which is a precursor of later work on the effects of mere categorization.

Reinforcement Theory

Levine and Campbell include reinforcement theory as one of their socio-psychological theories of intergroup hostility, which deals with the learning and generalization of aggressive responses. Those societies that are most likely to reinforce aggression against other in-group members should also be most likely to reinforce aggression against out-group members; moreover, a simple generalization rule suggests that out-groups most similar to the in-group are most likely to be the targets of aggression. It should be noted that Zawadski (1948) implicitly relied on a reinforcement principle to account for the maintenance of intergroup hostility, in which the dominant group benefits from the minority's disadvantaged condition.

TAJFEL'S COGNITIVE ASPECTS OF PREJUDICE

Levine and Campbell's discussion of the perception of group differences preceded much of the research in the 1970s and 1980s on cognitive processes in intergroup perception, yet it is obvious that many of their ideas are consonant with that research, particularly those of Wilder (1981) and Taylor (1981). If there is a single publication that marks the birth of the cognitive revolution in the intergroup area, however, it is Tajfel's article in the *Journal of Social Issues*. In it he criticized the contrasting views of the social and the physical worlds: "We have the rational model for natural phenomena; we seem to have nothing but a blood-and-guts model for social phenomena" (Tajfel, 1969, p. 80). Arguing that adaptive cognitive functioning exists in the social domain as well, he outlined the role of three important processes: categorization, assimilation, and search for conceptual coherence. He notes the simplifying function of *categorization* (N.B., Allport, 1954; Campbell, 1956), which often involves imposing dichotomies over continuous dimensions with the resultant accentuation of intercategory boundaries (Tajfel & Wilkes, 1963). *Assimilation* is the degree to which new information is structured by prior, learned expectancies (N.B., Lippmann's (1961/1922) view that "facts" are not independent of expectancy), and the causal attribution process that is central to our *search for coherence*. These three processes have received enormous attention by researchers over the past two decades. Even if the research was not stimulated directly by Tajfel's article, his thinking anticipated the direction of research on intergroup processes, and is still an inspiring source for ideas.

The 1970s and 1980s witnessed an explosion of research on the cognitive factors implicated in social perception and intergroup processes. This is not the place to review these contributions in detail, since the work relating most directly to prejudice and stereotyping is covered elsewhere in this volume. The volume edited by Hamilton, *Cognitive Processes in Stereotyping and*

Intergroup Behavior, provides a representative sample of some of the earlier work on illusory correlation (Hamilton, 1981), categorization (Taylor, 1981; Wilder, 1981), and memory and judgment (Rothbart, (1981), as these processes related to intergroup perception. An excellent recent summary can be found in Messick and Mackie (1989).

Earlier in this chapter, we suggested that the contribution of the cognitive perspective to intergroup relations resides, at least in part, on the metaphor of the human mind as a limited capacity system. To paraphrase Lippmann's eloquent statement, there is more subtlety and complexity in the world than we are able to comprehend. Reduction of complexity is achieved by a number of psychological mechanisms, the most prominent of which are outlined in Tajfel's 1969 paper: categorization, assimilation, and search for coherence. Space limitations do not allow us to do justice to the voluminous research in any one of these areas, so we will focus instead on a limited set of topics in the area of categorization: (1) social categorization and the minimal group paradigm, (2) the perception of intragroup variability, and (3) category-exemplar dynamics and its relation to the contact hypothesis.

SOCIAL CATEGORIZATION AND THE MINIMAL GROUP PARADIGM

Freud's description of the "narcissism of small differences" implies that conflict over trivial differences has its origins in processes other than the objective nature of the difference itself. Freud was not the first to make this suggestion. In Jonathan Swift's *Gulliver's Travels* (1735), enduring war is waged between two nations, the Big-Endians and the Little-Endians, in which the former prefers to break its eggs on the large, and the latter on the small, end of the egg. Swift's satire on the religious wars between Protestants and Catholics regarded religious preferences as comparable to the preferred side for breaking an egg. Of course, the combatants do not regard the differences as trivial, and can cite numerous reasons justifying the continuing hostility. In a sense the justifications may be correct. Even if a conflict is originally generated by negligibly small value differences, the consequences of sustained conflict may cease to be trivial. As a result of conflict, real differences can emerge, inequality may develop, and competition for limited resources is likely to occur. In real-world conflict, we can find evidence for almost all of the factors believed to be responsible for intergroup hostility. To determine which of these ingredients are necessary (or sufficient), it is obligatory to bring the problem under laboratory control, which is exactly what was done. Two critical experiments, one by Rabbie and Horwitz (1969), and the other by Tajfel (1970), will be considered in detail.

What were the minimal conditions necessary to establish preference for the in-group over the out-group? Rabbie and Horwitz attempted to answer this question by comparing two basic conditions: (1) a random categorization of subjects into "blues" and "greens" (the control condition), and (2) a random categorization condition augmented by "common fate." The principle of common fate is taken from the Gestalt literature, where commonality of movement is a powerful perceptual grouping principle. The common fate condition in Rabbie and Horwitz is not based on any inherent similarity within the blues or within the greens, nor is it based on any inherent difference between the blues and greens. The common fate is also not produced by any meaningful activity of either the blues or the greens. Specifically, subjects are told that as payment for the experiment, a limited number of inexpensive radios would be handed out; since there were only four radios for eight subjects, a rule would be used to distribute this limited resource. Under one of the main conditions, a coin toss determined whether the "blues" as a group, or the "greens" as a group, would receive the radios. Thus a common fate (receiving the radio or not) would be based on group membership, even though the allocation was randomly determined. The results of this experiment were clear: (1) random categorization alone did not result in differential evaluation of the in-group and out-group, but (2) the introduction of common fate led to more favorable evaluations of in-group than of out-group members.

Shortly after the Rabbie and Horwitz paper, Tajfel (1970) published his classic paper demonstrating that subjects classified on an apparently meaningless dimension (e.g., under- or overestimating dots, or preferring Klee vs. Kandinsky) would later allocate more resources to another in-group member over an out-group member. This would appear to conflict with Rabbie and Horwitz's null results in the control condition, but it should be recognized that in the subjects' minds, the dimensions in Tajfel's experiment may have been inferred to be meaningful; that is, subjects could plausibly infer that they are in fact more similar to, say, another (in-group) underestimator than they are to an (out-group) overestimator. A second important paper by Billig and Tajfel (1973) attempted to experimentally separate similarity from categorization, arguing that their results confirmed the categorization rather than the similarity explanation. However, their described procedures do not allow one to conclude with confidence that perceived similarity did not also continue to play a role. Thus, the Tajfel work, while demonstrating the power of highly arbitrary categorizations, cannot exclude perceived similarity as a causal factor in in-group bias.

The Rabbie and Horwitz experiments, by virtue of their reliance on a nonsimilarity manipulation for the induction of in-groups and out-groups, appear to demonstrate bias in the absence of perceived similarity of *dispositional* attributes. However, as Rabbie and Horwitz noted, their original common fate manipulation confounds competition with common fate, since the allocation of resources was zero sum. In a footnote, they describe a study in which allocation was based on independent coin tosses for each group separately, retaining common fate, and random generation of outcome *with-*

out competition, with similar results to their original data. It is unfortunate that these data were not also published, because it is the most convincing evidence for a very important idea.

One reason why the Rabbie and Horwitz findings are of interest is that they eliminate perceived similarity—at least perceived dispositional similarity—as a possible mechanism for in-group bias. It is, of course, possible that perceived similarity directly results from common fate itself (cf. Campbell, 1958), and that we prefer those who have similar experiences to our own. Horwitz and Rabbie (1989) indicate that by later increasing the sample size, they did find a bias favoring the ingroup in the control condition. Although this addendum reconciles the discrepancy with Billig and Tajfel (1973), it vitiates what may be the most important implication of the Rabbie and Horwitz experiments, that is, that common fate rather than arbitrary categorization is the necessary condition for intergroup bias.

At present there does not appear to be any single compelling explanation for in-group bias demonstrated in the minimal group paradigm. Although Social Identity Theory (SIT) has provided the most widely accepted account (Tajfel & Turner, 1986), it is not without its critics. One axiom of the theory is that people identify with groups in order to enhance their self-image (cf. the narcissism principle of Freud). This axiom produces two corollaries about the relationship between self-esteem and in-group identification: (1) group identification should lead to an enhancement of self-esteem, and (2) low self-esteem should lead to greater discrimination against out-groups (because of the desire for greater intergroup differentiation). Abrams and Hogg, in a review of the relevant literature, suggest that the empirical support for both of these hypotheses is tenuous. They say that SIT ". . . over-implicates self-esteem in intergroup behavior: self-esteem can, under some conditions, be incidental or even irrelevant" (Abrams & Hogg, 1988, p. 322).

Rabbie and Horwitz (1988) also comment:

> We find it implausible. . . to assume that social identity is implicated strongly or at all in causing ingroup favoritism in the minimal intergroup situation. There is no evidence to date that the experimenter's *ad hoc* classifications of subjects into Blues and Greens or Kandinskis and Klees were internalized by them into their self-concepts. If so, their self-concepts must be extraordinarily malleable. (p. 270)

In response, Turner (1988) suggests that the minimal group paradigm may not be the best arena in which to examine social identity processes.

There has been an enormous amount of research on in-group–out-group dichotomies since the original Rabbie and Horwitz and Tajfel studies. One of the most interesting studies has explored the implicit meaning of the we–they distinction. Perdue, Dovidio, Gurtman, and Tyler (1990) did a series of studies indicating that (1) nonsense syllables paired with *us, we*, or *ours* were judged more favorably than nonsense syllables paired with *them, they*, or *theirs*, and (2) when in-group and out-group pronouns served as masked primes in a category verification task (deciding whether trait adjectives were favorable or unfavorable), in-group pronoun primes speeded reaction times (RTs) to favorable traits and slowed RTs to unfavorable traits, whereas out-group primes had the reverse effects. Clearly, the implicit meaning of in-group pronouns are more favorable than out-group pronouns even in a context that is not intergroup in character.

Maass, Arcuri, and colleagues have also identified linguistic biases in the description of behaviors associated with in-group and out-group members (Maass, Salvi, Arcuri, & Semin, 1989; Maass & Arcuri, 1992). In a number of contexts they found that favorable in-group and unfavorable out-group behaviors are more likely to be described with abstract dispositional terms, whereas unfavorable in-group and favorable out-group behaviors are described at a more purely descriptive behavioral level.

In summary, although research on ethnocentrism in the context of the minimal group may have been stimulated in part by belief in the power of mere categorization, other, noncognitive processes, such as esteem enhancement may also be implicated. Whether or not noncognitive processes are involved, the importance of the minimal group research for understanding intergroup relations is enormous. First, this research extends the intellectual tradition of Swift, Freud, and Sherif in suggesting that intergroup bias resides, not in the content of intergroup differences, but in the in-group–out-group boundaries themselves. While there is some argument about the minimal conditions necessary for in-group favoritism, as in the discrepancy between the Rabbie and Horwitz versus Tajfel findings, with the possible exception of patently random pairings, almost any dimension capable of dichotomization can be used to induce a feeling of "us" versus "them," with the concomitant ethnocentric perceptions. In our view, attempts to explain real-world conflict by reference to the magnitude of "real" differences, such as Freud's statement that "greater differences should lead to an almost insuperable repugnance. . . ," mistakenly assume that the "reality" of group differences resides in the external world, rather than in the psychological meaning given to those differences. Religious differences may serve as the basis for barbaric interactions in one society and be treated as an inconsequential difference in another. Even within a society, a dimension that is meaningless at one time can become the basis for violent conflict at another time. One of the central messages of the minimal group research is that any dimension, however trivial, can serve as the kernel for generating intergroup division and conflict. We also suggest, without strong empirical evidence, that the opposite is also true, that is, a difference considered important at one time, can in principle lose its importance at another time, although the process, we suspect, is highly asymmetrical. It may be much more difficult to trivialize a dimension considered important than to create a psychologically important distinction out of a trivial one.

Second, and more generally, the minimal group research emphasizes the importance of category boundaries, consistent with the earlier suggestions of Allport, Campbell, Lippmann, and Tajfel. Categories serve to reduce the amount of information, and frequently function to map a large number of continuous values into a much smaller set of classifications. Dimensions such as under- or overestimation of dots are clearly continuous, and individuals who are barely at opposite sides of the under/over boundary are more similar to one another than is each to more polarized members of their own category. It is expected that when categorical information conflicts with actual similarity (i.e., for a given stimulus set, there is greater similarity across rather than within category boundaries), category information will be prepotent (cf. research on the group attribution error [Allison, Worth & King, 1990; Mackie & Allison, 1987]).

Third, we view the minimal group work as important, not because it is a self-contained explanation of intergroup hostility, but because in-group–out-group distinctions may be the nucleus around which other components of intergroup conflict can coalesce. For example, Howard and Rothbart (1980) found that subjects disproportionately remembered undesirable out-group behaviors following a minimal group manipulation, implying that even when the immediate effects of an ephemeral in-group–out-group distinction have faded, a "biased database" remains as a result of that classification. Consider how new, ambiguous behaviors can be assimilated to that set of memories, or how, in a competitive or conflict-ridden setting, unfavorable acts may become associated with the out-group category rather than with specific individuals. To the extent that people treat the in-group–out-group distinction as meaningful, it will also become a real basis for psychological and social grouping, and create a realistic basis for the distinction. Later, we elaborate on this developmental sequence.

PERCEPTION OF INTRAGROUP VARIABILITY

Given the importance and power of in-group–out-group dichotomies, and the Tajfel and Wilkes prediction that objects are perceived as more similar when categorized, we would expect differences in perceived intra-category variability for in-group and out-group. Attneave (1957) posed the question "why do all Orientals look alike?," and suggested that the more experience we have with a particular prototype, the more we are able to recognize deviations from that prototype. Using prototypes derived from geometric shapes, Attneave varied subjects' exposure to the prototypes and found support for his hypothesis.

The idea that we view the out-group as relatively undifferentiated goes back at least to Spinoza:

> If we have been affected with joy or sorrow by any one who belongs to a class or nation different from our own, and if our joy or sorrow is accompanied with the idea of this person as its cause, under the common name of the class or nation, we shall

not love or hate him merely, but the whole of the class or nation to which he belongs. (1930/1677, p. 161)

Since research in this area has already been nicely summarized (Park, Judd, & Ryan, 1991), we will not repeat those summaries here, but will focus instead on an interpretive issue. The issue concerns the mechanism underlying out-group homogeneity. The simplest interpretation was proposed by Attneave: experience and/or familiarity. It could be argued that blacks and whites (Linville & Jones, 1980) and Rutgers and Princeton students (Quattrone & Jones, 1980) are groups with rather little contact with one another, and lack of familiarity implies lack of differentiation. For this reason Park and Rothbart (1982) used men and women, since it is difficult to think of a clear social dichotomy with more contact than these two categories. They found evidence for out-group homogeneity, but also conceded that despite the magnitude of contact between men and women, there still may be differences in the nature or extent of information women have about women in comparison to men (and vice versa). For this reason, an experiment was conducted in which the information given to men and women about men and women was controlled (and equal) (Park and Rothbart, 1982, Experiment 4). The least differentiated information about a stimulus person (gender) was remembered equally well by in-group and out-group members, but the more differentiated information (occupation) was remembered substantially better by in-group than by out-group members.

The implications of these results are clear: even when the same information is available to in-group and out-group members, the information retained by in-group and out-group members is not the same. These results could nevertheless be handled by a familiarity model in that familiarity could promote a more differentiated cognitive structure of the in-group, whereby more differentiated information could be absorbed; the relatively undifferentiated structure associated with the out-group inhibits the incorporation of differentiated information.

More recently, Linville, Fischer, and Salovey (1989) have proposed an intuitive and straightforward explanation based on an aspect of familiarity: in-group members are encountered more frequently than out-group members, giving opportunity for the observation of a wider range of in-group traits/behaviors relative to the out-group. Since more (and more varied) members of the in-group are available relative to the out-group, judgments of the in-group variability are greater than those of the out-group. This explanation may be termed a "frequency" model because it proposes that greater perceived in-group variation is the result of more frequent and thus more varied encounters with in-group than with out-group members.

Linville et al. (1989) proposed a computer simulation to demonstrate the viability of their hypothesis. This computer simulation (known as PDIST) is conceptually very simple. Essentially, PDIST produces variance estimates that increase as the number of retrieved exemplars increases. Although not stated explicitly by Linville et al. (1989), the behavior of the model is precisely dictated by the statistical relation between the sample variance and the population variance. For small samples, the sample variance is too small to be a good estimate of the population variance, while for larger samples the sample variance approaches the population variance (Hays, 1988). PDIST essentially equates the out-group homogeneity effect with these known properties of the sample variance. In other words, PDIST implies that for in-groups, the sample of traits/behaviors, is large relative to that of out-groups, and because the sample of in-groups is larger, we produce a larger (and more veridical) variance estimate for in-groups than for out-groups.

However, is sample size all there is to the out-group homogeneity effect? A recent study by Judd and Park (1988) suggests that it is not. Judd and Park created minimal groups, where group members had the same amount of information about in-group members as about out-group members. Even under these conditions of minimal group membership, subjects judged the in-group to be more variegated than the out-group. Given that these groups had the same amount of contact with one another, a pure frequency/familiarity model appears untenable. This study, combined with a study showing that variance estimates of a group are sometimes stored on-line (Park & Hastie, 1987), suggest that a simple frequency explanation is not adequate to account for all of the out-group homogeneity effect.

Unfortunately, the Judd and Park findings leave us in a theoretical vacuum, because it is not clear what additional mechanism could account for out-group homogeneity in the minimal group setting. Judd and Park obtained two findings of immediate interest. First, using a global rating of similarity, out-group members were perceived to be more similar to one another than were in-group members. Second, an index of similarity derived from descriptions of each stimulus person where self was excluded did *not* show differences in perceived intragroup similarity as a function of in-group–out-group status. One possible explanation for the results using the global measure of similarity is that this measure, unlike the individual similarity measure, does not exclude the effects of self. It is possible that subjects see no differences in similarity between the out-group members and all in-group members minus the self. In other words, perhaps the greater perceived variability for in-group is really due to assumed differences between self and other in-group members.

One might salvage something akin to a strict frequency view by suggesting that we always have more information and thus more varied information about the in-group than about the out-group, even in minimal groups, because of the presence of the self as an in-group member. Judd and Park present some evidence supportive of the idea that reference to the self is more likely when thinking about the in-group than about the out-group, and future research will undoubtedly clarify the role of the self in the representation and judgments of group variability.

Research on perception of group variability has been of interest for a number of reasons. First, the tendency to view the out-group as less differentiated than the in-group seems to be independent of more affectively based intergroup processes, such as ethnocentrism (e.g., Park & Rothbart, 1982), and represents a contribution of the cognitive approach to intergroup perception. Second, the issue of perceptual complexity raises interesting issues about the nature of category differentiation. If the tendency to view the out-group as homogeneous exacerbates intergroup conflict, then the importance of changing stereotypes in the direction of greater complexity becomes paramount. How do we increase the complexity of our images of the out-group, particularly given the powerful tendency to assimilate new information to the existing stereotypes?

A number of interesting ideas have been suggested regarding stereotype change. Taylor (1981), Weber and Crocker (1983), and Crocker, Fiske, and Taylor (1984) suggest that subtyping is a way of creating a subordinate category that allows the superordinate category to remain unchanged. Thus, if we have a traditional view of women, and encounter a woman who is inconsistent with that stereotype, we, in effect, create a subcategory ("woman athlete," "woman executive," etc.), allowing the superordinate category to remain intact. Brewer and Miller (1988), however, suggest that by creating multiple subcategories, the usefulness of the superordinate category begins to diminish, and eventually disintegrates. These two perspectives are not inconsistent and may refer to different time periods in the developmental course of stereotype change. Meanwhile, the importance of perception of subgroups as a possible mediator of perceived variability was demonstrated by Park, Ryan, and Judd (1992).

Research on perception of variability raises basic questions about category structure and stereotype change, which in turn brings us to one of the most important potential sources of stereotype change—the contact hypothesis—which reintroduces familiarity and experience as the engine for change.

THE CONTACT HYPOTHESIS AND CATEGORY-EXEMPLAR DYNAMICS

Consistent with our theme that categorization, as a simplification mechanism, influences intergroup processes, we propose that an understanding of the ameliorative effects of intergroup contact is closely linked to the dynamic character of category-exemplar relations. In this section, we first discuss the contact hypothesis, and then examine the nature of exemplar-based change.

The idea that contact will lead to improved relations between groups is compelling, and early field researchers supported it strongly. For example, Deutsch and Collins (1952) interviewed a white woman about her experiences after moving into a racially integrated housing project:

> I started to cry when my husband told me we were coming to live here. . . I didn't want to. . . live here where there are so many colored people. . . but. . . there was no place else to go. . . Well, all that's changed. . . I've come to like [colored people] a great deal. . . I'd just as soon live near a colored person as a white; it makes no difference to me. (p. 655)

Unfortunately, the effectiveness of intergroup contact did not live up to the promise of the above interview. Allport and others produced a list of specifying conditions necessary for desirable effects of contact (i.e., equal status, accepting social atmosphere, voluntary vs. involuntary contact, etc., Allport, 1954; Cook, 1969, 1984), but even after satisfying these conditions, the sufficiency of contact as an amelioration for intergroup tensions remained unclear. Amir (1969), in a review of the literature, noted that the fulfillment of these conditions still did not guarantee positive attitude change; some studies showed reduced intergroup tensions through contact and other studies showed increased tensions through contact.

In 1976, Amir noted that little theorizing had at that time addressed the nature of the psychological processes involved in intergroup contact. A detailed understanding of the sociological conditions had been undertaken, but the psychological antecedents of effective intergroup contact had hardly been considered and were still virtually unknown. Social cognitive analysis of intergroup relations has, we believe, provided a useful framework for addressing some of Amir's concerns. This is supported by the recent surge of interest in the cognitive factors implicated in intergroup contact (e.g., Brewer & Miller, 1984; Brown & Turner, 1981; Hewstone & Brown, 1986; Rothbart & John, 1985).

A useful distinction coming from work on intergroup contact is made by Brown and Turner (1981), who distinguish between intergroup behavior and interpersonal behavior. Intergroup behavior, according to Brown and Turner, is characterized by acting in terms of the group, either collectively or individually, and is likely to show low intersubject variability. Interpersonal behavior, alternatively, is characterized by the individual's normal range of behavior and is determined not by group identification, but by individual personal relationships. For the purposes of understanding intergroup contact, if one accepts the distinction between interpersonal and intergroup behavior, the crucial question becomes: which kind of contact is likely to lead to more positive intergroup relations? We will consider in detail two of the more distinct views.

Brewer and Miller (1984) have articulated a theory, based on social identity theory (Tajfel, 1978), that argues for the efficacy of interpersonal contact as a means for improving face-to-face intergroup relations. They suggest the existence of three psychological modes of contact: category based, differentiation, and personalization. Brewer and Miller argue that contact will be effective as a means of improving group relations when it is at the level of differentiation or personalization (interpersonal rather than intergroup).

Category based, or intergroup, contact should not necessarily result in more positive intergroup relations because of the desire for group distinctiveness as posited by Social Identity Theory.

Clearly, there are two distinct stages in the process of contact-induced stereotype change. The first stage assumes that contact between group members occurs in a way that challenges existing group stereotypes. The second stage assumes generalization of the counterstereotypic information from the individual group members to the group as a whole. Some of the failures to find beneficial effects of contact represent failures at the first stage, while others represent failures at the second stage; that is, there is evidence that contact itself does not necessarily guarantee counterstereotypic, or even favorable, behaviors, as would be the case when there is a high level of conflict or competition between the groups. Many of the conditions that Allport, Cook, and Amir specify for amelioration address the conditions present during the first stage. For groups with a long history of enmity, it is no mean task to establish favorable interpersonal behavior, yet there is strong evidence that this can occur (e.g., Cook, 1969). Even if favorable interactions are generated in the first stage, there is still the difficult task of generalization to the group as a whole, to be addressed shortly.

Brewer and Miller (1984) make the interesting argument that the benefit of interpersonal contact on intergroup relations operates, not necessarily through generalization, but by altering the utility of the superordinate category: by coming to view group members in individuated ways rather than as exemplars of the category, the category itself comes to lose its predictive power, even though the content of the stereotype may remain unchanged. In an important study, Bettencourt, Brewer, Croak, and Miller (1992) compared the intergroup effects of interpersonal and intergroup orientation. Using the minimal group paradigm they first created two categories, with the correspondent in-group bias, then created four-person cooperative groups consisting of two in-group and two out-group members. The experimenters varied both the orientation of the group (interpersonal or task, where task was assumed to generate an intercategory perspective), and whether that group's relation to other groups was cooperative or competitive. They found, in comparison to a control condition, that interpersonal orientation lowered bias, whereas task orientation increased bias. The effects of intergroup cooperation and competition had roughly the same effects as interpersonal and task orientation, respectively. This research suggests that the effects of intergroup cooperation itself are mediated by a number of important variables, such as interpersonal orientation, and that categorization processes can hinder the beneficial effects of cooperation.

Although the contact hypothesis assumes that experiences with an individual from an outgroup should generalize to beliefs about the group as a whole, this does not appear to be an automatic process. The conditions necessary for generalization may be fairly restrictive, with group-level beliefs remaining somewhat autonomous from beliefs about the attributes of individual group members. Rothbart and John (1985) have suggested that generalization will occur only when exemplar attributes become associated with the category (i.e., when the category label is sufficiently activated).[4] If the category label is not activated, as would be the case with atypical exemplars, the attributes of category members will be functionally isolated from the perceived attributes of the group and exemplar-to-category generalization will not occur. This contention has been supported by findings from Rothbart and Lewis (1988) and Wilder (1984) as well as by research on categorization by Rips (1975). These studies found that generalization was dependent on the degree of fit between the attributes of the category member and the attributes of the category; generalization from the category exemplar to the category occurred most strongly when the exemplar was a "good fit," or "typical" example of the category. Recent research by Desforges et al. (1991) found evidence for generalization based on exposure to a single exemplar, presumably because the exemplar was typical of the category in some important ways.

It should be noted that the "discounting" of atypical exemplars constitutes a powerful mechanism for preserving the stability of stereotypic beliefs in the face of disconfirming information.[5] This process appears to be quite similar to the mechanism of compartmentalization, in which disconfirming information is isolated from the relevant concept, yet it is cognitively rather than affectively based. There is a strong irony in this process. It is exactly those exemplars who are most discrepant from the category that should place the greatest pressure on the category to change. Instead, these discrepant exemplars, by virtue of their atypicality, are unlikely to be encoded as category members. In our view, the circularity of this process, in which "challenging" exemplars are excluded from the category, is an example of the high "cost" of simplification. A prototype model of stereotyping allows for efficient categorization of exemplars on the basis of goodness of fit to the category, with the economy that such categorization affords (Smith, 1989), yet the goodness of fit principle is likely to exclude poorly fitting exemplars from the category, leaving the category insulated from change.

[4]As a historical note, the ideas about exemplar-category dynamics presented by Rothbart and John (1985) and Hewstone and Brown (1986) are not new. Lewin and Grabbe (1945), antedating Rothbart and John (1985) by 40 years in the same journal, published an article entitled, "Conduct, Knowledge, and Acceptance of New Values," in which they wrote: "Only if a psychological linkage is made between the image of specific individuals and the stereotype of a certain group, only when individuals can be perceived as 'typical representatives' of that group, is the experience with individuals likely to affect the stereotype." (p. 58)

[5]Rothbart and John (1993) found enormous stability in the ordering of stereotypic attributes over a four-year period. Using the mean test attributions for 14 different target groups at initial and final testing, they found an average $r = .92$ over a four-year period, compared to $r = .96$ over a one-week period.

These ideas suggest a paradoxical effect of contact. Although contact may lead to an exemplar becoming individuated, and thus differentiated from a category, the very process of individuation works against the generalization associated with the contact hypothesis. The same processes that make contact effective as a way of changing attitudes toward *members* of the category, may also work against generalization to the category as a whole.

Hewstone and Brown (1986) take these arguments to suggest that contact at an intergroup, rather than at an interpersonal, level is necessary for generalization to occur. It is of interest that Hewstone and Brown (1986), like Brewer and Miller (1984), base their ideas on Social Identity Theory. Whether the ability of SIT to generate two contradictory hypotheses is viewed as a strength or a weakness of the theory is left to the reader's judgment. They argue that category membership must be made salient throughout contact, or the experiences of the contact will fail to generalize to the entire group. Interpersonal encounters, because of their weak relationship to the category, may thus fail to modify group-level beliefs.

Lewis (1990) proposed that our idealized images of groups may, by virtue of their idealization, be particularly resistant to change. This is based in part on the previously discussed research by Krueger, and by Lewis, in which the representation of a category is more extreme than is justified by the exemplars themselves. To the extent that the mental representation of a category is idealized (i.e., displaced away from the actual central tendency), only a relatively small proportion of exemplars may constitute a good fit to the prototype. The large number of exemplars that fit the stereotype poorly may then be discounted, rather than accommodated, leaving the unrealistically extreme stereotype unchanged by disconfirming exemplars. Lewis's model, in short, suggests a mechanism whereby extreme stereotypes (i.e., stereotypes more extreme than warranted by the exemplars comprising the category) can resist modification.

Hewstone and Brown's (1986) book on the role of contact in intergroup conflict puts the issue of contact in stark relief. After considering the powerful social forces that spark social conflict in the Middle East, South Africa, Northern Ireland, and America's desegregated schools, it is clear that the ability of contact to ameliorate hostility in these settings is negligible. However, is the failure of contact in these settings an indictment of the contact hypothesis or, to paraphrase Hamlet only slightly "is there more in the heaven and earth of intergroup conflict than is embodied in the contact hypothesis?" Would even the strongest believer in the ameliorative effects of contact argue that it is strong enough to overcome, among other factors, direct and real competition over economic and political resources? Pettigrew's (1986) chapter in *Contact and Conflict in Intergroup Encounters* is a most thoughtful analysis of the limits of our ideas about the efficacy of contact, and perhaps more important, the inadequacy and vagueness of our current theories of intergroup conflict.

PROBLEMS AND PROSPECTS FOR THE COGNITIVE APPROACH TO INTERGROUP RELATIONS

If we consider the increase in the complexity of our ideas about intergroup hostility as we move, from the two-factor approach of Zawadski to the comprehensive assay of Levine and Campbell and to the recent work on social categorization, it becomes apparent that there is no "single, sovereign" principle to account for the complexity of intergroup processes. It is our view that most of the stated causes of group hostility have some validity under some circumstances, and the task is to try to understand the developmental nature of intergroup conflict, and the highly dynamic interplay that exists among causal factors. Consider two hypothetical cases. In Case 1, two societies differing in physical, linguistic, and value attributes develop independently and without knowledge of one another. After the two societies come in contact, there is friction because of different behavioral practices, and hostility increases. One society comes to dominate the other, and the relation shifts now to one of majority/minority relations, which in turn reflects unequal distribution of resources between the two groups, competition over resources, and the usual pattern of self- and other perception that occurs in minority–majority relations.

In Case 2, there are no physical, language, or value differences, but through essentially random factors, people in one region come to be treated differently from people in another region. This leads to political conflict, and although there are no readily apparent ways of physically identifying the different groups, the developing social importance of the distinction between, say, "Northerners" and "Southerners" means that people go to great lengths to determine which individuals are "on our side" and which ones are "on the other side."

These two scenarios are certainly not exhaustive of the near-infinite ways in which groups can develop into agonistic relations. They are merely meant to illustrate two ideas: (1) important differences (such as physical, language, or value differences) are not a necessary precursor to hostile attitudes, although differences can themselves develop in the course of interaction, which in turn can exacerbate conflict, and (2) social forces, such as externally imposed competition, cooperation, common and distinct fates, play an important role in defining and shaping in-group–out-group relations.

The first point illustrates the strength and importance of much of the research on intergroup processes from the cognitive perspective, in emphasizing the effects of categorization, establishment of mutually exclusive dichotomies, and the concomitants of that categorization. The second point illustrates the weakness of the purely cognitive perspective, given the impoverished way in which we conceptualize the nature of social forces. It is interesting to reflect that social psychology's most prominent cognitive theorist, Kurt Lewin, considered attractive and repellent forces to be of central importance in determining movement in the psychological field. Attempts to reduce these factors to cognitive processes, for example, chronic accessibility of constructs, seem limited either in being able to capture the forces that direct behavior, or in describing the dynamic interactions among conflicting groups.

To a large extent, the inadequacy of our models for thinking about the highly interactive and dynamic relations among groups is a problem for many different approaches to intergroup relations, and is not unique to the social cognitive perspective. The highly reductionist assumptions characteristic of much of social cognition make this approach particularly vulnerable in an area as complex and interdisciplinary as intergroup relations. We see value in models that emphasize the developmental nature of intergroup relations, as well as in models that view differing explanations as not necessarily mutually exclusive, but as representing causal factors present at different stages of the developmental chain. It may be useful in model building to import some of the ideas about nonlinear systems, and chaos theory, in which small initial causes may have disproportionately large effects at a later time (sensitivity to initial conditions).

It is appropriate to end this chapter with the customary admonition to recognize the importance of emotion in intergroup relations. Since other chapters deal with the relation among affect, emotion, and cognition, we confine ourselves to only one issue. An implicit, if not explicit, assumption of much of the cognitive work, particularly on the minimal group paradigm, is that the mild forms of affect generated in the laboratory, as a result of cognitive processes, differ in intensity, but not in kind from the violent forces that we often observe in real-life intergroup conflict. This assumption may be questionable. Although we assume that small differences in evaluation exist in continuous relation with intergroup violence, this assumption should be carefully examined. Dehumanization of the enemy and justification of violence against the outgroup based on a perceived history of injustice against the in-group seem to be common to most examples of real-life intergroup violence, but are not sentiments usually aroused in the laboratory. Perhaps general theoretical progress in intergroup relations will help identify the causes that generate intergroup violence, and these conditions are unlikely to be solely cognitive in character.

In reaching a general assessment of the cognitive contribution to intergroup relations, we may have a bias to focus on what has not yet been achieved rather than on what has been accomplished. Clearly the work of the last two decades has provided much substance to the earlier ideas of Lippmann, Allport, Campbell, Sherif, and Tajfel. It has enlarged the scope of our thinking about the nature of group processes well beyond the more limited ideas discussed by, say, Zawadski. The cognitive perspective has led to enormous progress, which we do not see abating. The only danger we sense is one of goals and proportions. One consequence of the cognitive revolution was to liberate us, at midcentury, from the hegemony of a single dominant model of intergroup relations. We now have a far more complex, and we believe more accurate, view of intergroup relations. The goal, however, is to understand intergroup relations, not to replace a limited psychodynamic perspective with a limited cognitive perspective. A major challenge remains to integrate our understanding of cognitive and affective processes, and to learn how powerful social forces are mediated by these two mechanisms.

ACKNOWLEDGMENTS

Myron Rothbart was supported in part by National Institutes of Mental Health Grant MH40662. We are deeply indebted to Mary Rothbart for her insightful comments, both substantive and stylistic. We are also grateful to Marilynn Brewer, Bernadette Park, and Mara Cadinu for their comments on an earlier draft.

REFERENCES

Abrams, D., & Hogg, M. A. (1988). Comments on the motivational status of self-esteem in social identity and intergroup discrimination. *European Journal of Social Psychology, 18*, 317–334.

Adorno, T. W., Frenkel-Brunswik, E., Levinson, D. J., & Sanford, R. N. (1950). *The authoritarian personality.* New York: Harper.

Allison, S. T., Worth, L. T., & King, M. W. C. (1990). Group decisions as social inference heuristics. *Journal of Personality and Social Psychology, 58*, 801–811.

Allport, G. W. (1954). *The nature of prejudice.* Cambridge, MA: Addison-Wesley.

Allport, G. W., & Postman, C. J. (1947). *The psychology of rumor.* New York: Henry Holt & Company.

Amir, Y. (1969). Contact hypothesis in ethnic relations. *Psychological Bulletin, 71*, 319–342.

Amir, Y. (1976). The role of intergroup contact in change of prejudice and ethnic relations. In P. Katz (Ed.), *Towards the elimination of racism.* New York: Pergammon Press.

Attneave, F. (1957). Transfer of experience with a class-schema to identification-learning of patterns and shapes. *Journal of Experimental Psychology, 54*, 81–88.

Bartlett, F. C. (1958). *Thinking: An experimental and social study.* London: Allen & Unwin.

Bettencourt, B. A., Brewer, M. B., Croak, M. R., & Miller, N. (1992). Cooperation and the reduction of intergroup bias: The role of reward structure and social orientation. *Journal of Experimental Social Psychology, 28*, 301–319.

Billig, M., & Tajfel, H. (1973). Social categorization and similarity in intergroup behavior. *European Journal of Social Psychology, 3*, 27–52.

Brewer, M. B., & Miller, N. (1984). Beyond the contact hypothesis: Theoretical perspectives on desegregation. In *Groups in contact: The psychology of desegregation*, Brewer & Miller (Eds.). New York: Academic Press.

Brewer, M. B., & Miller, N. (1988). Contact and cooperation: When do they work? In P. A. Katz & D. A. Taylor (Eds.), *Eliminating racism: Profiles in controversy* (pp. 315–326). New York: Plenum Press.

Brigham, J. C. (1971). Ethnic stereotypes. *Psychological Bulletin, 76*, 15–38.

Broadbent, D. E. (1958). *Perception and communication.* Oxford: Pergamon Press.

Brown, R. J., & Turner, J. C. (1981). Interpersonal and intergroup behavior. In J. C. Turner & H. Giles (Eds.), *Intergroup behaviour.* Chicago: University of Chicago Press.

Bruner, J. S., Goodnow, J. J., & Austin, G. A. (1962). *A study of thinking.* New York: Science Editions, Inc.

Campbell, D. T. (1956). Enhancement of contrast as composite habit. *Journal of Abnormal Psychology and Social Psychology, 53,* 350–355.

Campbell, D. T. (1958). Common fate, similarity, and other indices of the status of aggregates of persons as social entities. *Behavioral Science, 3,* 14–25.

Campbell, D. (1967). Stereotypes and the perception of group differences. *American Psychologist, 22,* 817–829.

Campbell, D. T. (1988). Introduction to *The Robbers' Cave experiment* (pp. xiii–xxi). Middletown, CT: Wesleyan University Press.

Cialdini, R. B., Borden, R. J., Thorne, A., Walker, M. R., Freeman, S., & Sloan, L. R. (1976). Basking in reflected glory: Three (football) field studies. *Journal of Personality and Social Psychology, 34,* 366–375.

Clarke, R. B., & Campbell, D. T. (1955). A demonstration of bias in estimates of Negro ability. *Journal of Social Issues,* 585–588.

Cook, S. W. (1969). Motives in a conceptual analysis of attitude-related behavior. In W. J. Arnold and D. Levine (Eds.), *Nebraska symposium on motivation.* Lincoln, NE: University of Nebraska Press.

Cook, S. W. (1984). Cooperative interaction in multiethnic contexts. In N. Miller & M. B. Brewer (Eds.), *Groups in contact: The psychology of desegregation* (pp. 155–185). New York: Academic Press.

Crocker, J., Fiske, S. T., & Taylor, S. E. (1984). Schematic bases of belief change. In J. R. Eiser (Ed.), *Attitudinal judgment* (pp. 197–226). New York: Springer-Verlag.

Dawes, R. M. (1964). Cognitive distortion. *Psychological Reports, 14,* 443–459.

Dawes, R. M. (1966). Memory and distortion of meaningful written material. *British Journal of Psychology, 57,* 77–86.

Dawes, R. M., Singer, D., & Lemons, F. (1972). An experimental analysis of the contrast effect and its implications for intergroup communication and the indirect assessment of attitude. *Journal of Personality and Social Psychology, 21,* 281–295.

Desforges, D. M., Lord, C. G., Ramsey, S. L., Mason, J. A., Van Leeuwen, M. D., West, S. C., & Lepper, M. R. (1991). Effects of structured cooperative contact on changing negative attitudes toward stigmatized social groups. *Journal of Personality and Social Psychology, 60,* 531–544.

Deutsch, M. (1990). Psychological roots of moral exclusion. *Journal of Social Issues, 46,* 21–25.

Deutsch, M., & Collins, M. E. (1952). The effect of public policy in housing projects upon interracial attitudes. In G. E. Swanson, T. M. Newcomb, and E. L. Hartley (Eds.), *Readings in social psychology* (rev. ed.). New York: Holt, Rinehart, and Winston.

Dollard, J., Doob, L. W., Miller, N. E., Mowrer, O. H., & Sears, R. R. (1939). *Frustration and aggression.* New Haven: Yale University Press.

Frazer, J. G., Sir (1919–1920). *The golden bough: A study in magic and religion.* London: Macmillan.

Freud, S. (1959/1926). *Group psychology and the analysis of the ego* (p. 33). New York: W. W. Norton & Co.

Hamilton, D. L. (1981). Stereotyping and intergroup behavior: Some thoughts on the cognitive approach. In D. L. Hamilton (Ed.), *Cognitive processes in stereotyping and intergroup behavior* (pp. 333–353). Hillsdale, NJ: Erlbaum.

Hays, W. L. (1988). *Statistics* (4th ed.). New York: Holt, Rinehart and Winston.

Hewstone, M., & Brown, R. (1986). Contact is not enough: An intergroup perspective on the "Contact Hypothesis." In M. Hewstone and R. Brown (Eds.), *Contact and conflict in intergroup encounters* (pp. 1–44). Oxford: Basil Blackwell.

Hewstone, M., & Brown, R. (Eds.). (1986). *Contact and conflict in intergroup encounters.* Oxford: Basil Blackwell.

Horwitz, M., & Rabbie, J. M. (1989). Stereotypes of groups, group members, and individuals in categories: A differential analysis. In D. Bar-Tal, C. F. Graumann, A. W. Kruglanski, & W. Strobe (Eds.), *Stereotyping and prejudice: Changing conceptions* (pp. 105–129). New York: Springer-Verlag.

Howard, J. W., & Rothbart, M. (1980). Social categorization and memory for in-group and out-group behavior. *Journal of Personality and Social Psychology, 38(2),* 301–310.

Judd, C. M., & Park, B. (1988). Out-group homogeneity: Judgments of variability at the individual and group levels. *Journal of Personality and Social Psychology, 54,* 778–788.

Judd, C. M., Ryan, C. S., & Park, B. (1991). Accuracy in the judgment of in-group and out-group variability. *Journal of Personality and Social Psychology, 61,* 366–379.

Krueger, J. (1992). On the overestimation of between-group differences. *European Review of Social Psychology, 3,* 31–56.

Krueger, J., Rothbart, M., & Sriram, N. (1989). Category learning and change: Differences in sensitivity to information that enhances or reduces intercategory distinctions. *Journal of Personality and Social Psychology, 56,* 866–875.

Levine, R. A., & Campbell, D. T. (1972). *Ethnocentrism: Theories of conflict, ethnic attitudes and group behavior.* New York: Wiley.

Lewin, K., & Grabbe, P. (1945). Conduct, knowledge, and acceptance of new values. *Journal of Social Issues,* 53–64.

Lewis, S. (1990). *Ideals as prototypes: The role of representational complexity.* Unpublished dissertation, University of Oregon, Eugene.

Linville, P. W., & Jones, E. E. (1980). Polarized appraisals of out-group members. *Journal of Personality and Social Psychology, 38,* 689–703.

Linville, P. W., Fischer, G. W., & Salovey, P. (1989). Perceived distributions of the characteristics of in-group and out-group members: Empirical evidence and a computer simulation. *Journal of Personality and Social Psychology, 57,* 165–188.

Lippmann, W. (1961/1922). *Public opinion.* New York: Macmillan.

Maass, A., & Arcuri, L. (1992). The role of language in the persistence of stereotypes. In G. R. Semin & K. Fiedler (Eds.), *Language, interaction and social cognition* (pp. 129–143). London: Sage.

Maass, A., Salvi, D., Arcuri, L., & Semin, G. (1989). Language use in intergroup contexts: The linguistic intergroup bias. *Journal of Personality and Social Psychology, 57,* 981–993.

Mackie, D. M., & Allison, S. T. (1987). Group attribution errors and the illusion of group attitude change. *Journal of Experimental Social Psychology, 23,* 460–480.

Medin, D. L. (1989). Concepts and conceptual structure. *American Psychologist, 44,* 1469–1481.

Medin, D., & Ortony, A. (1989). Psychological essentialism. In S. Vosnaidou & A. Ortony (Eds.), *Similarity and analogical reasoning* (pp. 179–195). Cambridge: Cambridge University Press.

Messick, D. M., & Mackie, D. M. (1989). Intergroup relations. *Annual Review of Psychology, 40,* 45–81.

Messick, D. M., & Thorngate, W. B. (1967). Relative gain maximization in experimental games. *Journal of Experimental Social Psychology, 3,* 85–101.

Miller, G. A. (1956). The magical number seven, plus or minus two. *Psychological Review, 63,* 81–97.

Park, B., & Hastie, R. (1987). Perception of variability in category development: Instance-versus abstraction-based stereotypes. *Journal of Personality and Social Psychology, 53,* 621–635.

Park, B. M., & Rothbart, M. (1982). Perception of out-group homogeneity and levels of social categorization: Memory for the subordinate attributes of in-group and out-group members. *Journal of Personality and Social Psychology, 42,* 1051–1068.

Park, B., Judd, C. M., & Ryan, C. S. (1991). Social categorization and the representation of variability in formation. In W. Stroebe and M. Hewstone (Eds.), *European review of social psychology* (Vol. 2, pp. 211–245). New York: Wiley.

Park, B. M., Ryan, C. S., & Judd, C. M. (1992). The role of meaningful subgroups in explaining differences in perceived variability for in-groups and out-groups. *Journal of Personality and Social Psychology, 63,* 553–567.

Peabody, D. (1968). Group judgments in the Philippines: Evaluative and descriptive aspects. *Journal of Personality and Social Psychology, 10,* 290–300.

Perdue, C. W., Dovidio, J. F., Gurtman, M. B., & Tyler, R. B. (1990). Us and them: Social categorization and the process of intergroup bias. *Journal of Personality and Social Psychology, 59,* 475–486.

Pettrigrew, T. F. (1986). The intergroup contact hypothesis reconsidered. In M. Hewstone and R. Brown (Eds.), *Contact and conflict in intergroup encounters* (pp. 169–195). Oxford: Basil Blackwell.

Posner, M. I., & Shulman, G. L. (1979). Cognitive science. In E. Hearts (Ed.), *The first century of experimental psychology* (pp. 371–405). New York: Halsted.

Quattrone, G. A., & Jones, E. E. (1980). The perception of variability within in-groups and out-groups: Implications for the law of small numbers. *Journal of Personality and Social Psychology, 38,* 141–152.

Rabbie, J. M., & Horwitz, M. (1969). Arousal of ingroup–outgroup bias by a chance win or loss. *Journal of Personality and Social Psychology, 13(3),* 269–277.

Rabbie, J. M., & Horwitz, M. (1988). Categories versus groups as explanatory concepts in intergroup relations. *European Journal of Social Psychology, 18,* 117–123.

Rips, L. J. (1975). Inductive judgments about natural categories. *Journal of Verbal Learning and Verbal Behavior, 14,* 665–681.

Rokeach, M. (1960). *The open and closed mind.* New York: Basic Books.

Rokeach, M., & Mezei, L. (1966). Race and shared belief as factors in social choice. *Science, 151,* 167–172.

Rothbart, M. (1981). Memory processes and social beliefs. In D. L. Hamilton (Ed.), *Cognitive processes in stereotyping and intergroup behavior.* Hillsdale, NJ: Erlbaum.

Rothbart, M., & Birrell, P. (1977). Attitude and the perception of facts. *Journal of Research in Personality, 11,* 209–215.

Rothbart, M., & John, O. (1985) Social categorization and behavioral episodes: A cognitive analysis of the effects of intergroup contact. *Journal of Social Issues, 41,* 81–104.

Rothbart, M., & John, O. (1993). Intergroup relations and stereotype change: A social–cognitive analysis and some longitudinal findings. In P. M. Sniderman, P. E. Tetlock, & E. G. Carmines (Eds.), *Prejudice, politics, and the American dream* (pp. 32–59, 307–332). Stanford, CA: Stanford University Press.

Rothbart, M., & Lewis, S. (1988). Inferring category attributes from exemplar attributes: Geometric shapes and social categories. *Journal of Personality and Social Psychology, 55,* 861–872.

Rothbart, M., & Taylor, M. (1992). Category labels and social reality: Do we view social categories as natural kinds? In G. R. Semin & K. Fiedler (Eds.), *Language, interaction and social cognition* (pp. 11–36). London: Sage.

Sherif, M., Harvey, O. J., White, B. J., Hood, W. R., & Sherif, C. W. (1988/1961). *The Robbers' Cave experiment: Intergroup conflict and cooperation.* Middletown, CT: Wesleyan University Press.

Simon, H. A. (1981). *The sciences of the artificial* (2nd ed.) (p. 36). Cambridge, MA: MIT Press.

Smith, E. E. (1989). Concepts and induction. In M. I. Posner (Ed.), *Foundations of cognitive science* (pp. 501–526). Cambridge, MA: MIT Press.

Spinoza, B. (1930/1677). The ethics. In J. Wild (Ed.), *Spinoza selections* (p. 249).

Sumner, W. G. (1906). *Folkways.* Boston: Ginn and Co.

Swift, J. (1977/1735). *Gulliver's travels.* New York: Oxford University Press.

Tajfel, H. (1969). Cognitive aspects of prejudice. *Journal of Social Issues, 25,* 79–98.

Tajfel, H. (1970). Experiments in intergroup discrimination. *Scientific American, 223,* 96–102.

Tajfel, H. (Ed.). (1978). Differentiation between social groups: Studies in the social psychology of intergroup relations. In *European monographs in social psychology, 14.* London: Academic Press.

Tajfel, H., & Turner, J. C. (1986). The social identity theory of intergroup behavior. In S. Worchel & W. G. Austin (Eds.), *Psychology of intergroup relations* (pp. 7–24). Chicago: Nelson-Hall.

Tajfel, H., & Wilkes, A. L. (1963). Classification and quantitative judgment. *British Journal of Social Psychology, 54,* 101–114.

Taylor, S. E. (1981). A categorization approach to stereotyping. In D. L. Hamilton (Ed.), *Cognitive approaches in stereotyping and intergroup behavior.* Hillsdale, NJ: Erlbaum.

Taylor, S. E., Fiske, S. T., Etcoff, N. C., & Ruderman, A. J. (1978). Categorical and contextual basis of person memory and stereotyping. *Journal of Personality and Social Psychology, 36,* 778–793.

Turner, J. C. (1982). Towards a cognitive redefinition of the social group. In H. Tajfel (Ed.), *Social identity and intergroup relations.* Cambridge and Paris: C. U. P. and Edition de la M. S. H., in press.

Turner, J. C. (1988). Comments on Doise's individual and social identities in intergroup relations. *European Journal of Social Psychology, 18,* 113–116.

Veblen, T. (1902). *A theory of the leisure class.* New York: Macmillan.

Weber, R., & Crocker, J. (1983). Cognitive processes in the revision of stereotypic beliefs. *Journal of Personality and Social Psychology, 45,* 961–967.

Wilder, D. A. (1981). Perceiving persons as a group: Categorization and intergroup relations. In D. L. Hamilton (Ed.), *Cognitive processes in stereotyping and intergroup behavior.* Hillsdale, NJ: Erlbaum.

Wilder, D. A. (1984). Intergroup contact: The typical member and the exception to the rule. *Journal of Experimental Social Psychology, 20,* 177–194.

Wills, T. A. (1981). Downward comparison principles in social psychology. *Psychological Bulletin, 90,* 245–271.

Zawadski, B. (1948). Limitations of the scapegoat theory of prejudice. *Journal of Abnormal and Social Psychology, 43,* 127–141.

Author Index

Abelson, R. P., 2, 7, 15, 17, 19–24, 26–27, 31–33, 35–36, 62, 70, 80–81, 89, 92, 98, 102, 105–106, 119, 130, 136, 205, 218, 234, 249, 256, 261, 266, 269, 281, 284, 287, 342
Abrams, D., 366, 378
Abramson, L. Y., 77, 102
Acorn, D. A., 95, 104
Adorno, T. W., 293, 316, 325, 342, 349, 358–359, 378
Agostinelli, G., 278, 287
Agustsdottir, S., 168, 191
Ajzen, I., 56, 59, 66, 68, 70, 196, 198, 207, 222–223, 228, 236, 249, 251, 268, 270, 281, 283
Alba, J. W., 152, 182, 184
Albright, J. S., 144, 149–150, 158, 167, 178–179, 184, 188
Alessi, C., 209, 252
Allen, V. L., 277, 281
Allison, S. T., 368, 378, 380
Allman, C., 56–57, 69
Allport, D. A., 81, 102
Allport, G. W., 9–10, 12, 55, 66, 109, 125–126, 136, 144–145, 148, 161, 184, 195, 249, 273, 281, 291, 294, 306, 311, 316, 324, 326, 328, 330, 334, 338, 341–342, 353, 363, 372, 378
Altemeyer, B., 325–326, 343
Altom, M. W., 155, 190
American Psychological Association, 79, 102
Amir, Y., 327, 343, 372, 378
Anastasio, R. A., 333, 343
Andersen, S. M., 51–52, 66, 147, 170, 184, 299, 316
Anderson, C. A., 42, 44, 66, 144, 151, 157, 161, 163, 166, 184
Anderson, H. H., 198, 219, 236, 250
Anderson, J. R., 21, 33, 82, 102, 161, 166, 184, 204, 209, 224, 232, 249
Anderson, N. H., 19, 33, 43, 55–56, 66, 119–120, 124, 136, 196, 198, 228, 249–250
Anderson, R. C., 116, 121, 137
Arcuri, L., 367, 380
Arkes, H. R., 272, 281
Aronson, E., 21, 27, 33, 218, 234, 249–250, 261, 281, 338, 343
Asch, S. E., 16, 18, 33, 40–41, 50, 66, 119, 125, 137, 261, 272–273, 275–277, 281
Ashmore, R. D., 126, 137, 292–293, 297, 316, 323–325, 334, 343
Asuncion, A. G., 229, 254, 266, 276, 278, 285–286
Attneave, F., 368, 378
Au, T. K., 90, 102
Augoustinos, M., 53–54, 66
Austin, G. A., 61, 67, 311, 317, 348, 379
Axsom, D., 277, 281

Backman, C. W., 132, 140, 167, 184
Baddeley, A. D., 214, 250

Bailey, J., 332, 344
Baillet, S. D., 135, 139, 173–174, 188
Baker, S., 231, 257
Baker, S. M., 299, 317
Banaji, M. R., 23–25, 33–34, 174, 182, 187, 231, 252
Bandura, A., 170, 184, 338, 343
Barclay, C. R., 181, 185
Bargh, J. A., 23, 25, 33, 36, 44, 49, 57, 60–61, 66, 69, 101–102, 115–116, 135, 137, 139, 144, 147, 153, 169, 172, 174–175, 179, 181–182, 185, 187, 225, 230, 250, 252, 265–267, 270, 281–282, 288, 306, 316
Baron, R. S., 314, 319
Barsalou, L. W., 52, 66, 144, 185, 212, 216, 250
Bar-Tal, D., 77, 104
Bartlett, F. C., 178, 185, 348, 378
Barton, J., 169, 185
Bassili, J. N., 84, 93–94, 100, 103, 118, 137
Batson, C. D., 62, 66
Baumeister, R. F., 159, 167, 185–186
Baumgardner, M. H., 232, 253
Beal, P., 334–335, 337, 345
Beattie, A. E., 56–57, 69
Beauvois, J. L., 62, 65, 66
Beck, A. T., 152, 166, 185
Beck, L., 42, 66–67
Bellezza, F. S., 176–177, 185
Belmore, S. M., 48, 67
Bem, D. J., 77, 103, 133, 137, 146, 167, 170, 185
Berglas, S., 167–168, 170, 188
Berkowitz, L., 11, 12
Bernstein, S., 147, 152, 169, 190
Berscheid, E., 129–130, 141, 301, 320
Bettencourt, B. A., 373, 378
Betz, A. L., 50, 73
Biernat, M., 301, 317
Billig, M., 323, 343, 365–366, 378
Billman, D., 216, 250
Birnbaum, M. H., 120, 137
Birrell, P., 350, 381
Bishop, G. D., 327, 345
Black, J. B., 131, 137
Blake, F., 63, 69
Blanchard, F. A., 337, 343
Blaxton, T. A., 231, 250
Block, J., 137
Bobo, L., 329, 345
Bodenhausen, G. V., 49, 74, 128, 137, 178, 193, 301, 306, 314, 317, 319
Boehm, L. E., 272, 281
Boettger, R., 60, 74
Bolland, J., 22, 35
Bond, R. N., 61, 66, 116, 135, 137, 160, 169, 185, 187, 230, 250
Borden, R. J., 358, 379
Borgida, E., 44, 53, 60, 63, 67, 71–72, 81, 106
Bower, G. H., 52, 71, 131, 135, 137, 147, 150, 175–176, 185, 208, 210, 252
Boyes-Braem, P., 217, 255
Bradburn, N., 201, 214, 221, 257, 288
Bradley, G. W., 146, 185
Braly, K. W., 64, 70, 126, 139, 296–299, 319
Branscombe, N. R., 231, 256
Breckler, S. J., 34–35, 148, 187, 206, 211, 222, 250, 262, 287
Brehm, J. W., 17, 33, 266, 268, 282, 287
Brekke, N., 53, 71
Brenner, M., 175, 185
Brewer, M. B., 25–26, 33, 55, 67, 80, 98, 106, 113, 140, 299, 303, 306, 311–312, 317, 371–373, 375, 378
Brewer, W. F., 98, 103
Brigham, J. C., 292, 296–298, 307–308, 317, 334, 343, 351, 378
Broadbent, D. E., 348, 378
Brock, T. C., 219, 227, 250, 255, 261, 266, 282, 284, 286
Bromley, S., 329, 343
Brown, J. D., 84, 104, 171, 192
Brown, M. M., 11, 12
Brown, N. R., 178, 185
Brown, P., 176, 185
Brown, R., 41, 67, 89–90, 98, 103, 107, 356, 372, 374–375, 379–380

Brown, R. J., 372, 379
Brown, Y., 275, 286
Brownfain, J. J., 145, 185
Bruner, J. S., 25–26, 33, 41–42, 60–61, 67, 137, 168, 185, 261–262, 287, 311, 317, 348, 379
Budesheim, T. L., 127, 141
Bugental, J.F.T., 145, 185
Burke, P. J., 149, 185
Burnstein, E., 235–236, 256–258, 268, 274, 282, 284
Burton, H. A., 135, 139, 153, 157–158, 176–177, 181, 188
Buss, A. H., 138, 146, 186
Butterfield, E. C., 197, 253

Cacioppo, J. T., 24, 35, 140, 210, 222, 235, 250, 255, 263, 265–267, 269, 273, 278, 282, 286
Caetano, A., 65, 67
Calder, B. J., 133, 140
Campbell, 275
Campbell, D. T., 297, 310, 317, 351–352, 355, 357, 360, 363, 366, 379–380
Campbell, E. Q., 330, 343
Campbell, J. D., 167, 171, 192, 275, 282
Cantor, N., 5, 12, 22, 33, 51, 67, 121, 137, 144, 149–150, 153–154, 158, 167–169, 178–179, 185, 188, 190–191, 212, 250, 299, 317
Cantril, H., 145, 191, 261, 287
Capella, J. N., 268, 282
Carbonell, J., 21, 33
Carlisle, C. J., 314, 319
Carlsmith, J. M., 18, 34
Carlston, D. E., 5, 9, 12, 44–45, 69, 73, 94, 103, 116, 120–122, 130–131, 137, 141, 143, 146, 176–178, 180, 182, 185–187, 193, 209, 212–213, 230, 232, 250–251, 255–257, 265, 288
Carpenter, S., 95, 104
Carpenter, S. L., 61, 67
Carroll, J. D., 20, 33
Carroll, J. S., 77, 104
Cartwright, D., 3, 12, 261, 282
Carver, C. S., 170, 176, 186
Cattell, R. B., 109, 137
Cauthen, N. R., 292, 296, 317
Cermak, L. S., 183, 186
Chacon, S., 170, 189
Chaiken, S., 82, 101, 103, 169, 190, 229, 251, 261–271, 277–278, 281–283
Chapin, W. F., 52, 67
Chase, W. G., 62, 67
Chassin, L., 169, 185–186, 278, 287
Chave, E. J., 288
Chein, I., 323, 325–327, 344
Cheng, P. W., 84, 86–88, 97, 103
Chew, B. R., 144, 149–150, 158, 167, 178–179, 186, 188
Chira, S., 25–26, 33
Cialdini, R. B., 275, 280, 282, 285, 358, 379
Clark, L. F., 94, 100, 105, 161, 164–166, 189
Clark, R. D., 275, 278, 285
Clarke, R. B., 361, 379
Clary, E. G., 301, 317
Clore, G. L., 11, 13, 134, 140, 267, 287
Clubb, B., 170, 189
Coffman, T. L., 296–297, 319
Cohen, A., 284
Cohen, A. R., 17, 33
Cohen, C. E., 58, 67, 125, 137, 301, 317
Cohen, L. H., 159, 192
Cohen, N. J., 209, 251
Cohen, O., 99, 107
Cohen, S., 332, 344
Collins, A., 11, 13
Collins, A. M., 224, 251
Collins, M. E., 371, 379
Combs, A. W., 148, 192
Conway, M., 167, 169–171, 177–178, 191
Cook, D., 335–336, 346
Cook, F. W., 327, 343
Cook, S. W., 372–373, 379
Cook, T. O., 209, 252

Cooley, C. H., 145, 149, 186
Cooper, C., 49, 71
Cooper, J., 18, 33, 234, 251, 264, 282, 301–302, 321
Cooper, L. A., 205, 256
Corey, S. M., 269, 282
Corkin, S., 231, 254
Cottrell, M. B., 235, 251
Cotty, E., 169, 186
Cox, M. G., 42, 68
Craik, F.I.M., 176, 183, 186
Crane, M., 147, 152, 169, 190
Crano, W. D., 278, 283
Crelia, R. A., 226–227, 230, 254
Croak, M. R., 373, 378
Crocker, J., 22–23, 30, 36, 95, 103, 371, 379, 382
Crockett, H. J., Jr., 26, 35
Crosby, F., 25–26, 33, 329, 343
Crutchfield, R. S., 3, 12, 261, 285
Cunniff, C., 92, 95, 107, 118–119, 141
Cunningham, J. D., 80, 106
Czapinski, J., 45, 72

d'Agostino, P. R., 93, 103
D'Andrade, R., 201, 214, 221, 257, 288
Darley, J. M., 60, 64, 67, 70, 301, 317
Davis, J. H., 274, 284
Davis, K. E., 77, 80–81, 105, 113–114, 139
Dawes, R. M., 307, 317, 361, 379
Dawson, V. L., 63, 67
Deaux, K., 149, 186
DeBono, K. G., 63, 67, 263, 267, 287
Deese, J., 19, 33
Define, P. G., 116, 138
Del Boca, F. K., 126, 137, 292–293, 297, 316, 323–325, 334, 343
de Montpellier, G., 58, 67
Dépret, E. F., 65, 67
Derry, P. A., 174, 189
Desforges, D. M., 170, 189, 374, 379
DeSoto, C. B., 111, 139
Deutsch, M., 273, 282, 359, 371, 379
Devine, P. G., 1, 10, 24–25, 28, 33, 59, 61, 67, 197, 226, 251, 265, 282, 299, 306, 317, 323, 325, 329–330, 333–338, 342–343, 345–346
Diehl, M., 303, 317
Di Giacomo, J. P., 54, 67
Dijker, A.G.M., 314, 317
Dishman, R. K., 209, 251
Dixon, T. M., 159, 186
Dodge, K. A., 11, 12
Dollard, J., 303, 317, 358, 379
Donders, F. E., 181, 186
Doob, L. W., 358, 379
Dorfman, D., 157–158, 174, 181, 187
Dovidio, J. F., 23, 25, 33, 309, 317, 325, 327, 329–330, 332–333, 336, 343–344, 366, 381
Downing, J. W., 213, 225, 253
Drake, R. A., 213, 225, 253
Dreben, E. K., 121, 138, 228, 251
Driscoll, D. M., 10, 50, 69, 213, 240, 256, 267, 287, 291
Dubois, N., 62, 65, 66
Duckitt, J., 323, 329, 344
Dudycha, G. J., 303, 317
Dugan, P. M., 46, 69, 305, 318
Dukerich, J. M., 232, 238, 253
Dull, V., 299, 317
Dumais, S. T., 334, 346
Duncan, B. L., 301, 317
Dunn, D. S., 28, 36, 200, 257
Durkheim, E., 53, 67
Duval, S., 146, 186, 338, 344
Duval, T. S., 338, 344
Duval, V. H., 338, 344
Dweck, C., 170, 186
Dyer, M. G., 22, 34

Eachus, H. T., 132, 140
Eagly, A. H., 82, 101, 103, 261–267, 269, 271, 278, 282–284, 310, 317
Ebbesen, E. B., 5, 12, 58, 67–68, 125, 137, 146, 187
Ebbinghaus, H., 181
Edwards, K., 251, 267, 283

Effrein, E. A., 167, 186
Ehrlich, H. J., 296, 318
Einhorn, H. J., 97, 103
Eiser, J. R., 266, 288
Elliot, A. J., 329–330, 335–336, 338, 343
Elliott, E. S., 170, 186
Ellsworth, P. C., 110, 140
Elster, J., 25, 34
Emory, G., 152, 166, 185
Erber, R., 56–57, 68
Esses, V. M., 314, 318
Etcoff, N. C., 360, 382
Etcoff, N. L., 113, 138
Evans, M., 49, 72
Evans, N., 309, 317
Evans, S., 84, 108
Eysenck, H. J., 109, 138
Eysenck, M. W., 138

Fairey, P. J., 275, 282
Falender, V. J., 167, 186
Farber, J., 332, 344
Farr, R. M., 54, 68
Fazio, R. H., 18, 23, 25, 33–34, 84, 103, 167, 186, 202, 206, 209–213, 217, 225, 228, 234, 238, 251–252, 258, 262–264, 266, 269 270, 282–284, 337, 344
Fenigstein, A., 138, 146, 186
Ferguson, T. J., 84, 96, 103, 176, 186
Festinger, L., 3, 12, 18, 34, 60, 68, 195, 234, 251, 261, 272–273, 276, 283, 338, 344
Fiedler, K., 46–47, 68, 90–91, 103, 106
Field, P., 284
Fincham, F. D., 85–86, 101, 103, 105
Fischer, G. W., 53, 71, 154, 189, 299–300, 319, 369–370, 380
Fischhoff, B., 85, 103
Fish, D., 89–90, 98, 103
Fishbein, M., 56, 68, 196, 198, 207, 228, 236, 249, 251, 268, 270, 283
Fiske, S. T., 1, 8, 12, 22–23, 25–26, 34, 39, 42–45, 49–51, 54–58, 60–63, 65, 67–69, 72–74, 84, 96, 98, 103, 107, 113–114, 121, 124, 138, 144, 147, 172, 182, 186, 208, 228, 239, 251, 261, 283, 306, 311–312, 314, 318, 360, 371, 379, 382
Flay, B. R., 209, 252
Fleming, D., 222, 251
Fletcher, G.J.O., 101, 103
Fong, G. T., 147, 186
Ford, T. E., 60, 73, 310, 314, 318, 320
Forgas, J. P., 11, 12, 314, 318
Fösterling, F., 86, 104
Fowles, D. C., 338, 344
Frazer, Sir J. G., 359, 379
Freeman, S., 358, 379
Frenkel-Brunswik, E., 293, 316, 325, 342, 349, 358–359, 378
Freud, S., 27, 34, 145, 186, 358, 379
Freund, T., 60, 69–70, 335, 345
Frey, D., 267, 283
Friberg, L., 209, 255
Friedman, A., 176
Friedrichs, R. W., 330, 344
Frieze, I. H., 77, 104
Fuhrman, R. W., 59, 67, 131, 140, 153, 178, 186, 189, 193
Fulero, S., 49, 72
Funder, D. C., 138

Gaertner, S. L., 23, 33, 309, 318, 325, 327, 329–330, 332–333, 336, 343–344
Ganellen, R. J., 176, 186
Gangestad, S., 46, 73
Gardner, R. C., 297, 318
Gastardo-Conaco, M. C., 276, 278, 286
Geen, T. R., 222, 250
Gentner, D., 22, 34
Gerard, H. B., 60, 70, 273, 282, 301, 321
Gergen, K. J., 114, 139, 144–149, 183, 186–187
Gersho, B. F., 314, 319
Geva, N., 232, 253
Gifford, R. K., 23, 34, 46, 69, 304, 318

Gilbert, D. T., 61, 69, 82, 94, 99, 104, 226–227, 251–252
Gilbert, G. M., 296–297, 303, 318
Gilligan, S. G., 135, 137, 147, 150, 175–176, 185, 208, 210, 252
Gilovich, T., 91, 104
Glass, D. C., 332, 344
Gleick, J., 241, 252
Glucksberg, S., 216, 253
Goethals, G. R., 41, 70, 278, 283
Goetz, E. T., 116, 137
Goffman, E., 146, 149, 187
Goldberg, L. R., 52, 67
Gollob, H. F., 235, 252
Gollwitzer, P. M., 60, 69
Goodman, M. E., 324, 344
Goodnow, J. J., 61, 67, 311, 317, 348, 379
Goodwin, S., 62
Gordon, C., 144–145, 147, 149, 183, 187
Gordon, P. C., 146, 188
Gordon, S. E., 58, 74, 117–118, 127, 131, 138, 141–142
Gorenflo, D. W., 278, 283
Gorkin, I., 169, 191, 335, 345
Govender, R., 270, 282
Grabbe, P., 374, 380
Graesser, A. C., 131, 138
Graham, E., 284
Graham, S., 84, 104
Gray, J. A., 338, 344
Gray, W., 217, 255
Greenberg, J., 338, 345
Greene, D., 147, 191, 277, 287
Greenwald, A. G., 24–25, 27, 33–35, 144–145, 147–148, 153, 161, 167, 171–172, 174–175, 177–178, 182, 187, 217, 228–229, 231, 252, 262–263, 266, 268–269, 283–284, 286–287
Grice, H. P., 90, 94, 104
Gross, P. H., 64, 67, 301, 317
Grubb, P. D., 95, 104
Gruder, C. L., 209, 252
Gschneidinger, E., 141, 149, 192
Gurtman, M. B., 366, 381
Haddock, G., 314, 318
Halamaj, J., 209, 252
Hamill, R., 44, 63, 69, 71, 147, 190
Hamilton, D. L., 1, 5, 10–11, 12, 23, 34, 41–42, 46, 50, 58, 69, 73–74, 84, 95, 100, 104, 117–118, 120, 127, 138, 146, 187, 291, 293, 296–298, 300–302, 304–307, 310, 313–316, 318–320, 326, 333, 342, 344, 364, 379
Hannah, D. B., 95, 103
Hanson, L. R., Jr., 45, 70
Hardin, C., 23, 33
Harding, J., 323, 325–327, 344
Harkins, S. G., 278, 284
Harter, S., 170, 187
Harvey, J. H., 91–92, 104
Harvey, O. J., 132, 138, 303, 319, 354, 381
Hasher, L., 152, 182, 184, 209, 252
Hass, R. G., 272, 284, 330–332, 335–336, 344–345
Hastie, R., 5, 11, 12–13, 23, 34, 44, 49, 52–53, 69, 72, 92, 95–96, 104, 121, 138, 146, 153, 177, 180, 187, 190, 209, 212, 219, 228, 251–252, 255, 300–301, 318–319, 370, 380
Hastorf, A. H., 110, 140
Haugtvedt, C., 268, 284
Hays, W. L., 370, 379
Heider, F., 3, 12, 17, 20, 34, 78, 89, 104, 113, 125, 138, 233–234, 252
Hemmeter, U., 47, 68
Hennigan, K. M., 209, 252
Henninger, M., 132, 141
Hepburn, C., 53, 71, 139
Herek, G. M., 25–26, 34, 262–263, 284
Herk, M., 341, 344
Herman, C. P., 146, 187
Herman, P. C., 5, 12
Hershey, L., 42, 66–67
Hewstone, M., 80, 82, 85–86, 89, 92, 94, 104–105, 356, 372, 374–375, 379–380

Higgins, E. T., 5, 12, 23, 34, 41, 44, 49, 61, 69–70, 96, 104, 111, 115–117, 132, 134, 138–139, 141, 144–146, 149, 153, 157–158, 160, 168–169, 172, 174, 179, 181–182, 187, 192, 225, 238, 252, 334–335, 344
Hilgard, E. R., 27, 34, 145, 187
Hillger, L. A., 90, 107
Hilton, D. J., 81, 84, 86–88, 90–91, 97, 104–105
Hilton, J. L., 60, 70
Himmelfarb, S., 262, 284
Hinsz, V. B., 274, 284
Hinton, G. E., 287
Hintzman, D. L., 154, 187
Hippler, H. J., 11, 12
Hixon, J. G., 61, 69, 94, 104
Hochschild, J. L., 341, 344
Hoffman, C., 59, 70
Hofmann, C., 47, 68
Hogan, R., 111, 139
Hogarth, R. M., 97, 103
Hogg, M. A., 366, 378
Holmes, D. S., 147, 188
Holyoak, K. J., 88, 103, 146, 188
Hood, W. R., 303, 319, 354, 381
Hopfield, J. J., 243, 248, 252
Horwitz, M., 364, 366, 380–381
House, P., 147, 191, 277, 287
Houston, D. A., 202, 252, 263, 269, 284
Hovland, C. I., 3, 12, 16–17, 34, 196, 199, 214, 248, 252, 256, 261, 266, 284, 287
Howard, J. W., 368, 380
Howes, P. W., 325, 346
Hu, L., 53, 71
Hubbard, M., 49, 72
Hubert, S., 121, 137, 228, 250
Huddy, L., 28, 36
Hull, J. G., 174, 188
Hutcherson, H. W., 94, 100, 105
Hymes, R. W., 221, 252

Iacobucci, D., 85, 105
Innes, J. M., 53–54, 66
Insko, C. A., 86, 106, 234–235, 252, 262, 284, 334, 346
Isenberg, D. J., 274, 284
Isham, J., 230, 256

Jackson, L. A., 314, 318
Jacoby, L. L., 81, 105
James, W., 132, 139, 144–145, 148–149, 161, 167, 188
Jamieson, D. W., 335, 344
Janis, I. L., 3, 12, 16, 34, 196, 199, 214, 248, 252, 261, 266, 284
Jaspars, J., 85–86, 104–105
Jennings, D. L., 91, 104
Jennings, S., 91, 104
Jodelet, D., 54, 70
John, O. P., 31, 35, 52, 67, 372, 374, 381
Johnson, B. T., 263, 265, 284
Johnson, C., 46, 71, 305, 319
Johnson, D., 217, 255
Johnson, M. K., 209, 252
Johnson-Laird, P. N., 78, 105
Jones, C. R., 23, 34, 41, 69, 96, 104, 115–117, 138
Jones, E. E., 16, 25–26, 34, 41, 60, 70, 77, 80–81, 97, 105, 113–114, 139, 146, 167–168, 170, 188, 259, 284, 369, 380–381
Jones, R. A., 302, 319
Jordan, N., 234, 252
Jourard, S. M., 145–146, 188
Jourden, F., 338, 343
Judd, C. M., 2, 13, 39, 47, 52, 63, 70–73, 111, 140, 143–144, 153, 169–170, 188, 191, 201–202, 213, 221, 225, 253, 270, 287, 330, 345, 361, 369–371, 380–381

Kahneman, D., 97, 105, 226, 257, 271–272, 284
Kallgren, C. A., 263, 288
Kalthoff, R. A., 159, 188

Kanouse, D. E., 45, 70, 77, 89, 105
Kaplan, M. T., 274, 284
Kardes, F. R., 34, 202, 251, 262, 283
Karlins, M., 296–297, 319
Kass, A., 24, 34
Kassin, S. M., 275, 284
Katz, A. N., 176, 188
Katz, D., 25–26, 34, 64, 70, 126, 139, 262, 268, 284, 296–299, 319
Katz, I., 330–332, 335–336, 344–345
Katz, L. B., 58, 69, 117–118, 138
Katz, P. A., 323–324, 334, 345
Keele, S. W., 153, 190
Keenan, J. M., 135, 139, 173–174, 176, 185, 188
Kelley, C. M., 81, 105
Kelley, H. H., 3, 8, 12, 16, 34, 46, 70, 77–78, 80–81, 85–88, 98, 105–106, 113, 132, 138–139, 261, 266, 276, 278, 284
Kelley, J. J., 196, 199, 214, 248, 252
Kelly, G. A., 145, 188
Kelman, H. C., 269, 273, 276, 278, 284
Kendzierski, D., 173, 188
Kenny, D. A., 84, 103
Kerlinger, F. N., 201, 253
Kiesler, C. A., 267, 284, 289
Kiesler, S. B., 284
Kihlstrom, J. F., 5, 12, 135, 139, 144, 149–150, 153–154, 158, 161, 167, 169, 173, 176, 178–179, 184, 188, 190
Kim, H.-S., 314, 319
Kim, M. P., 208, 253
Kinder, D. R., 25–26, 35, 63, 68, 330, 345
King, B., 284
King, G. A., 61, 70, 115, 138, 168–169, 187, 238, 252, 334–335, 344
King, M.W.C., 368, 378
Kintsch, W., 92, 105
Kirker, W. S., 135, 140, 147, 152–153, 158, 173–174, 176–177, 191
Kirscht, J. P., 270, 287
Kitayama, S., 152, 190, 268, 284
Klar, Y., 59, 70
Klatzky, R. L., 51–52, 66, 299, 316
Klein, R., 160, 187
Klein, S. B., 118, 122, 133–135, 139, 144, 149–150, 153, 155, 157–158, 167, 173, 176–179, 181, 188–189, 231, 253
Klinger, E., 116, 139
Klinger, M., 334–335, 337, 345
Knibbs, C. S., 81, 84, 88, 105
Knowles, E. S., 201, 253
Kosslyn, S. M., 205, 253
Kraft, D., 28, 36, 200, 257
Krauss, H. H., 292, 296, 317
Krech, D., 3, 12, 261, 285
Kriss, M., 84, 96, 106
Krosnick, J. A., 202, 213, 225, 253
Krueger, J., 360–361, 380
Kruglanski, A. W., 59–60, 69–70, 264, 269, 275, 277, 280, 285, 335, 345
Krull, D. S., 99, 104, 226–227, 252
Kuhn, M. H., 145, 189
Kuiper, N. A., 135, 140, 147, 152–153, 158, 173–177, 181, 189, 191
Kuklinski, J. H., 22, 35, 125, 140
Kulik, J. A., 201, 221, 253
Kumar, P. A., 23, 34, 49, 69, 95, 104
Kunda, Z., 167–168, 190, 301, 318
Kutner, B., 323, 325–327, 344

Lachman, J. L., 197, 253
Lachman, R., 197, 253
Lalljee, M., 80, 102
Lambert, A. J., 8–9, 109, 128, 139
Landman, J., 261, 285
Langer, E. J., 24–25, 35, 62, 70, 166, 189
LaPiere, R. T., 31, 35, 269, 285
Lapsley, D. K., 174, 181, 189
Larter, W. M., 63, 68
Latané, B., 24, 35, 247, 253–254
Lau, R. R., 25, 27, 36, 63, 68, 91, 105
Laufer, J. K., 113, 138
LeBon, G., 272, 285
Leddo, J., 80, 98, 105
Lee, D. J., 178, 193

Lee, D. J., 178, 193
Lehnert, W. G., 22, 35, 238, 253
Leippe, M. R., 232, 253
Leirer, V. O., 58, 69, 117–118, 138
Lemons, F., 361, 379
Lepper, M. R., 44, 49, 66, 72, 263, 270, 285, 374, 379
Lerner, M., 166, 192
Lesser, G., 284
Levin, S. R., 139
Levine, J. M., 285
Levine, R. A., 351, 355, 357, 360, 380
Levinson, D. J., 293, 316, 325, 342, 349, 358–359, 378
Levy, A. S., 174, 188
Lewenstein, M., 241, 254
Lewicki, P., 166, 189, 230, 253
Lewin, K., 16, 35, 243, 253, 374, 380
Lewis, S., 11, 52, 72, 347, 362, 374–375, 380–381
Leyens, J.-Ph., 8, 39, 42, 45–47, 62, 64–65, 70–71, 74
Liberman, A., 82, 101, 103, 263–264, 266–267, 269, 282
Lichtenstein, M., 58, 71, 73, 128, 137, 228, 256
Lightner, J. M., 91–92, 104
Lilly, T., 337, 343
Lingle, J. H., 178, 189, 199, 232, 238, 253, 265, 285
Linton, H., 284
Linville, P. W., 9, 22, 47, 53, 71, 143, 149–150, 154, 158–159, 161, 164–166, 168, 182, 186, 189, 299–300, 319, 369–370, 380
Lippmann, W., 291–294, 306, 319, 345, 351–352, 363, 380
Lisle, D. J., 28, 36, 200, 257
Locksley, A., 53, 71, 139
Lodge, M., 63, 69, 71
Loftus, E. F., 178, 189, 224, 251
Loftus, J. B., 118, 122, 133–135, 139, 153, 155, 157–158, 176–178, 181, 188–189, 231, 253
Logan, G. D., 225, 228, 253, 265, 285
Loken, B. A., 228, 253
Lombardi, W., 115–116, 135, 137, 139, 169, 187–188, 225, 252
Lombardi, W. J., 116, 139, 230, 250
Lombardi, W. L., 61, 66, 169, 185
Lord, C. G., 170, 176, 189, 263, 270, 285, 374, 379
Lucido, D. J., 332, 344
Lui, L., 299, 317
Lumsdaine, A. A., 261, 284
Lupfer, M. B., 94, 100, 105
Lusk, C. M., 47, 63, 70–71
Luskin, R. C., 22, 35

Maass, A., 275, 278, 285, 367, 380
Maccoby, N., 261, 283
Mackie, D. M., 9, 11, 12, 213, 229, 240, 254, 256, 259, 266–267, 269–270, 275–279, 285–287, 305, 313–314, 319–320, 364, 368, 380
Macleod, C. M., 230, 254
Macrae, C. N., 84, 106, 306, 319
Manis, M., 116, 139, 261, 285, 301, 317
Maoz, Y., 99, 107
Marburger, W., 178, 189
Marcus-Newhall, A., 101, 106
Markus, H., 39, 51, 61, 71, 134, 140, 143–144, 147, 149, 152, 158, 161, 165, 167–169, 175, 185–186, 189–190, 223, 258
Marques, J. M., 47, 71
Martin, L. L., 116, 140, 226–227, 230, 238, 254, 257
Marz, B., 62, 66
Mason, J. A., 374, 379
Mavin, G. H., 61, 70, 169, 187
Mayer, J. D., 52, 71
Mayseless, O., 60, 70, 275, 286
Mazze, K., 58, 70
McArthur, L. Z., 81, 88–89, 105
McCauley, C., 42, 66–67, 296, 310, 319
McClaskey, C. L., 11, 12
McClelland, J. L., 27, 36, 155, 189, 191, 204, 232, 239–240, 253, 256, 287
McCloskey, M. E., 216, 253
McConahay, J. G., 329–330, 345

McDaniel, M. A., 174, 181, 189
McFarland, C., 177, 189, 191
McGarvey, W., 235, 252
McGill, A. L., 85, 91, 97, 105
McGillis, D., 25–26, 34, 80, 105
McGuire, C. V., 133, 139
McGuire, W. J., 3, 12, 16–17, 21, 27, 33, 35, 39, 71, 133, 139, 145, 167–169, 189, 198–199, 214, 220, 222, 233–234, 248–249, 254, 261, 263, 265–268, 281, 285, 287
McKenzie-Mohr, D., 60, 71
McKoon, G., 24, 36, 93, 106, 225, 255, 266, 287
McLachlan, A., 277, 286
McLaughlin, J. P., 309, 318
McMillan, D., 49–50, 73, 228, 231, 235, 257, 301, 320
McPartland, T. S., 145, 189
Mead, G. H., 132, 140, 145, 149, 167, 190
Medin, D. L., 54, 71, 153–155, 190, 192, 212, 236, 256, 354, 380
Meneses, B. F., 314, 319
Mervis, C. B., 217, 255
Messick, D. M., 279, 286, 359, 364, 380
Mezei, L., 362, 381
Michela, J. L., 78, 80, 105
Mickler, 275
Miki, H., 56–57, 73
Milberg, S. J., 56–57, 69
Milgram, S., 272, 286
Millar, M. G., 200, 254, 270, 286
Miller, A. G., 292–293, 319
Miller, C. E., 274, 284
Miller, D. T., 81, 97, 105–106, 271, 284
Miller, F. D., 80, 84, 92, 94, 96–97, 107
Miller, G. A., 348, 380
Miller, N., 314, 320, 371–373, 375, 378
Miller, N. E., 358, 379
Milne, A. B., 306, 319
Milner, B., 231, 254
Milstead, M., 174, 181, 189
Minsky, M., 21–22, 27, 35
Mischel, W., 22, 33, 51, 58, 67, 70, 121, 137, 212, 250, 299, 317
Mittal, B., 210, 254
Monteith, M. J., 10, 323, 329–330, 335–336, 338–340, 342–343, 345–346
Moore, L., 332, 344
Moreland, R. L., 61, 71
Mori, D., 169, 190
Moscovici, S., 53–54, 68, 71, 274–276, 286
Mowrer, O. H., 358, 379
Moylan, S. J., 314, 318
Mueller, J. H., 147, 190
Mulilis, J., 338, 344
Mullen, B., 46, 49, 53, 71, 305, 319
Murphy, G. L., 54, 62–63, 71, 74
Murphy, T. D., 155, 190
Myers, D. G., 327, 345
Myrdal, G., 327–328, 330, 338, 345

Nakamura, G. V., 98, 103
Nebergall, R. E., 198, 256
Nedler, L. M., 314, 319
Neely, J. H., 230, 254, 334, 345
Neimeyer, R. A., 159, 188
Neisser, U., 146, 178, 190
Nelson, C., 18, 35, 41–42, 72
Nelson, R., 278, 283
Nelson, T. E., 116, 139
Nelson, T. F., 301, 317
Nelson, T. O., 230, 254
Nemeroff, C., 25–26, 35
Nemeth, C., 274–275, 286
Neuberg, S. L., 25–26, 34, 49, 55–57, 59, 68–69, 71–72, 124, 138, 213, 254, 306, 311–312, 318
Newcomb, T. M., 21, 27, 33, 234, 249, 254, 261, 272, 281, 286
Newell, A., 17, 21, 35, 81, 106, 207, 254
Newman, L. S., 84, 93, 106
Niedenthal, P. M., 144, 149–150, 158–159, 167–169, 178–179, 185, 188, 190

Nisbett, R. E., 15, 35, 44, 49, 53–54, 67, 69, 72, 77, 81, 97, 105–106, 130, 140, 166, 190
Norman, D., 21, 35
Nosofsky, R. M., 154–155, 190, 212, 254
Novick, L. R., 84, 86–88, 97, 103
Nowak, A., 9, 24, 35, 195, 234, 241, 245, 247, 253–254, 257
Nunn, C. Z., 26, 35
Nurius, P., 149, 168, 185, 190
Nuttin, J. M., Jr., 175, 190
Nyberg, S. E., 174, 193

Oberlander, L., 146, 192
O'Brien, M., 310, 319
Olshavsky, R. W., 169, 186
Ortiz, V., 53, 71, 139
Ortony, A., 11, 13, 236, 257, 354, 380
Orvis, D., 80, 106
Osborne, R. E., 226, 251
Osgood, C. E., 19, 35, 195, 208, 254–255
Ostrom, T. M., 1, 5, 9, 12, 24, 35, 39, 43–44, 48, 72–73, 80, 82, 85, 106, 146, 178, 180, 187, 189–190, 195, 197, 199, 210, 219, 222, 232–233, 238, 251, 253, 255, 261, 265–266, 268, 282, 284–286
Ottati, V. C., 125, 140

Padawer-Singer, A., 133, 139, 145, 169, 189
Page, R., 297, 320
Paivio, A., 205, 209, 255
Park, B. M., 2, 13, 39, 42, 46, 52–53, 70, 72–73, 96, 104, 111, 140, 143–144, 153, 169–170, 188, 190–191, 228, 252, 270, 287, 300, 319, 330, 345, 361, 369–371, 380–381
Patnoe, S., 16, 35
Pavelchak, M. A., 55, 68, 124, 138
PDP Research Group, 27, 36, 204, 232, 239–240, 253, 256
Peabody, D., 360, 381
Peak, H., 268, 286
Peeters, G., 45, 72
Peitgen, H.-O., 244, 247, 255
Pelham, B. W., 99, 104, 172, 190, 226–227, 252
Pennington, N., 11, 13, 219, 255
Pepitone, A., 60, 75
Perdue, C. W., 366, 381
Pere, G., 170, 189
Personnaz, B., 275, 286
Pettigrew, T. F., 49, 72, 301, 319, 324, 345, 375, 381
Pettit, G. S., 11, 12
Petty, R. E., 24, 35, 140, 196, 210, 219, 222, 227, 235, 250, 255, 261, 263, 265–269, 273, 278, 282, 284, 286
Picek, J. S., 235–236, 255
Pietromonaco, P., 61, 66, 116, 137, 230, 250
Pilkonis, P. A., 267, 289
Pittman, T. S., 167, 188
Pliner, P., 169, 190
Plog, A. E., 181, 189
Posner, M. I., 153, 190, 334, 345, 348, 381
Postman, C. J., 353, 378
Potts, G. R., 176, 185
Powell, M. C., 34, 202, 251, 262, 283
Pratkanis, A. R., 34–35, 144–145, 148, 153, 161, 172, 174, 178, 187, 200–201, 208–210, 212, 214, 221, 255, 262, 267, 286–287
Pratto, F., 56–57, 69, 267, 270, 282, 288
Preisler, R. M., 263, 288
Prentice, D. A., 26, 33
Pressly, S. L., 335–336, 338, 345
Presson, C. C., 169, 185–186, 278, 287
Priester, J. R., 196, 255
Proshansky, H. M., 323–327, 334, 344–345
Pruitt, D. J., 86, 106
Pryor, J. B., 84, 96, 106
Pullyblank, J., 176

Pylyshyn, Z. W., 82, 106, 209, 255
Pyszczynski, T., 338, 345

Quattrone, G. A., 99, 106, 369, 381

Rabbie, J. M., 364, 366, 380–381
Racine, J. P., 84, 103
Rainio, K., 16, 35
Ramsey, S. L., 374, 379
Rasinski, K. A., 11, 13, 201, 212, 214, 221, 238, 257, 265–266, 288
Ratcliff, R., 24, 36, 93, 106, 225, 255, 266, 287
Raymond, P., 61, 66
Read, S. J., 80, 85, 88–89, 98, 101, 106
Reber, A. S., 230, 255
Reder, L. M., 210, 255
Reed, S. K., 153, 191, 212, 255
Reeder, G. D., 45, 72, 80, 98, 106, 113, 140
Regan, D., 113, 140
Reichel, L. D., 314, 319
Rempel, J. K., 199, 258, 262, 265, 289
Reynolds, R. E., 116, 137
Rhodewalt, F. T., 167–168, 170, 188, 191
Rholes, W. S., 23, 34, 41, 69, 96, 104, 106, 115–117, 138
Riesbeck, C., 30, 35
Rife, D., 284
Riggle, E. D., 125, 140
Rips, L. J., 178, 185, 211, 256, 374, 381
Rizzo, N., 332, 344
Robinson, I. E., 292, 296, 317
Rocher, S., 64, 74
Rodeach, M., 327–328, 345
Rogers, C. R., 145, 148, 191
Rogers, J. P., 153, 191
Rogers, T. B., 135, 140, 147–148, 152–153, 158, 167, 173–177, 189, 191
Rojahn, K., 49, 72, 301, 319
Rokeach, M., 268, 287, 338, 341–342, 362, 381
Roland, P. E., 209, 255
Roney, C.J.R., 172, 192
Ronis, D. L., 270, 287
Rosch, E. H., 217, 255, 299, 319
Rosenberg, M. J., 17, 20–21, 27, 33, 35, 149, 170, 191, 205, 234, 236, 249, 261, 266, 281, 287
Rosenberg, S., 18, 35, 41–42, 72, 125, 140, 208, 253
Ross, L., 15, 35, 44, 49, 54, 62, 66, 72, 81, 106, 114, 130, 140, 147, 170, 184, 191, 263, 277, 285, 287
Ross, M., 81, 106, 171, 177–178, 189, 191
Rothbart, M., 11, 31, 35, 46, 49, 52, 58, 72–73, 228, 256, 312, 319, 347, 350, 354, 361, 364, 368–369, 371–372, 374, 380–381
Rothman, A. J., 23, 33
Rozin, P., 25–26, 35
Ruble, D. N., 50, 58, 60, 63, 72–73
Ruderman, A. J., 360, 382
Rudman, L., 60, 67
Rule, G. R., 176, 186
Rumelhart, D. E., 21, 27, 35–36, 155, 189, 191, 204, 232, 239–240, 253, 256, 287
Ruscher, J. B., 56–57, 68, 73, 314, 318
Rush, A. J., 152, 166, 185
Russell, D., 91, 105
Russo, E. M., 285
Ruvolo, C. M., 301–302, 318
Ryan, C. S., 361, 369, 371, 380–381

Sabonmatsu, D. M., 202, 251
Sagar, H. A., 301, 318
Salancik, G. R., 133, 140, 167, 169–170, 191
Salovey, P., 53, 71, 154, 189, 299–300, 319, 369–370, 380
Salvi, D., 367, 380
Sanbonmatsu, D. M., 34, 46, 73, 262, 283
Sanford, R. N., 293, 316, 325, 342, 349, 358–359, 378
Sanitioso, R., 333, 343

Santa, J. L., 209, 256
Saxe, L., 329, 343
Schachtel, E. G., 182, 191
Schacter, D. L., 230, 256
Schadron, G., 64, 70, 73–74
Schaffer, L. G., 28, 36
Schaffer, M. M., 154, 190
Schaller, M., 310, 319
Schallert, D. L., 116, 137
Schank, R. C., 21–22, 24, 30, 35–36, 81, 89, 92, 98, 106, 218, 256
Scheier, M. F., 138, 146, 170, 186
Schelling, T., 25, 36
Schlenker, B. R., 167, 191
Schneider, D. J., 3, 13, 42, 73, 110, 125, 140, 146, 177, 180, 191, 270, 287
Schneider, W., 25, 36, 225, 232, 256, 265, 287, 334, 345–346
Schofield, J. W., 301, 318
Schroth, H. A., 314, 319
Schuman, H., 329, 345
Schuster, H. G., 241, 256
Schwarz, N., 11, 12–13, 125, 134, 139–141, 149, 192, 201, 256, 267, 287
Scott, C. K., 131, 140
Seago, D. W., 303, 319
Sears, D. O., 25–28, 35–36, 330, 345
Sears, R. R., 358, 379
Secord, P. F., 132, 140, 167, 184
Sedikides, C., 42, 48, 59, 66–67, 73, 213, 256
Sedlak, A., 42, 72, 125, 140
Segal, M., 42, 66–67
Seifert, C. M., 24, 36
Seligman, M.E.P., 77, 102
Semin, G. R., 90–91, 103, 106
Sentis, K. P., 134, 140, 147, 167, 175, 190, 235, 256
Sermat, V., 19, 33
Sermin, G., 367, 380
Seta, C. E., 122, 140
Seta, J. J., 122, 140, 226–227, 230, 254
Setterlund, M. B., 159, 190
Shaffer, D. R., 261–263, 265, 269, 288
Shannon, L., 50, 73
Shapiro, M. M., 132, 138
Shapiro, P., 314, 321
Sharkey, N., 24, 36
Shavitt, S., 26, 36, 262–263, 287
Shaw, 17
Shaw, B. F., 152, 166, 185
Shedler, J., 116, 139
Sheffield, F. D., 261, 284
Shefrin, H. M., 25, 36
Shephard, R. N., 205, 256
Shepherd, J. W., 84, 106
Sherif, C. W., 31, 36, 198, 256, 265, 287, 303, 319, 354, 381
Sherif, M., 31, 36, 145, 191, 196, 198, 256, 261, 265, 272–273, 287, 303, 319, 354, 381
Sherman, J. W., 275, 286, 293, 300–302, 315–316, 318–319
Sherman, R. C., 95, 106
Sherman, S. J., 2, 13, 39, 46, 73, 111, 140, 143–144, 169–170, 185–186, 191, 213, 235–236, 240, 255–256, 265–267, 270, 278, 287, 301, 305–306, 318, 330, 335, 345
Sherman-Williams, B., 301, 318
Shevell, S. K., 178, 185
Shiffrin, R. M., 25, 36, 225, 232, 235–236, 255–256, 265, 287, 334, 345–346
Shoben, E. J., 178, 193, 211, 256
Showers, C., 149–150, 160, 191
Shpitizajzen, A., 60, 69
Shulman, G. L., 348, 381
Shustack, M. W., 85, 106
Sidera, J., 267, 282
Sigall, H., 297, 320
Siladi, M., 147, 152, 169, 190
Simon, H. A., 17, 21, 35, 62, 67, 81, 106, 207, 254, 352, 381
Singer, D., 361, 379
Skelly, J. J., 9, 259, 276, 278, 286
Skelton, J. A., 167–168, 170, 188
Skowronski, J. J., 9, 45, 50, 73, 94, 103, 121–122, 137, 178, 186, 193, 195, 213, 230, 232, 250–251, 256
Sloan, L. R., 358, 379

Slugoski, B. R., 86–87, 91, 97, 105, 107
Smith, E. E., 8, 153–155, 192, 211–212, 236, 256, 353, 374, 381
Smith, E. R., 24, 36, 47, 52–53, 73–74, 77, 80–82, 84–85, 92, 94, 96–97, 101, 107, 115, 128, 140–141, 154–155, 166, 192, 207, 209, 231, 256, 300, 306, 312, 320–321
Smith, H. S., 159, 192
Smith, J., 61, 71
Smith, M., 261–262, 287
Smith, M. C., 93, 103, 118, 137
Smith, R. A., 63, 68
Smolensky, P., 287
Snyder, C.R.R., 334, 345
Snyder, M., 46, 60, 73, 129–130, 141, 146, 192, 200, 256, 263, 267, 287, 301, 320
Snygg, D., 148, 192
Solano, C., 111, 139
Songer, E., 235, 252
Sorrentino, R. M., 111, 141, 172, 192
Souppe, D., 244, 247, 255
Spielman, L. A., 267, 288
Spinoza, B., 368–369, 381
Squire, L. R., 209, 251
Sriram, N., 361, 380
Srull, T. K., 1, 5, 11, 13, 23, 37, 39, 43, 49, 58, 71, 73–74, 82, 101, 107–108, 111, 115–118, 120–121, 127, 130–131, 135, 141–144, 146, 149, 151, 169, 176–178, 189, 192–193, 204, 208, 214, 228, 230, 235, 256–257, 310, 320
Staats, A. W., 208, 257
Staats, C. K., 208, 257
Stangor, C., 49–50, 58, 60, 63, 72–73, 228–229, 231, 235, 251, 257, 261, 266, 282, 301, 310, 314, 318, 320
Stasser, G., 277, 288
Steeh, C., 329, 345
Steffen, V. J., 310, 317
Steiner, I. D., 132, 141
Stephan, C. W., 314, 320
Stephan, W. G., 302, 314, 320, 323, 326–327, 346
Sternberg, R. J., 85, 106
Stevens, S. S., 197, 257
Stitt, C. L., 296, 310, 319
Stone, M., 238, 257
Stoner, J.A.F., 274, 288
Storms, M., 113, 141
Strack, F., 11, 13, 141, 149, 192, 238, 257
Strauman, T. J., 160, 187, 192
Street, R. L., 268, 282
Stroebe, W., 334, 346
Stroessner, S. J., 10, 291, 305–306, 312–314, 320
Stryker, S., 149, 192
Subramaniam, G., 181, 185
Suci, G. J., 19, 35, 208, 255
Sudman, S., 11, 12, 201, 256
Sullivan, L. A., 314, 318, 320
Sumner, W. G., 357
Swann, W. B., 73, 129, 141, 200, 256
Swann, W. B., Jr., 46, 73, 167, 171, 192
Swift, J., 364, 381
Szamrej, J., 24, 35, 247, 254

Tagiuri, R., 41–42, 67
Tajfel, H., 55, 73–74, 126, 141, 303, 320, 326, 346, 351, 356–358, 360, 363–366, 372, 378, 382
Tanke, E. D., 129–130, 141, 301, 320
Tannenbaum, P. H., 19, 21, 27, 33, 35, 195, 208, 234, 249, 254–255, 261, 281
Tannenbaum, P. II, 268, 288
Taylor, D. A., 146, 192
Taylor, M., 312, 319, 354, 381
Taylor, S. E., 1, 12, 23, 34, 39, 43–45, 49, 51, 56, 60–61, 68, 74, 84, 96, 98, 103, 107, 113–114, 138, 144, 147, 171–172, 186, 192, 208, 239, 251, 261, 283, 304, 320, 351, 360, 363–364, 371, 379, 382
Teasdale, J. D., 77, 102

Tesser, A., 47, 74, 167, 171, 192, 200, 213, 243, 254, 257, 261–263, 265, 270, 275, 282, 286, 288, 301, 317
Tetlock, P. E., 60, 74
Teuber, H. L., 231, 254
Thaler, R. H., 25, 36
Thein, R. D., 23, 33
Thoits, P. A., 149, 192
Thomas, W. I., 195, 257
Thompson, C. P., 50, 73, 178, 193
Thompson, S. C., 45, 74
Thorne, A., 358, 379
Thorngate, W. B., 359, 380
Thurstone, L. L., 195, 198, 257, 288
Titus, W., 95, 106, 277, 288
Tomkins, S. S., 23, 36
Tota, M. E., 61, 66, 116, 135, 137, 169, 181, 185, 230, 250
Totten, J., 113, 140
Tourangeau, R., 11, 13, 201, 212, 214, 221, 238, 257, 265–266, 288
Town, J. P., 92, 104
Trabasso, T., 81, 107
Trafton, J. G., 153, 189
Trolier, T. K., 46, 69, 95, 104, 127, 138, 302, 305, 318, 333, 344
Trope, Y., 98–99, 107, 117, 141, 171–172, 193, 226, 257, 274, 282
Trudeau, J. V., 167, 191
Trzebinski, J., 42, 74
Tulving, E., 147, 176, 178, 186, 193, 200, 206, 257
Turnbull, W., 91, 107
Turner, J. C., 274, 276–280, 288, 358–359, 366, 372, 379, 382
Turner, T. J., 131, 137
Tversky, A., 226, 257, 272, 284
Tyler, R. B., 309, 317, 366, 381

Uleman, J. S., 25, 36, 57, 74, 92, 95, 107, 118–119, 141
Unverzagt, W. H., 127, 142

Vala, J., 65, 67
Valins, S., 77, 105
Vallacher, R., 234, 245, 257
Van den Broek, P., 81, 107
Van der Kloot, W. A., 42, 74
van der Pligt, J., 266, 288
van Dijk, T. A., 92, 105
Van Hook, E., 157–158, 174, 181, 187
van Kleeck, M. H., 89–90, 103, 107
Van Leeuwen, M. D., 374, 379
Vanman, E. J., 314, 320
Van Manen, S., 56–57, 73
Van Mechelen, I., 42, 74
Vaughn, L. A., 337, 343
Veblen, T., 359, 382
Vinacke, W. E., 297, 320
Vinokur, A., 274, 282
Vivekananthan, P. S., 18, 35, 41–42, 72
Von Hendy, H. M., 57, 68
von Hippel, W., 231, 257
Vosniadou, S., 236, 257
Voter, J., 90, 107

Wackenhut, J., 330–332, 335, 345
Walker, M. R., 358, 379
Walters, G., 296–297, 319
Warren, R. E., 175, 193
Watson, S. F., 120, 142
Weary, G., 146, 185
Weber, R., 22–23, 30, 36, 95, 103, 371, 382
Weber, S. J., 269, 288
Webster's New World Dictionary of the American language, 43, 74
Wegener, D. T., 196, 227, 255
Weigel, R. H., 325, 346
Weiner, B., 77, 105, 107
Wells, G. L., 84, 95–96, 103, 107
West, S. C., 374, 379
West, S. G., 275, 285
Westie, F. R., 330, 346
Wherry, M. B., 159, 190
White, B. J., 303, 319
White, R., 261–262, 287
White, R. K., 30, 36
Wicker, A. W., 269, 288
Wicklund, R. A., 146, 186, 338, 344

Wiggins, E. C., 206, 211, 250
Wilder, D. A., 31, 36, 278–279, 288, 314, 320–321, 363–364, 374, 382
Wilkes, A. L., 74, 360, 363, 382
Willemsen, T. M., 42, 74
Williams, C. J., 202, 251
Williams, J. A., 26, 35
Williams, R. M., Jr., 326–327, 346
Wills, T. A., 359, 382
Wilson, T. D., 28, 36, 44, 69, 166, 190, 200, 257
Winter, L., 92, 95, 107, 118–119, 141
Wishner, J., 41, 74, 119, 141
Wolfson, M. R., 132, 141
Wood, W., 263, 269, 278, 283, 288
Word, C. O., 301–302, 321
Worth, L. T., 50, 69, 276, 278, 286, 368, 378
Wright, J. C., 62–63, 67, 71, 74
Wrightsman, L. W., 275, 284
Wu, C., 269, 288
Wurf, E., 61, 71, 144, 149, 161, 165, 167–168, 175, 190
Wyer, R. S., 82, 85, 101, 107–108, 111, 115–118, 120–121, 125, 127–128, 130–132, 135, 137–142, 146, 187, 265, 288
Wyer, R. S., Jr., 1, 5, 8–9, 12–13, 23, 37, 39, 43, 49, 58, 73–74, 109, 143–144, 146, 149, 151, 168–169, 176–178, 186, 192–193, 204, 208, 212–214, 225, 228, 230, 235, 256–257
Wylie, R., 145, 148, 193

Xu, G., 272, 281

Yarkin, K. L., 91–92, 104
Yates, D., 277, 281
Yates, J. F., 270, 287
Yi, Y., 271, 288
Yzerbyt, V. Y., 45–47, 64, 70–71, 73–74

Zadny, J., 301, 321
Zajonc, R. B., 3, 13, 24–25, 37, 39, 51, 71, 143, 190, 223, 229, 235–236, 257–258, 261, 267, 288–289
Zanna, M. P., 5, 12, 41–42, 60, 69, 71, 74, 120, 138, 146, 187, 191, 199, 206, 251, 258, 262, 265, 267, 269, 283, 289, 301–302, 314, 318, 321, 335, 344
Zárate, M. A., 52, 73–74, 101, 107, 128, 141, 154–155, 192, 300, 306, 312, 320–321
Zavalloni, M., 274, 286
Zawadski, B., 348, 350, 363, 382
Zechmeister, E. B., 174, 193
Zeitz, C. M., 63, 67
Zelen, S. L., 145, 185
Znaniecki, F., 195, 257
Zuckerman, M., 84, 108
Zukier, H., 40, 50, 60, 66, 75
Zuroff, D. C., 53, 75
Zuwerink, J. R., 10, 323, 329–330, 335–338, 342–343, 345–346

Subject Index

Accessibility, 61, 200–203, 213, 262, 269–270
  chronic and contextual construct accessibility, 168
ACT* model, 21, 161, 164
Accuracy, 171
Affect, 78, 207
Aggression, 11, 349
Analogue representations, 205, 222
Algorithm, 82–84
American Creed, 327
Anchor-and-adjust heuristic, 226
ANOVA model, 8, 88, 97–98
Assimilation 196, 353, 363
Associative network, 143, 147, 212, 233, 150
Attention decrement hypothesis, 48
Attitude, (*see* Chapter 7), 9, 195
  conceptions of attitude, 196–203
    dimensional vs multidimensional structure, 220–223
  attitude behavior consistency, 200
  attitude functions, 26, 262–265, 342
Attitude change, 261, 265, 275
Attribution, (*see* Chapter 4), 8, 17, 113
  internal vs external, 77, 79
  dispositional vs situational, 77, 79, 95, 99, 113–114
  linguistic and conversational influences, 89–91
  schematic and sequential-stage models, 98–100
Attributional ego defensiveness, 146
Availability, 262, 270
Authoritarian personality, 293, 325, 349, 358–360
Automatic processing, 62, 225–228, 306, 334
Autobiographical memory, 177–180

Base-rate, 60
Behaviorism, 15–18, 145, 354
Bin model, 151
Bottom-up processing, 62, 225

Categorization, 200, 211, 291, 311–315, 353–354, 363–368, 371, 374
Category-based expectancies, 26
Central route processing, 268
Central traits, 18, 41, 42, 119
Centrality, 149
Coacting central subsystems,
  deliberate vs spontaneous, 24–29
  automatic vs controlled, 24–29
  intended vs unintended, 24–29
  explicit vs implicit, 24–29
  cooperative vs antagonistic parallel processing, 24–29
Cognitive consistency theories, 348
  balance theory, 17, 21, 233–236, 268
  congruity theory, 21, 195, 363
  dissonance theory, 17–18, 21, 195, 269
Collective self, 148

Competition, 356
Compliance, 273–274
Confrontation technique, 327, 341
Cognitive responses, 196, 261
Cognitive revolution, 347–348
Conformity, (*see* Chapter 7), 9, 260, 273–277, 279–280
Conceptual dependency system, 21
Consensus information, 81, 85, 275–278
Consistency information, 85
Construal, 54
Contact hypothesis, 11, 371–375
Continuum model, 55–57
  category- vs attribute (piecemeal)-based processes, 123–124
  theory- vs data-driven processes, 123–124
Contrast, 196
Controlled processing, 61, 225–228, 334
Conversion, 275
Cooperation, 356
Correspondent inference, 77, 80, 81, 100
Covariation-based approach, 80
Covariation information, 85
Cued-recall method, 92

Declarative knowledge, 9, 148, 161–166
Dehumanization, 377
Depth of processing, 176
Diagnosticity, 45
Diffuse self, 148
Disconfirmation, 45
Discounting, 374
Discrepancies, 337–338
Discrimination, 349
Displacement, 354
Distinctiveness, 85, 169
Distinctiveness hypothesis, 48
Distributed networks, 204
Dynamical systems, 241–248
  intrapsychic dynamical attitude systems, 245–247
  interpersonal dynamical attitude systems, 247–248

Ego, 145
Ego defense, 268
Elaboration likelihood model, 196
Encoding, 44
Encoding specificity, 181
Episodic memory, 178, 182
Ethnocentrism, 351, 357
Exemplars, 52, 81, 212, 216, 371, 375
Exemplar models, 153, 300
Expectancy value theory, 56
Expertise, 62–63
Explicit memory, 229–231

False consensus effect, 277
Fan effect, 225
Frames, 22, 130
Frustration, 349
Frustration-aggression hypothesis 354
Frustration-aggression-displacement theory, 358–360
Fundamental attribution error, 62, 81

Gestalt, 40, 42, 47–48, 57, 234
Group decision making, 11
Group narcissism, 358
Group polarization, 274
  persuasive arguments explanation, 274

Halo effect, 125, 127
Heuristic processing, 269
Hierarchical structure, 178, 215–218, 299
Hypothesis, 46

Identification, 273
Inference rules, 81
Illusory correlation, 46–47, 53
Implementation, 82–84

Implicit memory, 229–231
Implicit personality theory 41–42, 52–55, 125
Impression formation, (*see* Chapter 3), 8, 79, 119–122
Impression management, 167
Impression sensitivity hypothesis, 48
Information integration theory, 57, 237–239
In-group, 278–279, 293, 303–305, 352, 360, 364–371
In-group favoritism, 367
Inhibition, 337
Inoculation theory, 268
Intergroup conflict, 375
Intergroup hostility, 348–349, 350, 353,355, 357
Intergroup relations, (*see* Chapter 11), 10–11, 347–348, 354–355, 372, 378
Internalization, 273, 275
Interpersonal attraction, 78
Interpersonal orientation, 373

Judgmental confidence, 264–265

Learned helplessness, 78
Learning theory, 271
Life space, 16, 78, 80
Linguistic biases, 367
Logical Model, 86
Logtropism, 18–19

Majority influence, 274–275
Material self, 148
Meaning change, 41
Memory,
  episodic, 200, 206, 222
  semantic/conceptual, 200, 206
Memory-based processing, 62, 228–229
Memory set, 58
MINERVA model of exemplar memory, 157
Minimal group, 11, 304, 356, 367–369, 373
Minority influence, 274
Motivation, 78, 82, 263, 271
  accuracy and defense motivation, 264
Multiple exemplar models, 154–155
Multiple selves, 148–151, 157

Neats vs Scruffies, 7, 23–24, 32
Negative interdependence, 355
Negativity, 45
New Look in perception, 61
Next-in-line effect, 175
Noncommon effects, 80
Normative models, 81
Novice, 63

Observational goals,
  memory set, 58–60
  accuracy, 58–60
  impression formation, 58–60
On-line processing, 62, 228–229
Out-group, 278–279, 293, 303–305, 352, 360, 364–371
Out-group homogeneity, 53, 369–370

Parallel processing, 231–233
Parallel distributed processing, 101, 155–157, 239–241
Particularization, 356
Perceived freedom, 268
Peripheral traits, 41
Person memory, 44, 47, 50
Person memory model, 122, 126–127
Person perception, *see* Impression formation
Personality, 42, 109, 143
Personal construct theory, 145
Persuasion, 9, 17, 196, 259–272, 273, 279–280
  elaboration likelihood model, 196, 266
  heuristic-systematic model, 266
  information processing analysis, 199

Positive interdependence, 355
Pragmatics, 65
Prejudice, (*see* Chapter 10), 10, 28–32, 125, 323, 349
  prejudice reduction, (Chapter 10), 10, 326–328, 342
  modern forms, 10, 328–335
    ambivalence, 10, 331–332, 335, 341
    aversive racism, 332–333, 335, 226, 341
    dissociation model, 333–335
  old-fashioned prejudice, 329
Prejudice reduction, (*see* Chapter 10), 10, 326–328, 342
Primacy effect, 41, 48
Priming, 60–61, 96–97, 160, 181, 201, 213
Private self, 148
Proactive interference, 181
Procedural knowledge, 9, 144, 148, 161–166
Production systems, 163, 184, 206
Projection, 359
Propaganda, 326
Propositional network models, 21
Propositional units, 204, 210, 222
Prototypes, 52, 81, 143, 146–147, 182, 212, 299, 368, 374
Prototype models, 153
Psychoanalytic approach, 145, 293, 325, 348
Public self, 148

Realistic conflict model, 355, 357–358
Reinforcement theories, 363
Representativeness, 169
Response-time methodology, 92
Robbers' Cave experiment, 354–357

Salience, 44, 96
Scapegoating, 348, 359
Schema, 22, 51–53, 81, 134, 143, 146–147, 182
Scripts, 18, 80, 81, 146–147, 222
Self, (*see* Chapter 6), 9, 264, 269
  actual, ideal, ought, 143
Self-appraisal, 159
Self-awareness, 200
Self-complexity, 158–160
Self-concept, 132, 143, 145, 148, 167, 169, 263
  spontaneous self-concept, 145
Self-consistency, 171
Self-consciousness, 146
Self-disclosure, 146
Self-discrepancy, 160, 169
Self-enhancement, 82, 148, 171
Self-esteem, 145, 159–160, 366
Self-evaluation, 131, 162
Self-focused attention, 170, 338
Self-fulfilling prophecy, 302, 306
Self-identity, 148
Self-knowledge, 133, 170
Self-monitoring, 146
Self-perception, 131, 146
Self-presentation, 82, 146, 162, 167
Self-reference, 173–174, 176–177
Self-regulatory processes, 165, 170, 338–340
Self-schema, 152, 169
Self-serving biases, 81
Semantic differential, 19
Semantic memory, 134–135, 182
Semantic network, 151
Serial processing, 231–233
Set size, 49
Social categorization, 364–368
Social comparison, 162
Social identity theory, 11, 358, 366, 372–373, 375
Social influence, (Chapter 8), 9, 259, 277, 280
Social learning, 324
Social perception, 110
Social self, 148
Social judgability hypothesis, 64
Sociocultural perspective, 293, 316
Spiritual self, 148
Spontaneous attribution, 91, 101
Spreading activation, 151, 224, 162

Stereotype, (*see* Chapter 9), 10, 45, 47, 50–54, 57, 64, 125–129, 333, 350–353, 373–374
  conceptions of stereotypes,
    faulty reasoning process, 295
    kernel of truth, 295, 297, 310
    overgeneralizations, 295
  content, 309–311
Stereotype assessment,
  Katz and Braly method, 296–298, 308–309
  consensual beliefs, 296–298, 308–309
  validity, 296–298, 308–309
Stereotype change, 314–315, 371
Stereotype formation, 303–305
Story model, 219
Stroop task, 175, 181
Subjective validity, 264–265, 272
Subtyping, 23
Sufficiency threshold, 264
Survey methodology, 11
Symbolic nodes, 204
Systematic processing, 268
Subcategory, 371
Subordinate category, 371
Subjectivism, 15
Superordinate category, 371
Superordinate goals, 356

Task orientation, 373
Target-based expectancies, 26
Thematic affect units, 22
Therapeutic techniques, 327
Top-down processing, 62, 225
Traits, 47, 51, 79, 110
Trait-behavior cluster, 122–123, 126
Trait inferences, (*see* Chapter 4), 8, 94, 100

Well-earned reputation theory, 348–349
Word-fragment completion, 93
Working memory, 214, 162

Validity, 276–278,
Vividness, 44